Auburn Speech + Hearing Clinic

Screening Children *for* Auditory Function

edited by
Fred H. Bess
and
James W. Hall III

Bill Wilkerson Center Press
Nashville, Tennessee

SCREENING CHILDREN FOR AUDITORY FUNCTION

Copyright © 1992 by Bill Wilkerson Center Press

Proceedings of the International Symposium on Screening Children for Auditory Function held June 27-29, 1991, in Nashville, Tennessee, cosponsored by the Bill Wilkerson Center and the Division of Hearing and Speech Sciences Vanderbilt University School of Medicine.

Library of Congress Catalog Card Number: 92-70246
ISBN 0-9631439-0-5

This book was manufactured in the United States of America
on recycled, acid-free paper.

Contents

Foreword vii
Preface ix
Contributors xiii

PART I. Description of the Problem

Chapter 1 1
Screening in the 1990s: Some Principles and Guidelines
John W. Feightner

Chapter 2 17
Changing Demographics of Infants in the Neonatal Intensive
Care Unit: Impact on Auditory Function
Jayant P. Shenai

Chapter 3 31
Epidemiology and Natural History of Otitis Media
Jerome O. Klein

Chapter 4 39
Special Issues Concerned with Screening for Middle Ear
Disease in Children
Jerry L. Northern

Chapter 5 61
Controversies in the Screening of Central Auditory Processing
Disorders
Brad A. Stach

Chapter 6 79
Prevalence Rates and Cost-Effectiveness of Risk Factors
Robert G. Turner and Barbara K. Cone-Wesson

Chapter 7 105
Newborn Hearing Screening—Education of the Medical Profession
Stephen Epstein

Chapter 8 111
Policy Formulation: A Real World View
Alfred A. Baumeister

PART II. Screening Newborns for Auditory Function

Chapter 9 127
Auditory Brainstem Response (ABR) in Infants: Screening
and Diagnostic Applications
Deborah Hayes

Chapter 10 145
Newborn Hearing Screening with Auditory Brainstem Response
(ABR): Experience with 1982 Versus 1990 Joint Committee
Risk Criteria
James W. Hall III and Charlotte H. Prentice

Chapter 11 163
A Model for Neonatal Hearing Screening
M. Wende Yellin and Faith C. Wurm

Chapter 12 171
Infant Hearing Screening in Ohio
Gayle Riemer and Susan Farrer

Chapter 13 181
Orienting as a Means of Assessing Hearing in Newly Born Infants
Richard S. Bernstein and Judith S. Gravel

Chapter 14 191
Otoacoustic Hearing Screening in Newborns: Optimization
G. Salomon, B. Anthonisen, J. Groth, and P.P. Thomsen

Chapter 15 207
Neonatal Hearing Screening Using Evoked Otoacoustic Emissions:
The Rhode Island Hearing Assessment Project
Karl R. White, Antonia B. Maxon, Thomas R. Behrens,
Peter M. Blackwell, and Betty R. Vohr

Chapter 16 229
Sensorineural Hearing Loss in High-Risk Infants
Diane L. Sabo, David R. Brown, and Jon F. Watchko

PART III. Screening Infants and Young Children for Auditory Function

Chapter 17 243
Screening for Hearing Loss: Behavioral Options
Allan O. Diefendorf

Chapter 18 261
The Infant Hearing Program (IHP) of Arkansas: Its Past,
Present, and Future
Terrey Oliver Penn

Chapter 19 273
Screening the Preschool-Age Child
Thomas Mahoney

Chapter 20 287
Cheers for Ears: A Community Immittance Screening Program
for Preschoolers
Nancy E. Harrison and Barbara J. Price

PART IV. Screening School-Age Children for Auditory Function

Chapter 21 297
Screening School-Age Children
Jackson Roush

Chapter 22 315
Sensitivity, Specificity, and Predictive Value of Immittance
Measures in the Identification of Middle Ear Effusion
Robert J. Nozza, Charles D. Bluestone, and David Kardatzke

Chapter 23 331
Hearing Screening in Montana: A Public/Private Partnership
*Michael K. Wynne, Mary Jo Grote, Susan A.W. Toth, and
Merle DeVoe*

Chapter 24 361
The Selective Auditory Attention Test (SAAT): A Screening Test for
Central Auditory Processing Disorders in Children
Rochelle Cherry

Chapter 25 373
    Screening for Auditory Disorders in Psychiatric Hospitals
    Judith A. Marlowe, Tamara Lewis Engels, and Robert W. Keith

PART V. Intervention

Chapter 26 385
    Current Issues in Early Intervention
    Donald B. Bailey, Jr.

Chapter 27 399
    Birth to Five: The Important Early Years
    Marie Thompson

Chapter 28 435
    An Ecological and Developmental/Contextual Approach to
    Intervention with Children with Chronic Otitis Media
    Lynne V. Feagans, Kristi Hannan, and Elizabeth Manlove

Chapter 29 463
    Parent-Infant Intervention Strategies: A Focus on Relationships
    Nancy Rushmer

Chapter 30 477
    Hearing-Impaired Children in the Schools: Integrated or Isolated?
    Pamela E. Montgomery and Noel D. Matkin

Appendix 1 495
    Joint Committee on Infant Hearing 1990 Position Statement

Appendix 2 507
    Consensus Statement—Screening Children for Auditory Function

Appendix 3 511
    Newborn Hearing Screening with Auditory Brainstem Response:
    Programs and Protocols
    James W. Hall III and Charlotte H. Prentice

Author Index 529

Subject Index 531

Foreword

The voices that are heard in this volume come from the mouths of giants in the fields of pediatric audiology, otolaryngology, speech-language pathology, and education of the hearing impaired—experts who have opened up a new world of screening, testing, diagnosis, and habilitation for children. Through them we know how best to use auditory brainstem response (ABR) to screen for hearing loss at birth; we know how to use ABR and visual response audiometry for detailed auditory testing at older ages; we know what methods will best habilitate the infant or child with hearing deficit; we know how to identify the child who is at risk for language delays due to recurrent otitis media and how to treat those problems. Yet this enormous reservoir of knowledge seems to have a disappointing impact on the general population and the medical community. The only encouraging news is that at the present time a bill has been introduced into the House of Representatives that mandates universal hearing screening of *all* newborns. This author feels strongly that the time has come to insist on the screening of *all* babies, not just those at risk. One survey after the other has revealed that around 50% of hearing-impaired babies are missed by dependence on the high-risk register. Whatever the course of this bill, it will create an awareness of the need for this screening that is long overdue.

The fact remains that the recent public health document recommending goals for the nation for the year 2000 (*Healthy People 2000*) did *not* list newborn hearing screening as an objective; it merely proposed to "reduce the average age at which children with significant hearing impairment are identified to no more than twelve months." The rationale for overlooking newborns was that baseline data for newborn screening were not available. The same document did, however, urge that 80% of providers of primary care for children routinely screen infants and children for impairments of speech and language. It is probably a reasonable estimate that less than 10% of newborns are presently screened for hearing, and fewer than 1% of infants and children are screened in physicians' offices. These figures illustrate the discrepancy between knowledge and application in the realm of screening.

The faculty/staff in the Division of Hearing and Speech Sciences at Vanderbilt University School of Medicine and the Bill Wilkerson Center have recognized that we are having difficulty in selling our programs to those who can implement them. They have shrewdly invited, in addition to the array of other experts, two speakers for the philosophy of influencing public policy and for the kind of evidence our research must present in order to achieve policy implementation. Their chapters are well worth careful study and contemplation. Dr. Feightner analyzes research on screening and states that acceptance of new programs is now subject to an increasing demand that their effectiveness be demonstrated with high quality evidence. Dr. Baumeister points out the well-studied ways to impact public policy, including influencing the Congress—an essay that we should all take to heart.

The above reports inform us how to get access to the power brokers in whose hands public policy lies. The expertise to accomplish our goals is available, and all the necessary knowledge is assembled, as exemplified in this book. It remains for us to learn how to implement it.

As Dr. Baumeister points out, children are too often the helpless victims of a system that responds only to powerful interests. Children are our future; we must invest in it!

Thank you, Vanderbilt University and Bill Wilkerson Center, for helping us find the way to do it.

Marion P. Downs, D.H.S.

Preface

Due to the undaunted and persistent efforts of such pioneers as the Ewings (Irene R. and Alex W.G.) of England and Marion P. Downs of the United States, the importance of early detection of hearing loss in young children has been acknowledged for more than four decades. In fact, by the early 1960s Downs (1967) had developed a comprehensive early identification program for all newborns in the Denver area and had screened more than 10,000 babies using the so-called arousal test. Despite the recognized value of early identification, we have been slow to develop hearing screening programs in the United States, especially for newborns. Less than 3% of all newborns in the United States are screened for hearing impairment, and consequently, the average age of identification for hearing loss is unacceptably high—above 2½ years. It appears that those of us in hearing health care have convinced ourselves of the necessity for early identification, however, we have not yet convinced those groups that are in positions to influence public policy.

As we enter into the 1990s, we have witnessed a renewed interest in early identification of hearing loss. The former Surgeon General, C. Everett Koop, established early identification as a priority area in health care; the American Academy of Audiology recently developed a position statement on early detection of hearing loss in children (1988); the Joint Committee on Infant Hearing (1991) recently revised the high-risk register; and the American Academy of Otolaryngology-Head and Neck Surgery developed a partnership with the Alexander Graham Bell Association for the Deaf for the purpose of promoting the importance of early identification and for developing model screening programs for states. Much of this focused energy on early identification has been brought about in an effort to realize an ambitious goal set forth by *Healthy People 2000* (1990)—to reduce the average age of identification of hearing loss in children from 2½ years to 12 months. Despite the widespread enthusiasm for early identification, there are many unanswered questions concerning the screening process for children of all ages.

The renewed impetus for early identification, and the need to answer and clarify numerous questions on early detection of hearing loss, prompted the organization of an international symposium on screening children for auditory function. Sponsored by the Division of Hearing and Speech Sciences of Vanderbilt University School of Medicine and the Bill Wilkerson Center, this important meeting was designed as a forum for presentation of state-of-the-art information on early identification of auditory dysfunction in children. We made a special effort to address screening issues for children of all ages. In addition, a call for papers was circulated well before the meeting in order to assure the inclusion of recent research efforts. About 300 participants from the United States, Canada, and several European countries attended the conference, which was held on June 27-29, 1991, in Nashville, Tennessee. The conferees included audiologists, otolaryngologists, pediatricians, speech-language pathologists, educators of the hearing impaired, and public health officials. This book represents the proceedings from that international meeting.

The book is divided into five sections. Part I offers a description of some of the critical problems facing those of us involved in screening children. Part II addresses issues, techniques, and model programs associated with newborn screening. Parts III and IV examine important issues concerned with screening infants and preschool- and school-age children. Finally, Part V focuses on some of the intervention issues and strategies appropriate for children of different age groups. A consensus statement on screening children for hearing loss was also developed and appears in Appendix 2. The statement was developed by representatives of several professional organizations including the American Academy of Audiology, the American Academy of Pediatrics, the Alexander Graham Bell Association for the Deaf, and the American Academy of Otolaryngology—Head and Neck Surgery.

The symposium and book would not have been possible without the generous support of the Maternal and Child Health Bureau (MCHB). We are especially grateful to James Papai, Elizabeth Brannon, and Aaron Favors of MCHB for recognizing the timely need for developing a state-of-the-art meeting on screening children for hearing loss. We also acknowledge the sponsoring institutions, the Bill Wilkerson Center and

Vanderbilt University School of Medicine. Numerous other individuals contributed to the success of the meeting and this book. As Coordinator of the newly established Bill Wilkerson Center Press, Mary Sue Fino-Szumski typed and formatted the chapters, coordinated manuscript preparation, and oversaw the entire publication process. Kathy Hollis played an invaluable role throughout all phases of the meeting including local arrangements, schedules, budgets, and correspondence. We are also grateful for the assistance of Susan Logan, Jeanne Dodd, Dorothy Adams, Kathryn Carney, Janey Gleaves, and the staff of the Bill Wilkerson Center Hearing Clinic.

Fred H. Bess and James W. Hall III, Editors

REFERENCES

American Academy of Audiology. 1988. Early identification of hearing loss in infants and children. *Audiology Today* 2:8-9.

Downs, M.P. 1967. Testing hearing in infancy and early childhood. In F.E. McConnell and P.H. Ward (eds.), *Childhood deafness*. Nashville, Tenn.: Vanderbilt University Press.

Joint Committee on Infant Hearing. 1991. 1990 position statement. *Audiology Today* 3:14-17.

U.S. Department of Health and Human Services, Public Health Service. 1990. *Healthy people 2000: National health promotion and disease prevention objectives*. Washington, D.C.: U.S. Government Printing Office.

Contributors

B. Anthonisen, M.Sc.
Department of Audiology
Gentofte University Hospital
Hellerup, Denmark

Donald B. Bailey, Jr., Ph.D.
Frank Porter Graham Child
    Development Center
University of North Carolina at
    Chapel Hill
Chapel Hill, North Carolina

Alfred A. Baumeister, Ph.D.
Department of Psychology
Vanderbilt University
Nashville, Tennessee

Thomas R. Behrens, Ph.D.
U.S. Department of Education
Washington, D.C.

Richard S. Bernstein, Ph.D.
Department of Otolaryngology
Albert Einstein College of Medicine
Rose F. Kennedy Center
Bronx, New York

Fred H. Bess, Ph.D.
Division of Hearing and Speech
    Sciences
Vanderbilt University School of
    Medicine and
Bill Wilkerson Center
Nashville, Tennessee

Peter M. Blackwell, Ph.D.
Rhode Island School for the Deaf
Providence, Rhode Island

Charles D. Bluestone, M.D.
Department of Pediatric Otolaryngology
Children's Hospital of Pittsburgh and
Department of Otolaryngology
School of Medicine
University of Pittsburgh
Pittsburgh, Pennsylvania

David R. Brown, M.D.
Department of Pediatrics
Division of Neonatology
School of Medicine
University of Pittsburgh
Pittsburgh, Pennsylvania
current affiliation:
Division of Neonatal Medicine
Newark Beth Israel Medical Center
Newark, New Jersey

Rochelle Cherry, Ed.D.
Department of Speech
Brooklyn College
City University of New York
Brooklyn, New York

Barbara K. Cone-Wesson, Ph.D.
Department of Otolaryngology
University of Southern California
Los Angeles, California

Merle DeVoe, M.S.
Educational Hearing Conservation
    Program
Office of Public Instruction
State Capital
Helena, Montana

Allan O. Diefendorf, Ph.D.
Audiology and Speech-Language
    Pathology
Department of Otolaryngology-Head
    and Neck Surgery
Indiana University School of Medicine
Indianapolis, Indiana

Marion P. Downs, D.H.S.
Department of Otolaryngology
University of Colorado
Health Sciences Center
Denver, Colorado

Tamara Lewis Engels, M.S.
Ear Institute of Indiana
Indianapolis, Indiana

Stephen Epstein, M.D.
The Ear Center
Wheaton, Maryland

Susan Farrer, M.A.
Children's Hospital Medical Center
Cincinnati, Ohio

Lynne V. Feagans, Ph.D.
Department of Human Development and
    Family Studies
The Pennsylvania State University
University Park, Pennsylvania

John W. Feightner, M.D.
Department of Family Medicine
McMaster University
Hamilton, Ontario
Canada

Judith S. Gravel, Ph.D.
Department of Otolaryngology
Albert Einstein College of Medicine
Rose F. Kennedy Center
Bronx, New York

Mary Jo Grote, M.A.
Communicative Disorders and Sciences
The Wichita State University
Wichita, Kansas

J. Groth, M.A.
Department of Audiology
Gentofte University Hospital
Hellerup, Denmark

James W. Hall III, Ph.D.
Division of Hearing and Speech
    Sciences and
Department of Otolaryngology
Vanderbilt University School of
    Medicine
Nashville, Tennessee

Kristi Hannan, M.A.
Department of Human Development and
    Family Studies
The Pennsylvania State University
University Park, Pennsylvania

Nancy E. Harrison, M.S., CCC-A
Wood County Office of Education
Bowling Green, Ohio

Deborah Hayes, Ph.D.
Audiology, Speech Pathology, and
    Learning Services
The Children's Hospital
Denver, Colorado

David Kardatzke, B.S.
Department of Biostatistics
Graduate School of Public Health
University of Pittsburgh
Pittsburgh, Pennsylvania

Robert W. Keith, Ph.D.
Division of Audiology
University of Cincinnati Medical Center
Cincinnati, Ohio

Jerome O. Klein, M.D.
Department of Pediatrics
Boston University School of Medicine
and Division of Pediatric Infectious
    Diseases
Boston City Hospital
Boston, Massachusetts

Thomas Mahoney, Ph.D.
Bureau of Communicative Disorders
Family Health Services Division
Utah Department of Health
Salt Lake City, Utah

Elizabeth Manlove, Ph.D.
Department of Human Development and
    Family Studies
The Pennsylvania State University
University Park, Pennsylvania

Judith A. Marlowe, Ph.D.
Judith A. Marlowe Ph.D. Audiology
    Associates
Winter Park, Florida

Noel D. Matkin, Ph.D.
Hearing and Speech Sciences
University of Arizona
Tucson, Arizona

Antonia B. Maxon, Ph.D.
Department of Communication Sciences
University of Connecticut
Storrs, Connecticut

Pamela E. Montgomery, M.S.
Tucson Medical Center
Tucson, Arizona

Jerry L. Northern, Ph.D.
Audiology Division
University Hospital and
Department of Otolaryngology
Department of Pediatrics
University of Colorado School of
    Medicine
Denver, Colorado

Robert J. Nozza, Ph.D.
The Audiology Center
Children's Hospital of Pittsburgh
and Department of Otolaryngology
School of Medicine
University of Pittsburgh
Pittsburgh, Pennsylvania

Terrey Oliver Penn, M.S.
Hearing, Speech, & Vision Services
Arkansas Department of Health
Little Rock, Arkansas

Charlotte H. Prentice, M.S.
Newborn Hearing Screening Program
Division of Hearing and Speech
    Sciences
Department of Otolaryngology
Vanderbilt University Medical Center
Nashville, Tennessee

Barbara J. Price, M.S., CCC-A
Lucas County Office of Education
Toledo, Ohio

Gayle Riemer, M.A.
Children's Hospital Medical Center
Cincinnati, Ohio

Jackson Roush, Ph.D.
Division of Speech and Hearing
    Sciences, School of Medicine
University of North Carolina
Chapel Hill, North Carolina

Elizabeth S. Ruppert, M.D.
Department of Pediatrics
Medical College of Ohio
Toledo, Ohio

Nancy Rushmer, M.A.
Infant Hearing Resource
Portland, Oregon

Diane L. Sabo, Ph.D.
The Audiology Center
Children's Hospital of Pittsburgh
and Department of Otolaryngology
School of Medicine
University of Pittsburgh
Pittsburgh, Pennsylvania

**Gerhard Salomon, M.D.,
    Dr.med.Sc.**
Department of Audiology
Gentofte University Hospital
Hellerup, Denmark

Jayant P. Shenai, M.D.
Department of Pediatrics
Vanderbilt University School of
    Medicine
Nashville, Tennessee

Brad A. Stach, Ph.D.
Audiology and Speech Pathology
    Services
The Methodist Hospital and
Department of Otorhinolaryngology and
    Communicative Sciences
Baylor College of Medicine
Houston, Texas

Marie Thompson, Ph.D.
College of Education
Speech and Hearing Sciences
Early Childhood Special Education
University of Washington
Seattle, Washington

P.P. Thomsen, B.Sc.
Madsen Electronics
Herlev, Denmark

Susan A.W. Toth, M.A.
Institute for Human Resources
University of Montana
Missoula, Montana

Robert G. Turner, Ph.D.
Department of Otolaryngology
University of California
San Francisco, California

Betty R. Vohr, M.D.
Women and Infants' Hospital of
    Rhode Island and
Brown University Program of Medicine
Providence, Rhode Island

Jon F. Watchko, M.D.
Department of Pediatrics
Division of Neonatology
School of Medicine
University of Pittsburgh
Pittsburgh, Pennsylvania

Karl R. White, Ph.D.
Early Intervention Research Institute
Utah State University
Logan, Utah

Faith C. Wurm, M.S., CCC-A
UT Southwestern Medical Center at
    Dallas
Dallas, Texas
current affiliation:
Division of Hearing and Speech
    Sciences
Vanderbilt University School of
    Medicine
Nashville, Tennessee

Michael K. Wynne, Ph.D.
Communicative Disorders and Sciences
The Wichita State University
Wichita, Kansas

M. Wende Yellin, M.S., CCC-A
Communicative and Vestibular
    Disorders
UT Southwestern Medical Center at
    Dallas
Dallas, Texas

In dedication to the pioneers of early identification:

Marion P. Downs,

Irene R. Ewing,

and

Alex W.G. Ewing

PART I.

Description of the Problem

Chapter 1

Screening in the 1990s:
Some Principles and Guidelines

John W. Feightner

INTRODUCTION

Screening, or early detection, of disorders has received increasing attention in health care over the last quarter century. While initially supported more by enthusiasm than science, this picture has changed. Principles for screening have gained wider acceptance and have evolved over the past two decades. But the statement of principles is just the beginning. Perhaps of greater importance is the gradual acceptance that *evidence* of a screening procedure's performance, derived from rigorous evaluation techniques, should play a key role in the rational application of such guidelines and should guide our subsequent policies. This gradual evolution in screening concepts has been bolstered by two further developments. As a result of appropriately designed research studies, higher quality data have become increasingly available in many areas. Second, the theoretical understanding and methodological strategies for evaluating screening tests have become more sophisticated. While advances continue at a fairly rapid pace, the field of screening is, in many ways, still in its early stages. The quality of evidence across different screening efforts varies considerably. Hence, guidelines that focus on the evaluation of available evidence of screening performance, using specific key dimensions, can aid in drawing careful conclusions for clinical actions and policies. Before discussing these guidelines and

1

principles, it is important to consider screening efforts within an historical context and to clarify some commonly used terms.

EARLY DETECTION: THE EVOLUTION OF A CONCEPT

Screening has generated increasing interest in medicine, particularly in the postwar era. The general premise for screening, or early detection, clearly makes sense. Treating a health problem or disease only after it is creating hardship for an individual, the family, and society is insufficient. Early detection offers the opportunity to recognize the condition before symptoms appear, and to prevent or diminish suffering. The groundwork for much of the initial efforts in this area was laid through increased understanding of disease mechanisms and the technology explosion that followed World War II. With this technology came advanced treatments and more sophisticated tests. At the same time, technology created enthusiasm for prevention, mainly through immunization, and when prevention was not possible, early detection. An example is promotion of the annual complete physical examination, particularly during the 1960s and 1970s. Other efforts included mass population screening and the mushrooming of multiphasic screening strategies. Screening became a rallying concept in the battle against ill health and also developed into a booming industry.

The historical roots for such an approach, in fact, go back at least 70 years. In 1922, the American Medical Association, convinced that the annual checkup has long-term benefits, officially and enthusiastically endorsed this approach and encouraged its implementation (Emerson 1923). Others have argued that this approach actually originated as early as the mid 1800s (Shattuck 1948). The 1970s and 1980s were decades of transition. Support for early detection efforts continued as people recognized the limitations of curative medicine. However, the need to incorporate critically appraised evidence to guide our screening policies and actions was also recognized (Canadian Task Force on the Periodic Health Examination 1979; Sackett 1975). As technology became more advanced and sophisticated, so did our understanding of techniques to evaluate test performance. The randomized controlled trial was applied more frequently to evaluate the effectiveness of therapeutic interventions and, on occasion, to evaluate programs of prevention. Finally, with the dawning of the 1990s has come the recognition that economic factors and strategies for implementation must also be incorporated into the evaluation of screening activities and decisions regarding screening policy. Hence, the age of screening development, with its technology imperative, has evolved to what might be viewed as an age of screening evaluation.

The Canadian Task Force on the Periodic Health Examination and its sister organization, the U.S. Preventive Services Task Force (subsequently the Expert Panel on Preventive Services), have provided invaluable leadership in the careful evaluation of early detection actions. These bodies have developed an approach to the careful evaluation of evidence relating to screening and early detection and have undertaken careful review of a significant number of health conditions (Canadian Task Force on the Periodic Health Examination 1979 and updates; U.S. Preventive Services Task Force 1989). These two organizations have, to a large extent, provided the foundation for the principles and guidelines that will be discussed in this article.

CLARIFYING SOME SCREENING TERMS AND CONCEPTS

The term *screening* is often used as an all-encompassing term for efforts aimed at the early detection of a condition. In the early stages, most screening efforts involved distinguishing an asymptomatic volunteer from the general public, which created few problems. Assessing volunteers in supermarkets and shopping malls is but one historical example. However, as the field evolved, other strategies for early detection emerged. Examples of such strategies include efforts by family physicians to assess blood pressure in their office on a regular basis, or to carry out Pap smears for the early detection of carcinoma of the cervix.

Sackett and Holland, in an early paper (1975), argued for a more careful definition and application of these terms and for consideration of the subsequent implications for test performance. They suggest that *screening* should apply to those activities that separate, from the general population, healthy volunteers into groups with high and low probability for a particular disorder. On the other hand, *case finding* should refer to testing of patients who have sought health care for disorders that may be completely unrelated to the early detection effort. Classically, a screening test would apply to those efforts aimed at general populations whereas case finding would occur most commonly in a family physician's office as part of overall patient care. The early detection of hearing deficits may fall into either category. In the newborn infant population, early detection may more closely approximate screening. Efforts aimed at early identification of a disorder in children within the community, however, might fit either the screening or case finding definition. For simplicity, the term *screening* will be used in this paper. In any event, the objective is the early identification and diagnosis of hearing deficits in "asymptomatic" children of unsuspecting parents.

Screening tests differ from diagnostic tests. Screening tests are, by definition, not diagnostic. Therefore, children with a positive screening outcome must be considered "at risk" for the problem until careful diagnostic testing can establish the presence or absence of the disorder. Strategies for evaluating the performance of screening tests and calculating the impact of their imperfections will be discussed later in the chapter. Also, screening tests, unlike diagnostic tests, are generally applied to populations with a very low likelihood of the disorder. This is often true even in so-called high-risk groups. Tests that perform well in diagnostic settings may be ill-suited for screening purposes. Moreover, it may be necessary to develop a sequential screening program, where a less expensive initial screen is used to increase the likelihood of the condition existing in the group receiving the second test. The beneficial and detrimental implications of such an approach are discussed later.

PRINCIPLES AND GUIDELINES

In the late 1960s, the World Health Organization (WHO) espoused a set of principles for screening for disease (World Health Organization 1971). These principles have formed the basis of subsequent recommendations for a rational approach to screening. Since the initial WHO guidelines, a great deal has been learned about how to cogently apply such principles. Perhaps the most significant advance is the growing acceptance that evidence that withstands critical scrutiny should guide our actions. The Canadian Task Force on the Periodic Health Examination and the U.S. Preventive Services Task Force have contributed significantly to advancing an evidence-based approach. Both organizations have, using rigorous evaluation strategies, provided careful reviews of evidence relating to dozens of early detection efforts (Canadian Task Force on the Periodic Health Examination 1979 and updates; U.S. Preventive Services Task Force 1989). As the field develops further, even more methodologically sophisticated evaluations can be expected, such as formal overview analysis and economic evaluation techniques.

Careful reviews and the research required to provide high quality evidence may be viewed as a delay in the implementation of policy and action. Can we afford to be so demanding about high quality evidence? Can we not take what we know about a condition and about a particular screening maneuver, combine it with logic and common sense, and develop a reasonable policy? For example, if lung cancer can be detected early by a chest X ray, why not routinely do chest X rays on smokers? The test is simple, is not invasive, and seems capable of early detection. Unfortunately, careful trials of such efforts have proven our logic wrong (Canadian Task Force on the Periodic Health Examination 1990 update). A similar situation exists in preschool screening for developmental health problems. Preschool screening is a major health concern and the focus of intensive effort, both in test development and in interventions. The early detection of problems that can affect school performance and learning makes a good deal of sense. Regrettably, careful evaluation of such efforts has demonstrated no benefit (Cadman et al. 1987; Feightner 1990). Indeed, the only significant outcome was increased concern and anxiety for parents of children with problems. Such experiences are humbling. They argue strongly for careful guidelines in screening and the careful review of evidence when formulating screening policies. The successful efforts to reduce stroke through the early detection and treatment of hypertension demonstrate clearly that beneficial results can be achieved.

Perhaps the strongest argument for evidence-guided actions is what might be called the ethical imperative of screening. When patients come to the health care system with a problem, there are both explicit and implicit requests for help. While providing the best available treatment for their problems is essential, they approach the system recognizing, hopefully, the potential limits and imperfections of curative medicine. However, with screening, the providers of care within the system search out the individual. It is implied that such actions will result in more good than harm to an unsuspecting and unrequesting patient. Hence, the demand for high quality evidence is even greater in the field of screening and early detection than in clinical care of symptomatic disease (Sackett and Holland 1975).

In reviewing the evidence for specific screening efforts, six important questions can guide our decisions about clinical policies and actions.

1. Is the burden of the problem significant to the individual and to society?
2. Is there acceptable evidence of effective treatment once the problem is detected?
3. Has the screening test been properly evaluated, and has it demonstrated acceptable performance in the screening setting?
4. Is there evidence that a screening program, with subsequent treatment, is of greater benefit than waiting until symptoms develop?
5. Have the important cost issues been considered and evaluated?
6. Are there plausible strategies and sufficient resources to ensure implementation?

The application of these questions to the early detection of hearing deficits is extremely relevant. Although drawing heavily on valuable contributions from the past, they are an attempt to express the key principles of screening in the context of the 1990s.

Is the burden of the problem significant? While advocates of particular screening efforts may feel the significance of the condition's burden is obvious, it must still be demonstrated as objectively as possible. Simple proof of prevalence is insufficient. The additional demonstration of actual impact measured in an acceptable fashion is essential. Burden is most commonly considered from the perspective of the individual, particularly in terms of pain and suffering. There is, as well, a population or societal perspective, which considers the impact on society of such factors as early death and loss of time from work.

Early efforts in screening tended to focus on the early detection of conditions where mortality and classic disease morbidity were the outcomes of interest. The intensive efforts to develop strategies for early detection and subsequent treatment of high blood pressure and the development of the Pap smear for the early detection of carcinoma of the cervix are but two examples. Burden, however, can have many dimensions. More recently, concerns have been increasingly focused on such factors as loss of function, loss of income, and loss of opportunity. For example, outcomes such as problems with learning secondary to vision or hearing deficits have begun to receive our attention. Over time, our view of pain and suffering has expanded to incorporate important new dimensions.

The careful measurement of such expanded definitions of burden can present problems and, in some cases, may require the development of new instruments and the generation of previously unavailable data. Other factors influencing the evaluation of burden include the age of onset of the problem and its duration. The frequency of the condition of interest interacts with its severity in evaluating burden. Common problems of little significance are unlikely to receive our attention, whereas even relatively rare phenomena that carry disastrous outcomes may be the subject of intensive effort. Finally, the burden of suffering can be considered in relative terms so that, in a state of limited resources, the hierarchy of priorities will be established.

Is there acceptable evidence of effective treatment once the problem is detected? Rarely does screening in itself benefit the individual. Indeed, labeling an individual as having a disease can have harmful effects even in the context of effective therapy (Feldman 1990). Hence, it is incumbent on those providing a screening program to ensure that individuals ultimately diagnosed as having the condition can be provided effective treatment.

Evidence supporting the effectiveness of the available therapy must be of appropriate quality. Some research designs, though widely used, can only provide relatively weak evidence of effectiveness. An established hierarchy of strength of evidence has been widely accepted (Sackett et al. 1985). The research design providing the strongest evidence for effectiveness is the randomized controlled trial (RCT). While often more expensive and time consuming than other designs, RCTs provide the best protection against biases that might result in misleading conclusions. The RCT design has been successfully deployed to evaluate a wide range of interventions, including counseling and programs of clinical care.

Unfortunately, evidence from a proper RCT may not be available or feasible. In such cases, nonrandomized controlled trials and cohort studies can provide evidence for the effectiveness of therapy. Other study designs such as case-control studies and before-after designs provide weaker evidence and generally play a supplementary role in evaluating effectiveness. Again, is it unrealistic to demand such high quality evidence? The answer is arguably no. Recent history provides us with many examples where therapy, after receiving an initial enthusiasm, has been demonstrated to be of no benefit.

Wrong conclusions lead to wasted resources, a situation that the current health care system cannot tolerate. This is particularly important when evaluating therapy for individuals who are identified as a result of a screening program. Screening programs create significant increases in the demand for subsequent investigations and therapy. Thus, evidence for effectiveness of therapy is an important principle.

Has the screening test been properly evaluated, and has it demonstrated acceptable performance in the screening setting? With the increasing availability of new technology, the demand for careful evaluation of screening test performance is clearly a central principle. Advances in the evaluation of test performance and the impact of such performance have provided the opportunity for more cogent decisions. The assessment of screening tests should incorporate two broad dimensions. First is the evaluation of test performance itself with the identification of the test's sensitivity, specificity, and calculation of its predictive value in relevant populations. Second, studies that evaluate new screening tests must be appropriately designed and executed. There are certain criteria for assessing design. Examples would be ensuring that the test was compared in a blinded fashion to an acceptable gold standard, that it was evaluated on an appropriate spectrum of patients, and that it was assessed in terms of its reproducibility and observer variation (Sackett et al. 1985).

The *sensitivity* of the test defines the percentage of people with the disease of interest who test positive (figure 1). Sensitivity can also be described as the true positive rate. A test's *specificity* defines the number of people without the disease who test negative. This has also been referred to as the true negative rate. A false positive rate can be calculated by the formula "1 − specificity." While sensitivity and specificity can, in fact, change somewhat in different populations, they are generally regarded as relatively stable test characteristics. However, a test's sensitivity and specificity will change as a function of the threshold for defining a positive test. For example, the sensitivity and specificity of an auditory brainstem response (ABR) will differ for a 40 dB HL versus 30 dB HL stimulus. For practical purposes, these characteristics move in opposite directions as the definition of a positive

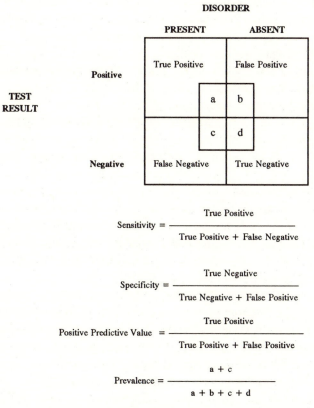

Figure 1. This figure illustrates the method used to calculate the test characteristics: sensitivity, specificity, positive predictive value, and prevalence.

outcome changes. If sensitivity is raised, specificity is lowered, and vice versa.

The predictive value of a test reflects the percentage of individuals who test positive and, in fact, have the disease. Similarly, predictive value of a negative test reflects the percentage of people testing negative who are truly free of the disease. This concept is useful in the clinical setting where one must work with a positive or negative test result for an individual patient. The predictive value of the test is dependent on its sensitivity and specificity. However, it is also affected, often dramatically, by a change in prevalence. Hence, a test that is useful in a population with a moderate to high prevalence of the disorder may be of little value in low prevalence situations (e.g., screening). The implications of the above must be taken into account when evaluating the quality of performance for any given screening test.

Generally, screening tests should have a high sensitivity so that a smaller percentage are missed on the initial screen. However, in a low prevalence screening situation, even a test with a relatively high specificity may generate a large number of false positive results. If the implications of labeling are significant, or if follow-up investigations are risky or expensive, a significant number of false positives can be a problem. This is sometimes dealt with by using a two-stage screening process, where a low-risk, less expensive second screening test is applied before moving to diagnostic investigations. Alternatively, the threshold for a positive test can be raised to increase the specificity and, hence, reduce the number of false positives. However, this will in turn increase the number of false negatives (because sensitivity will decrease) and must be done in light of the implications of false reassurance for individuals who screen negative despite having the disorder.

Because the test characteristics for screening procedures can have a profound impact on screening programs and on the individuals screened, this dimension requires careful scrutiny in any evaluation of a screening effort. Regrettably, studies that purport to evaluate test performance often suffer from significant methodological flaws. Two problems arise with remarkable frequency. First, sensitivity and specificity are either improperly defined or improperly calculated. Second, follow-up evaluation is often inadequate. If only those individuals testing positive are followed and retested, sensitivity and specificity cannot be calculated. While positive predictive value can be calculated in such circumstances, it provides no reflection of how many individuals with the condition are missed by the screening test. If follow-up for all patients (those screened positive and negative) is attempted but falls below 80%, significant biases can influence the results and significantly limit the value of any calculations.

Is there evidence that a screening program, with subsequent treatment, is of greater benefit than waiting until symptoms develop? While not always available, such studies provide the strongest evidence on which to base screening actions. They answer the central question, Do asymptomatic individuals who are screened and subsequently receive treatment fare better than individuals in an unscreened control group?

Randomized controlled trials play an even more significant role in the evaluation of screening programs. An RCT is the only design that can effectively rule out the many biases inherent in other designs that attempt to compare screened and unscreened populations. Cadman and colleagues (1984) have outlined the way in which such community-based trials of programs differ from those traditionally evaluating pharmacologic agents. Studies evaluating such programs should have as their initial target the full population at risk, not simply a selected high-risk subpopulation. Moreover, outcome should include all relevant short- and long-range outcomes. For example, in assessing the impact of screening for hearing loss, important outcomes might include developmental progress and school performance. Follow-up should be on all individuals who enter the study and not just those who fully receive treatment. Finally, the difference in outcome between screened and control groups must be of significance to society and not merely statistically significant.

This approach is particularly important when attempting to screen for conditions that may follow a fluctuating course rather than a continuous progressive one. For example, Shapiro et al. (1987), using a randomized controlled design, were unable to demonstrate any benefit from routine screening for depression and anxiety in the ambulatory care setting. This finding contradicted earlier reports from non-RCTs, which suggested the promising potential for such endeavors.

Have the important cost issues been considered and evaluated? Issues of screening cost versus screening impact will receive increasing emphasis during the 1990s. There are many important dimensions to cost. When evaluating screening programs, four dimensions are important. Risks of test side effects and labeling directly affect the patient, whereas costs and cost related to impact are more commonly viewed from a societal or system perspective.

The first issue to consider is whether the risks of the test, subsequent investigations, and treatment have been considered. Screening tests that identify patients who must go on to further complicated and invasive testing procedures may be of limited value. This is true even if the screening procedure may in itself be quick and inexpensive. Screening for carcinoma of the colon using stool for occult blood is but one example. Many individuals screened for carcinoma of the colon will be older and, in some cases, somewhat frail. Subsequent diagnostic tests carry significant risks for the elderly patient. Such risks are true for patients who have the condition, but at least they stand the chance of receiving benefit from subsequent treatment. The situation is worse still for patients falsely labeled and for whom the only outcomes of being incorrectly labeled by the screening process are the risks associated with further investigations.

The second significant cost issue is the impact of labeling. Initially considered of limited importance, studies in the field of hypertension as well as preschool screening have confirmed that labeling can indeed have an impact (Feldman 1990). Workers labeled as hypertensive miss more time from work than their unlabeled colleagues. Parents of children labeled as having developmental problems have increased concerns and anxieties. Clearly, this dimension must be taken into account when evaluating the overall cost of screening programs.

Third, traditional or simple costs must also be considered. These may be costs borne directly by the individual or more broadly by the health care system. Such costs include the cost of the screening program, the cost of the time spent with the patient by health professionals, the cost to the patient of time away from work or other activities, the cost of subsequent diagnostic tests and treatment if the patient has the condition, and costs for any additional tests and treatments that may arise from unexpected findings from the initial investigations.

Finally, one reflection of the magnitude of costs is to calculate the cost per case presented. While helpful, such analyses are limited, and more sophisticated approaches that take into account impact, as well as cost, provide more valuable data. In an economic analysis of screening, the task is to determine not whether screening is more economical than cure but whether early detection will save lives and improve health in a more economic fashion than treating the established disease (Weinstein 1990). In simplest terms, economic evaluation looks at the impact of outcome in terms of the quantity and quality of life. Such economic analyses fall into three paradigms: cost-effectiveness (the simplest and most limited comparison), cost-benefit, and cost-utility.

In each approach, costs are extensively evaluated in the broadest dimension and incorporate many of the items discussed earlier. However, for each approach, the outcome component differs. Cost-effectiveness looks at the cost in comparison to the outcome of interest, often lives saved. This strategy makes it difficult to compare the economic impact across programs where outcomes may vary. As a result, cost-benefit and cost-utility analyses have been developed as strategies for converting outcomes into consistent units across programs to allow such comparisons. Cost-benefit analysis instruments exist that can capture the expression of benefit in dollar terms. Cost-utility analysis strategies measure outcome in terms of quality as well as duration of life. While such economic evaluations generate controversy and need to be further refined, they represent an area of growing significance in the assessment of screening efforts.

Are there plausible strategies and sufficient resources to ensure implementation? The best-tested and most effective screening effort can have an impact only if it reaches the population for which it is intended. In addition to ensuring that screening is offered to those who can benefit, a high percentage of those for which it is intended must actually receive the screening procedure. Then, those who screen positive must link with further diagnostic and treatment efforts. To be successful, programs must be feasible, have sufficient resources, and have effective links across the stages from screening to treatment. Screening for hypertension in shopping malls looked promising because both the test and the access were feasible. However, enthusiasm waned when studies identified that a significant proportion of individuals identified as possibly hypertensive did not effectively link with follow-up assessment and treatment.

The challenge, then, is to ensure that a screening program is effective and that it can be implemented. There must be compliance from both the provider and the receiver. Programs that can be executed through institutions are more likely to be successfully implemented than those that occur in the community. However, implementation in institutions may be impractical, costly, or untimely, and the implementation of programs or recommended policies in the community can be a slow and difficult process. Extensive data exist to accentuate how challenging such efforts can be (Inui et al. 1981; Carter et al. 1981). While barriers to implementation have been well delineated, the development of successful implementation strategies has been slow. Implementation in the community may become more effective as information systems become more sophisticated and more easily managed. Such advances will also provide opportunities for audit and feedback, strategies that show some promise for effecting behavior change. Involving respected individuals as "educational influentials" has been proven to be effective for the acceptance and uptake of some recommendations (Lomas et al. 1991). Such techniques, however, will need continued development and evaluation. In the meantime, the evaluation of screening efforts must take into consideration the likelihood of successful implementation. Efforts that seem feasible and have been proven effective will require the commitment of sufficient resources to enhance the likelihood of successful implementation.

Hence, an important principle in evaluating screening activities is to determine whether strategies have been developed to disseminate and facilitate implementation of the new knowledge and whether the resources exist to support such implementation.

SUMMARY

Asking the six questions presented above can focus the review of existing evidence to determine whether a screening program would do more good than harm. When sufficient evidence exists to support such programs, it can provide a strong argument for the funding of such activities. Often evidence of acceptable quality is incomplete or, in certain cases, severely lacking. Drawing such conclusions after reviewing the evidence can be discouraging. However, this need not be the case. Identifying important gaps in evidence can guide needed research, which can, in turn, contribute substantially to advances in the field. Moreover, valuable health care resources will not be wasted on useless efforts and can be channeled instead into areas where effectiveness is well proven. In the short term, such a careful approach may seem less expedient. However, in the long run, demanding rigorous assessment of existing evidence and high quality data to guide policy will provide ultimate benefit to the population served by the health care system.

REFERENCES

Cadman, D., Chambers, L., Feldman, W., and Sackett, D. 1984. Assessing the effectiveness of community screening programs. *Journal of the American Medical Association* 251(12):1580-1585.

Cadman, D., Chambers, L.W., Walter, S.D., et al. 1987. Evaluation of public health preschool child developmental screening: The process and outcome of a community program. *American Journal of Public Health* 77:45-51.

Canadian Task Force on the Periodic Health Examination. 1979. The periodic health examination. *Canadian Medical Association Journal* 121:1123-1254.

Canadian Task Force on the Periodic Health Examination. 1984. The periodic health examination: 2. 1984 update. *Canadian Medical Association Journal* 130:1278-1285.

Canadian Task Force on the Periodic Health Examination. 1986. The periodic health examination: 2. 1985 update. *Canadian Medical Association Journal* 134:721-729.

Canadian Task Force on the Periodic Health Examination. 1988. The periodic health examination: 2. 1987 update. *Canadian Medical Association Journal* 138:618-626.

Canadian Task Force on the Periodic Health Examination. 1989. The periodic health examination: 1989 update parts 1 and 2. *Canadian Medical Association Journal* 141:205-216.

Canadian Task Force on the Periodic Health Examination. 1989. The periodic health examination: 1989 update part 3. *Canadian Medical Association Journal* 141:1136-1140.

Canadian Task Force on the Periodic Health Examination. 1989. The periodic health examination: 1989 update part 4. *Canadian Medical Association Journal* 141:1233-1240.

Canadian Task Force on the Periodic Health Examination. 1990. The periodic health examination, 1990 update: 1. Early detection of hyperthyroidism and hypothyroidism in adults and screening of newborns for congenital hypothyroidism. *Canadian Medical Association Journal* 142(9):955-961.

Canadian Task Force on the Periodic Health Examination. 1990. The periodic health examination, 1990 update: 2. Early detection of depression and prevention of suicide. *Canadian Medical Association Journal* 142(11):1233-1238.

Canadian Task Force on the Periodic Health Examination. 1990. The periodic health examination, 1990 update: 3. Interventions to prevent lung cancer other than smoking cessation. *Canadian Medical Association Journal* 143(4):269-272.

Canadian Task Force on the Periodic Health Examination. 1990. The periodic health examination, 1990 update: 4. Well-baby care in the first 2 years of life. *Canadian Medical Association Journal* 143(9):867-872.

Canadian Task Force on the Periodic Health Examination. 1991. The periodic health examination, 1991 update: 1. Screening for cognitive impairment in the elderly. *Canadian Medical Association Journal* 144:425-431.

Canadian Task Force on the Periodic Health Examination. 1991. The periodic health examination, 1991 update: 2. Administration of pneumococcal vaccine. *Canadian Medical Association Journal* 144:665-671.

Carter, W.B., Belcher, D.W., and Inui, T.S. 1981. Implementing preventive care in clinical practice. II. Problems for managers, clinicians and patients. *Medical Care Review* 38:195-216.

Emerson, H. 1923. Periodic medical examinations of apparently healthy persons. *Journal of the American Medical Association* 81:1376-1381.

Feightner, J.W. 1990. Preschool screening: A review of the evidence. In R.B. Goldbloom and R.S. Lawrence (eds.), *Preventing disease: Beyond the rhetoric*. New York: Springer-Verlag.

Feldman, W. 1990. How serious are the adverse effects of screening? *Journal of General Internal Medicine* 5:S50-53.

Inui, T.S., Belcher, D.W., and Carter, W.B. 1981. Implementing preventive care in clinical practice. I. Organizational issues and strategies. *Medical Care Review* 38:129-154.

Lomas, J., Enkin, M., Anderson, G.M., Hannah, W., et al. 1991. Opinion leaders vs. audit and feedback to implement practice guidelines. *Journal of the American Medical Association* 265(17):2202-2207.

Sackett, D.L. 1975. Laboratory screening: A critique. *Clinical Laboratory Developments, Federation Proceedings* 34(12):2157-2161.

Sackett, D.L., and Holland, W.W. 1975. Controversy in the detection of disease. *Lancet* 1:357.

Sackett, D.L., Haynes, R.B., and Tugwell, P. 1985. *Clinical epidemiology: A basic science for clinical medicine*. Boston: Little, Brown and Co.

Shapiro, S., German, P.S., Skinner, E.A., et al. 1987. An experiment to change detection and measurement of mental morbidity in primary care. *Medical Care* 25:327-339.

Shattuck, L. 1948. *Report of the sanitary commission of Massachusetts, 1850*. Reprinted. Cambridge: Harvard University Press.

U.S. Preventive Services Task Force. 1989. *Guide to preventive clinical services: An assessment of the effectiveness of 169 interventions*. Baltimore: Williams and Wilkins.

Weinstein, M.C. 1990. Economics of prevention: The costs of prevention. *Journal of General Internal Medicine* 5:S89-92.

World Health Organization. 1971. Public Health Papers no. 45: "Mass Health Examinations." Geneva 81-82.

Chapter 2

Changing Demographics of Infants in the Neonatal Intensive Care Unit: Impact on Auditory Function

Jayant P. Shenai

INTRODUCTION

In recent years, advances in science and technology have increased the chances for survival of very-low-birth-weight (VLBW) neonates and other severely compromised newborns. These infants are at an increased risk for sensorineural hearing loss in addition to other sequelae. Early detection of hearing loss in children is essential in order to initiate the medical and educational intervention critical for their optimal development. In this chapter, I discuss the status of neonatal intensive care, its impact on survival and morbidity in VLBW infants, and changes in the prevalence of certain neonatal conditions and their impact on auditory function.

NEONATAL INTENSIVE CARE

Regionalization of perinatal care is recognized as a potential means of reducing perinatal mortality and morbidity (Lucey 1973; Killam, Barrett, and Cotton 1981; Johnson 1982; McCormick, Shapiro, and Starfield 1985). The concept involves implementation of a care system within a region that includes designation of a regional perinatal center, assessment of care levels at all perinatal facilities in the region, and establishment of a network of perinatal services. These services include education for physicians, nurses, and other health care providers; consultation and communication; site visits for evaluation of needs; provision of specialized equipment; and high-risk patient referral including transport. These services are provided with the expectation that the perinatal health care providers in the region will improve their abilities to anticipate complications, to identify high-risk maternal and neonatal patients, and to optimally deliver their care.

Regionalization of perinatal care was initiated in Tennessee in 1972. The neonatal component of the program was formally established in 1974 and the obstetric component in 1977. Currently, the program is served by five designated regional perinatal centers located in the metropolitan cities of Nashville, Memphis, Knoxville, Chattanooga, and Johnson City. There are approximately 100 community hospitals with perinatal services in the state. The annual number of births in the state has ranged from 64,154 in 1974 to 77,678 in 1989. The regionalization during its first decade of implementation has been successful in improving perinatal care in the state as indicated by favorable changes in referral patterns and improved outcome of transported neonates (Shenai et al. 1991).

The designated regional perinatal center for Middle Tennessee is located at Vanderbilt University Medical Center in Nashville. The neonatal intensive care unit (NICU) at Vanderbilt is a 48-bed unit with 24 intensive and 24 intermediate care beds. Approximately 850 newborn infants needing specialized care are admitted to the NICU annually. Approximately 220 of these infants are of the VLBW (< 1500 g birth-weight) category, and among these, approximately 90 infants are of the ultra-low-birth-weight (ULBW) (< 1000 g birth-weight) category.

The VLBW neonates typically have multiple problems associated with immaturity of various organ systems. These problems include difficulties with thermoregulation, respiratory insufficiency from hyaline membrane disease, pulmonary edema from symptomatic patent ductus arteriosus, hyperbilirubinemia, and increased susceptibility to bronchopulmonary dysplasia (BPD), sepsis, periventricular-intraventricular hemorrhage (P-IVH), perinatal asphyxia, and retinopathy of prematurity. A prolonged hospital course is typical in these infants. Because of the potential exposure of these infants to one or more risk factors associated with sensorineural hearing loss, auditory screening is recommended before their discharge from the NICU (Joint Committee on Infant Hearing 1991). In addition to this screening, a detailed

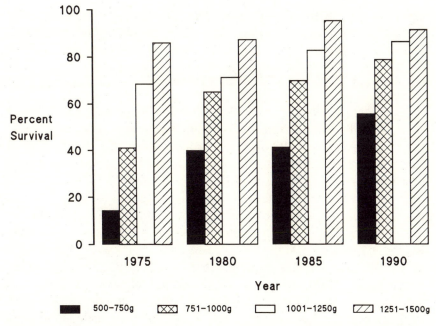

Figure 1. Percent survival of very-low-birth-weight (VLBW) neonates admitted to Vanderbilt NICU between 1975 and 1990.

evaluation of auditory function and speech and language development is performed in all high-risk infants enrolled in the Vanderbilt newborn follow-up clinic.

SURVIVAL OF VLBW NEONATES

The percent survival of VLBW neonates admitted to Vanderbilt NICU during the years between 1975 and 1990 is shown in figure 1. During this period, there has been a progressive increase in the percentage of VLBW neonates discharged alive at the end of their first hospitalization in the NICU. The increase in survival has been particularly impressive among the ULBW neonates. Similar trends in survival have been observed by others (Stewart, Reynolds, and Lipscomb 1981). The improved survival of VLBW neonates is attributed to advances in the knowledge of pathophysiology of various neonatal diseases, technologic advances made possible by miniaturization of equipment to evaluate and treat very small subjects, and enhanced expertise in the delivery of neonatal care not only at the regional center but also at other facilities within the referral network (Stahlman 1989; Shenai et al. 1991).

MORBIDITY AMONG VLBW SURVIVORS

The incidence of major handicaps in VLBW neonates born between 1976 and 1985 and discharged alive from Vanderbilt NICU is shown in table 1 (Grogaard et al. 1990). Major handicaps characterized by cerebral palsy, mental retardation, retinopathy of prematurity, and sensorineural hearing loss were present in more than 5% of the VLBW survivors. Approximately 18% of the survivors had at least one handicap, and among these, about one-third of the children had two or more handicaps. For most handicaps, there was an inverse correlation between the birth weight and incidence of the handicap. A similar incidence of handicaps in VLBW survivors has been reported by others (Fitzhardinge 1976; Saigal et al. 1982). Although the prevalence of neurodevelopmental handicaps among VLBW survivors appears to be decreasing with evolving neonatal intensive care, the VLBW infants remain about three times as likely as normal newborn infants to have an adverse neurodevelopmental outcome, and the risk increases with decreasing birth weight (Papile, Munsick-Bruno, and Schaefer 1983; McCormick 1985). Poor cognitive function, academic achievement, and behavior at school age are characteristic of the adverse neurodevelopmental outcome in VLBW survivors, particularly in those with evidence of perinatal growth failure (Hack et al. 1991).

VLBW NEONATES AND HEARING LOSS

The number of admissions to Vanderbilt NICU of ULBW neonates has doubled from approximately 6% of all admissions in 1976 to 12% in 1989. During the same period, the number of NICU beds assigned for the care of a ULBW neonate has more than quadrupled as evidenced by an increase in the bed occupancy rate from approximately 8% in 1976 to 34% in 1989. These increases in the ULBW patient care needs reflect the trend during recent years in neonatal intensive care in which smaller and more immature newborn infants are being successfully resuscitated and supported. Immaturity is a common denominator among several studies examining the neonatal risk factors for sensorineural hearing loss

Table 1
Major Handicaps in VLBW Survivors*

Birth weight (g)	Total group	500-750	751-1000	1001-1250	1251-1500
Admissions[1] (No.)	1919	230	453	540	696
Discharged alive (No.)	1411	70	281	427	633
Discharged alive (% Admissions)	74	30	62	79	91
Followed (No.)	632	35	132	220	245
Cerebral palsy (% Survivors)	7.6	14.3	7.9	8.9	5.2
Mental retardation[2] (% Survivors)	6.5	11.5	7.5	7.0	4.7
Retinopathy[3] (% Survivors)	5.5	17.1	12.1	4.1	1.6
Hearing loss[4] (% Survivors)	5.4	3.8	4.7	5.1	6.4
Any handicap (% Survivors)	18.0	26.9	23.4	17.8	13.4
Multiple handicaps[5] (% Survivors)	6.7	11.5	8.4	7.2	4.7

* Modified from Grogaard, J.B., et al. (1990).
[1] Data from Vanderbilt NICU during study period 1976 through 1985.
[2] Intelligence quotient $\leq$ 70 at $\geq$ 18 months of corrected age.
[3] Severe retinopathy of prematurity (cicatricial or blindness).
[4] Hearing loss evaluated with $\geq$ 18 months of follow-up.
[5] Two or more handicaps .

(Duara et al. 1986; Halpern, Hosford-Dunn, and Malachowski 1987; Salamy, Eldredge, and Tooley 1989). It stands to reason, therefore, that with decreasing gestational age of patients in the NICU, a concomitant increase in the incidence of sensorineural hearing loss can be expected to occur. These observations support the need for a program of systematic sequential evaluation of auditory function as a critical component of neonatal intensive care and follow-up.

Why is immaturity an important neonatal risk factor for sensorineural hearing loss? The possible reasons become evident when one examines the neonatal conditions commonly associated with a low gestational age.

BRONCHOPULMONARY DYSPLASIA

BPD, a form of chronic lung disease, occurs commonly in VLBW neonates, particularly in those requiring supplemental oxygen therapy and mechanical ventilation for respiratory failure in the early postnatal period. The development of BPD in these infants is believed to be influenced by lung immaturity and factors promoting injury and those inhibiting repair of tissues involving the lung and tracheobronchial tree (Northway, Rosan, and Porter 1967). The diagnosis of BPD is based on the triad of supplemental oxygen need, respiratory symptoms, and characteristic chest radiographic abnormalities that persist beyond 28 days of postnatal age.

The incidence of BPD at Vanderbilt NICU is estimated to be 32% among VLBW survivors and as high as 60% among the ULBW infants of this group (Hazinski 1990). Based on the data from the regional perinatal centers, it is estimated that annually there are 175 new cases of BPD in Tennessee, making BPD the leading cause of chronic lung disease in children.

In addition to the supplemental oxygen therapy, the management of infants with BPD often includes fluid restriction and diuretic treatment. Furosemide, a potent loop diuretic, is commonly used for its beneficial diuretic and nondiuretic pulmonary effects (Englehardt, Elliott, and Hazinski 1986). Furosemide elimination by the kidney is decreased in VLBW neonates relative to older infants and children, resulting in potentially toxic accumulation of furosemide in the tissues with long-term administration (Mirochnick et al. 1988). The potential ototoxicity of loop diuretics, altered pharmacokinetics of these medications secondary to immaturity, and their frequent long-term use in management of chronic lung disease account for the increased risk for sensorineural hearing loss in infants with BPD.

NEONATAL SEPSIS

Infections are a major cause of mortality and morbidity in the newborn infants. Based on the time of onset of infection, neonatal sepsis is classified as congenital (or intrauterine), perinatal (acquired around birth), or postnatal (acquired after birth).

The common organisms for congenital sepsis include *Toxoplasma gondii*, rubella virus, cytomegalovirus, herpes simplex virus, and *Treponema pallidum* (McIntosh 1984). Mucocutaneous, eye, and bone lesions, hepatosplenomegaly and jaundice, intracranial calcifications and microcephaly, and malformations including congenital heart disease are the common manifestations of congenital sepsis. The incidence at Vanderbilt NICU of proven congenital sepsis has ranged from approximately 0.4% to 1.0% of all admissions during the period 1980 through 1990, making this form of sepsis rare relative to the other forms. Despite advances in antimicrobial therapy, the outcome for infants with congenital sepsis remains poor as evidenced by a high incidence of sequelae including sensorineural hearing loss, blindness, and mental retardation.

The common organisms for perinatally acquired sepsis include Group B beta-hemolytic streptococcus, *Escherichia coli*, gram-negative enteric bacteria, *Haemophilus* species, and *Listeria monocytogenes* (Harris and Polin 1983; Bortolussi 1990). The spectrum of perinatally acquired infections varies from asymptomatic bacteremia to overwhelming sepsis including disseminated intravascular coagulopathy and meningitis. The neurologic sequelae, including sensorineural hearing loss, occur in 30% to 50% of survivors with neonatal meningitis (Siegel 1985).

Coagulase-negative staphylococcus is currently the most prevalent pathogen associated with postnatally acquired sepsis (St. Geme and Harris 1991). Infections due to this organism are particularly common in chronically hospitalized VLBW infants and are often associated with the presence of foreign bodies such as central vascular catheters and endotracheal tubes. Coagulase-negative staphylococcus can result in both systemic and focal infections. The systemic infection with meningitis is associated with mortality as high as 15% and significant morbidity including sensorineural hearing loss among the survivors. Although the hospital-borne coagulase-negative staphylococcus is resistant to antibiotics such as penicillin, oxacillin, and gentamicin, most species of the organism remain sensitive to vancomycin. Vancomycin is therefore the antibiotic of choice for both prophylaxis and treatment of suspected or proven coagulase-negative staphylococcal sepsis. Vancomycin elimination by the kidney is correlated inversely with gestational and chronological age, resulting in the increased risk for tissue accumulation, and nephrotoxicity and ototoxicity in young VLBW infants (Schaad, McCracken, and Nelson 1980).

The incidence at Vanderbilt NICU of proven perinatal or postnatal bacterial sepsis during the period 1980 through 1990 has remained birth-weight specific, ranging from approximately 11% to 17% among ULBW infants, from 4% to 7% among larger VLBW infants (1001-1500 g birth weight), and from 2% to 4% among other infants (>1500 g birth weight). The potential ototoxicity of antimicrobial agents such as aminoglycosides and vancomycin, altered pharmacokinetics of these medications secondary to immaturity, and their frequent repeated use for both prophylaxis and treatment of recurrent sepsis account for the increased risk for sensorineural hearing loss in infants with neonatal sepsis and meningitis.

PERIVENTRICULAR-INTRAVENTRICULAR HEMORRHAGE

P-IVH is the most common type of neonatal intracranial hemorrhage and is characteristic of the VLBW infant (Volpe 1989). The site of origin of P-IVH characteristically is the subependymal germinal matrix, and extension of hemorrhage into the ventricular system and brain parenchyma can occur. Intravascular factors such as altered cerebral blood flow, vascular factors such as tenuous capillary integrity, and extravascular factors such as deficient connective tissue support are implicated in the pathogenesis of P-IVH. Ultrasonography is the diagnostic procedure of choice and allows grading of the severity of P-IVH (Papile et al. 1978).

The incidence of P-IVH at Vanderbilt NICU has been birth-weight specific, ranging from approximately 35% to 38% among ULBW infants, and from 22% to 28% among larger VLBW infants (1001-1500 g birth weight) (Hutchison, Barrett, and Fleischer 1982). More severe grades of P-IVH are typically seen in the ULBW infants. The most critical determinant of long-term neurologic outcome is the degree of brain parenchymal injury (Volpe 1989). Among infants with severe grades of P-IVH, neurologic sequelae including major motor deficits and poor cognitive development are seen in more than 70% of the survivors. Sensorineural hearing loss is most likely to be present in these infants.

NEONATAL HYPERBILIRUBINEMIA

Hyperbilirubinemia in the VLBW neonates results from transient deficiencies in hepatic bilirubin uptake, intracellular transport, and conjugation mechanisms compounded by increased enterohepatic circulation of the pigment (Rodgers and Stevenson 1990). In addition, bilirubin production in the neonate is twofold to threefold greater on a per body-weight basis than in the adult. Increased breakdown of heme from senescent red blood cells in extravascular sites of blood collection, such as in P-IVH, adds to the bilirubin pool.

Bilirubin neurotoxicity is largely determined by the serum concentration of unconjugated bilirubin, albumin-binding of bilirubin, and integrity of the blood-brain barrier (Cashore 1990). Bilirubin neurotoxicity is typically characterized by yellow staining of the basal ganglia and nuclear areas of the brain (kernicterus) seen at autopsy. Sick VLBW neonates are at an increased risk for kernicterus because of the longer duration of hyperbilirubinemia, lower concentration of serum albumin, more cardiovascular instability, and vulnerable blood-brain barrier. Although the typical clinical neurologic manifestations of kernicterus are rarely seen, the possibility of subtle neurotoxicity remains a major concern in the VLBW neonates. The risk of a neuro-developmental handicap including sensorineural hearing loss has been shown to be associated with a serum total bilirubin concentration as low as 6 mg/dl in the VLBW neonates (Van de Bor et al. 1989). This risk is estimated to increase by 30% for each 2.9 mg/dl increase of maximal serum total bilirubin concentration. Palmer and Smith (1990) have suggested that the serum bilirubin concentrations alone may not be sufficient for prediction of kernicterus in the VLBW neonates and that other rapid noninvasive measurements of energy metabolism, such as by nuclear magnetic resonance spectroscopy, may be needed for detection of impending or actual brain cell injury induced by bilirubin.

At Vanderbilt NICU the number of patients treated with one or more exchange transfusions for the exclusive indication of severe hyperbilirubinemia has not exceeded ten per year during the period 1980 through 1990. Conversely, nearly 100% of the VLBW neonates are treated with phototherapy for lesser degrees of hyperbilirubinemia. The neonatal risk criterion of "hyperbilirubinemia at a level exceeding indication for exchange transfusion" as specified by the Joint Committee on Infant Hearing (1991) is therefore based on an intervention that is rarely performed in the NICU. This criterion may need to be modified to include other VLBW neonates with lesser degrees of hyper-bilirubinemia and with susceptibility to more subtle forms of bilirubin neurotoxicity.

SUMMARY

Modern intensive care has increased the chances for survival of VLBW neonates and other severely compromised newborns. The increase in survival has been particularly impressive among the ULBW neonates. Despite these advances, the VLBW neonates remain about three times as likely as normal newborn infants to have an adverse neurodevelopmental handicap in the form of cerebral palsy, mental retardation, retinopathy of prematurity, and sensorineural hearing loss. Furthermore, the risk increases with decreasing birth weight. With decreasing gestational age of patients in the NICU and a concomitant increase in the prevalence of certain neonatal conditions such as BPD, sepsis, P-IVH, and hyperbilirubinemia, the overall incidence of sensorineural hearing loss in the NICU patient population is expected to increase. A program of systematic sequential evaluation of auditory function is therefore a necessary component of neonatal intensive care and follow-up.

THE FUTURE

The prevention of prematurity needs to be the primary focus in the perinatal health care delivery of the future. In addition to further improvement in survival with advances in the intensive care capabilities, the prevention of morbidity among the survivors needs to be the major goal of the neonatal care of the future. Early detection of abnormalities and appropriate timely intervention need to be continued for the promotion of optimal development in the future survivors of neonatal intensive care.

REFERENCES

Bortolussi, R. 1990. Neonatal listeriosis. *Seminars in Perinatology* 14 (Suppl. 1):44-48.

Cashore, W.J. 1990. The neurotoxicity of bilirubin. *Clinics in Perinatology* 17:437-447.

Duara, S., Suter, C.M., Bessard, K.K., and Gutberlet, R.L. 1986. Neonatal screening with auditory brainstem response: Results of follow-up audiometry and risk factor evaluation. *Journal of Pediatrics* 108:276-281.

Englehardt, B., Elliott, S., and Hazinski, T.A. 1986. Short- and long-term effects of furosemide on lung function in infants with bronchopulmonary dysplasia. *Journal of Pediatrics* 109:1034-1039.

Fitzhardinge, P.M. 1976. Follow-up studies of the low birth weight infant. *Clinics in Perinatology* 3:503-516.

Grogaard, J.B., Lindstrom, D.P., Parker, R.A., Culley, B., and Stahlman, M.T. 1990. Increased survival rate in very low birth weight infants (1500 grams or less): No association with increased incidence of handicaps. *Journal of Pediatrics* 117:139-146.

Hack, M., Breslau, N., Weissman, B., Aram, D., Klein, N., and Borawski, E. 1991. Effect of very low birth weight and subnormal head size on cognitive abilities at school age. *New England Journal of Medicine* 325:231-237.

Halpern, J., Hosford-Dunn, H., and Malachowski, N. 1987. Four factors that accurately predict hearing loss in "high risk" neonates. *Ear and Hearing* 8:21-25.

Harris, M.C., and Polin, R.A. 1983. Neonatal septicemia. *Pediatric Clinics of North America* 30:243-258.

Hazinski, T.A. 1990. Bronchopulmonary dysplasia. In V. Chernick and E.L. Kendig, Jr. (eds.), *Disorders of the respiratory tract in children* (pp. 300-320). Philadelphia: Saunders.

Hutchison, A.A., Barrett, J.M., and Fleischer, A.C. 1982. Intraventricular hemorrhage in the premature infant. *New England Journal of Medicine* 307:1272-1273.

Johnson, K.G. 1982. The promise of regional perinatal care as a national strategy for improved maternal and infant care. *Public Health Report* 97:134-139.

Joint Committee on Infant Hearing. 1991. 1990 position statement. *Asha* 33(Suppl. 5):3-6.

Killam, A.P., Barrett, J.M., and Cotton, R.B. 1981. The impact of a tertiary perinatal center on survival of the very low birth weight infant. *Journal of Tennessee Medical Association* 74:870-872.

Lucey, J.F. 1973. Why we should regionalize perinatal care. *Pediatrics* 52:488-491.

McCormick, M.C. 1985. The contribution of low birth weight to infant mortality and childhood morbidity. *New England Journal of Medicine* 312:82-90.

McCormick, M.C., Shapiro, S., and Starfield, B.H. 1985. The regionalization of perinatal services: Summary of the evaluation of a national demonstration program. *Journal of the American Medical Association* 253:799-804.

McIntosh, K. 1984. Viral infections of the fetus and newborn. In M.E. Avery and H.W. Taeusch, Jr. (eds.), *Diseases of the newborn* (pp. 754-768). Philadelphia: Saunders.

Mirochnick, M.H., Miceli, J.J., Kramer, P.A., Chapron, D.J., and Raye, J.R. 1988. Furosemide pharmacokinetics in very low birth weight infants. *Journal of Pediatrics* 112:653-657.

Northway, Jr., W.H., Rosan, R.C., and Porter, D.Y. 1967. Pulmonary disease following respirator therapy of hyaline-membrane disease: Bronchopulmonary dysplasia. *New England Journal of Medicine* 276:357-368.

Palmer, C., and Smith, M.B. 1990. Assessing the risk of kernicterus using nuclear magnetic resonance. *Clinics in Perinatology* 17:307-329.

Papile, L-A., Burstein, J., Burstein, R., and Koffler, H. 1978. Incidence and evolution of subependymal and intraventricular hemorrhage: A study of infants with birth weights less than 1,500 gm. *Journal of Pediatrics* 92:529-534.

Papile, L-A., Munsick-Bruno, G., and Schaefer, A. 1983. Relationship of cerebral intraventricular hemorrhage and early childhood neurologic handicaps. *Journal of Pediatrics* 103:273-277.

Rodgers, P.A., and Stevenson, D.K. 1990. Developmental biology of heme oxygenase. *Clinics in Perinatology* 17:275-291.

Saigal, S., Rosenbaum, P., Stoskopf, B., and Milner, R. 1982. Follow-up of infants 501 to 1,500 gm birth weight delivered to residents of a geographically defined region with perinatal intensive care facilities. *Journal of Pediatrics* 100:606-613.

St. Geme III, J.W., and Harris, M.C. 1991. Coagulase-negative staphylococcal infection in the neonate. *Clinics in Perinatology* 18:281-302.

Salamy, A., Eldredge, L., and Tooley, W.H. 1989. Neonatal status and hearing loss in high-risk infants. *Journal of Pediatrics* 114:847-852.

Schaad, U.B., McCracken, Jr., G.H., and Nelson, J.D. 1980. Clinical pharmacology and efficacy of vancomycin in pediatric patients. *Journal of Pediatrics* 96:119-126.

Shenai, J.P., Major, C.W., Gaylord, M.S., Blake, W.W., Simmons, A., Oliver, S., and DeArmond, D. 1991. A successful decade of regionalized perinatal care in Tennessee: The neonatal experience. *Journal of Perinatology* 11:137-143.

Siegel, J.D. 1985. Neonatal sepsis. *Seminars in Perinatology* 9:20-28.

Stahlman, M. 1989. Implications of research and high technology for neonatal intensive care. *Journal of the American Medical Association* 361:1791.

Stewart, A.L., Reynolds, E.O.R., and Lipscomb, A.P. 1981. Outcome for infants of very low birthweight: Survey of world literature. *Lancet* 1:1038-1041.

Van de Bor, M., Van Zeben-van der Aa, T.M., Verloove-Vanhorick, S.P., Brand, R., and Ruys, J.H. 1989. Hyperbilirubinemia in preterm infants and neurodevelopmental outcome at 2 years of age: Results of a national collaborative survey. *Pediatrics* 83:915-920.

Volpe, J.J. 1989. Intraventricular hemorrhage and brain injury in the premature infant: Neuropathology and pathogenesis. *Clinics in Perinatology* 16:361-386.

Chapter 3

Epidemiology and Natural History of Otitis Media

Jerome O. Klein

INTRODUCTION

Otitis media is one of the most common infectious diseases of infants and children. The epidemiology and natural history have been studied extensively, providing data about the incidence of the disease, risk factors associated with severe and recurrent infection, and the morbidity and sequelae. After every episode of acute otitis media (AOM), middle ear effusion (MEE) persists for variable periods of time, often weeks to months. *Acute otitis media (AOM)* is effusion in one or both middle ears accompanied by one or more signs of acute illness including earache, otorrhea, ear tugging, fever, irritability, lethargy, anorexia, vomiting, or diarrhea. *Asymptomatic middle ear effusion (MEE)* is liquid in one or both ears in a well child; diagnosis of MEE requires visualization of a gas-liquid mixture, otorrhea, or marked reduction in mobility of the tympanic membrane to positive and negative pressure. Conductive hearing loss usually accompanies MEE. Because of the frequency of AOM, the persistence of MEE, and the accompanying hearing loss, pediatricians have been concerned that children who have severe and recurrent middle ear disease might also suffer from delay or impairment of speech, language, or cognitive abilities. The purpose of this review is to present selected information to guide the interested health professional in identifying features of children who are at risk for severe and recurrent otitis media. I will present data from studies of the Greater Boston Otitis Media Study Group (Teele et al. 1989; Teele et al. 1990).

Incidence of Acute Otitis Media

Otitis media is the most frequent reason, after well-baby examinations, for office visits to physicians responsible for child care. By 3 years of age children may be categorized into three groups of approximately equal size relative to acute infections of the middle ear: one group is free of otitis media, a second group has occasional episodes, usually associated with an upper respiratory infection, and the third group has severe and recurrent disease. The frequency of the disease is a significant cost for parents and is associated with extensive usage of antibiotics. Investigators at the Food and Drug Administration found that otitis media was the diagnosis for 42% of the 44.5 million courses of antibiotics prescribed for children less than 10 years of age in 1986 (Nelson et al. 1987).

Risk Factors Associated with Acute Otitis Media

AGE

Otitis media may begin in early infancy. In the greater Boston study of 877 children followed from birth, 9% of children had an episode of AOM by 3 months of age (Teele et al. 1989). The peak age-specific incidence of AOM occurred in the second half of the first year of life. By 1 year of age more than 60% of the children had at least one episode of AOM, and 17% had three or more episodes. By 3 years of age, more than 80% of the children had experienced AOM, and over 40% had three or more episodes.

SIBLING HISTORY

A sibling history of recurrent AOM was the strongest predictor of recurrent otitis media in the greater Boston studies. Such a history raised the risk for recurrent AOM more than twofold. The specific reason is unknown, but a genetic predisposition based on anatomic, physiologic, or immunologic factors is likely. Environmental factors in the household may play a role in increased incidence of AOM in families.

GENDER

Male gender is associated significantly with increased risk for AOM. The gender difference has been identified in other bacterial and viral infections including neonatal sepsis, bacterial and aseptic meningitis, and croup.

BREAST-FEEDING

Breast-fed infants are at lower risk than infants who are exclusively bottle fed. In the greater Boston studies, the protective effect did not increase with increased duration of breast-feeding. The effect of 3 months of breast-feeding was similar to that of 12 months. The mechanism for the protective effect of breast milk or a harmful effect of cow or formula milk is not known. The hypothesis that an immune factor in breast milk is responsible for protection is supported by studies of special feeding bottles for infants with cleft palate. Infants who were fed with a bottle containing breast milk had fewer days of MEE than infants fed with a bottle containing formula, suggesting that protection was due to a constituent of the breast milk rather than position or other features of the technique of feeding (Paradise and Elster 1984).

AGE AT FIRST EPISODE

First episode of AOM early in life appears to be a risk factor for severe and recurrent disease. Boston children who experienced a first episode during the first 6 months of life were more likely to have two or more additional episodes during the next two years than children whose first AOM occurred after the first birthday. These data suggest that early infection identifies an underlying factor in the patient that leads to severe and recurrent disease. These data add support for the concept that genetic predisposition based on anatomic, physiologic, or immunologic factors is significant in the child's experience with AOM.

DAY CARE

Infants and children in group day care have frequent exposures to infectious agents. The close contact of children, each of whom brings the microbiologic experience of the household to the group, and the crowding in many centers and socialization of young are responsible for a high incidence of infectious events. Wald and colleagues followed children prospectively from birth to determine the incidence of AOM.

Myringotomy and placement of ventilating tubes were far more frequent in children in day care (21% by the second year of life) than in children who were in home care (3%) (Wald et al. 1988).

PERSISTENT MIDDLE EAR EFFUSION

Fluid persists in the middle ear for varying periods of time after AOM. The signs of acute infection resolve with appropriate antibiotic therapy, but the MEE, now sterile in the cases of bacterial infection, persists. The type of antibiotic does not appear to influence the duration of MEE. At the conclusion of a 10-day course of antibiotic therapy, approximately 70% of the Boston children still had MEE, 40% had effusion at one month, 20% had effusion at two months, and 10% had effusion at three months. The reasons for prolonged duration of MEE after episodes of AOM are still uncertain. The most likely explanation appears to be a persistent inflammatory reaction due, perhaps, to microbial antigens that remain after the organism has been killed. The antigens may act on the secretory glands resulting in continuous excretion of fluid into the middle ear. Rational management of persistent MEE awaits further elucidation of the pathogenesis.

NATURAL HISTORY OF OTITIS MEDIA AND HEARING LOSS

Audiograms of children with MEE usually indicate a mild-to-moderate conductive hearing loss. The median loss is approximately 25 dB (Fria et al. 1985). Conductive hearing loss due to MEE appears to be influenced by the volume of the fluid partially or completely filling the middle ear space rather than the quality of the fluid (serous, mucoid, or purulent). The hearing impairment associated with MEE is reversed with resolution of the MEE.

Sensorineural hearing loss is uncommonly associated with otitis media. Some investigators have described a permanent sensorineural loss presumably as a result of invasion of microorganisms or inflammatory mediators through the round window membrane or due to a suppurative complication of AOM such as labyrinthitis. Permanent deafness may also result from inflammatory changes that result from adhesive otitis media or ossicular discontinuity.

Few studies of hearing have been performed during episodes of AOM. To my knowledge, only Olmstead and coworkers have documented the hearing status of children during and following an acute episode (Olmstead et al. 1964). They identified moderate hearing loss in children throughout a six-month period of observation. Thus, data about concern for hearing loss during and following acute infection are extrapolated from data developed in audiologic studies of children with MEE of long duration (usually obtained prior to placement of ventilating tubes). Hearing loss during AOM may be different and data are needed to document the course of hearing loss during acute infection and the MEE that follows.

SUPPURATIVE COMPLICATIONS OF OTITIS MEDIA

Intracranial complications of otitis media including meningitis, brain abscess, and lateral sinus thrombosis are relatively uncommon today. Intratemporal complications, those that occur in the aural cavity and adjacent areas of the temporal bone including chronic suppurative otitis media, mastoiditis, and petrositis, are more common. The suppurative complications are usually managed with systemic and local antibiotic therapy but on occasion require surgical incision, drainage, or debridement. In developing countries and areas with limited medical facilities, mastoiditis and purulent draining ears remain common and are a continuing cause of deafness.

NONSUPPURATIVE COMPLICATIONS OF OTITIS MEDIA

Conductive hearing loss is the most frequent complication of otitis media today. Recent studies indicate that children who had recurrent episodes of otitis media or prolonged time spent with middle ear effusion perform less well on tests of speech and language than do their disease-free peers. The Greater Boston Otitis Media Study Group evaluated at age 7 years children who had been observed for ear disease from birth (Teele et al. 1990). After controlling for confounding variables, estimated time spent with MEE during the first 3 years of life was significantly associated with lower scores on tests of cognitive ability, speech and language, and school performance at age 7 years. After considering time spent with MEE during the first 3 years of life, time spent after age 3 years was not a significant predictor of scores on any of the tests administered.

Results of this investigation, and others, suggest that children who suffer from recurrent otitis media in the first years of life were measurably different from disease-free peers at age 7 years. Otitis media and the accompanying MEE appear likely to present impediments to reception or interpretation of auditory stimuli and may have adverse effects on development in infancy.

Summary

Acute otitis media (AOM) is a disease of early infancy: the peak age-specific attack rate is during months 7 through 12; first episodes are very uncommon after 3 years of age. By age 3 years more than two-thirds of children have had at least one episode of AOM, and one-third have had three or more episodes. Epidemiologic data identify children at risk for recurrent AOM: males more than females; infants who have a first episode early in life; children with siblings or parents with histories of severe and recurrent otitis media; children who are not breast-fed; and children who attend day care.

Suppurative complications of AOM are now relatively uncommon. The most frequent complication is the conductive hearing loss that accompanies fluid that persists in the middle ear for weeks to months after every episode of AOM. The median hearing loss for children with middle ear effusion is approximately 25 dB. The results from recent studies suggest that children with recurrent AOM and prolonged time spent with middle ear effusion have lower scores on tests of cognitive abilities, speech and language, and school performance.

References

Fria, T.J., Cantekin, E.I., and Eichler, J.A. 1985. Hearing acuity of children with otitis media with effusion. *Archives of Otolaryngology* 111:10-16.

Nelson, W.L., Kuritsky, J.N., Kennedy, D.L., et al. 1987. Outpatient pediatric antibiotic use in the US. Trends and therapy for otitis media 1977-1986. In program and abstracts of the 27th Interscience Conference on Antimicrobial Agents and Chemotherapy. Washington, D.C.: American Society for Microbiology.

Olmstead, R.W., Alvarez, M.C., Moroney, J.D., and Eversden, M. 1964. The patterns of hearing following acute otitis media. *Journal of Pediatrics* 65:252-255.

Paradise, J.L., and Elster, B.A. 1984. Breast milk protects against otitis media with effusion. *Pediatric Research* 18:283A.

Teele, D.W., Klein, J.O., Rosner, B., and the Greater Boston Otitis Media Study Group. 1989. Epidemiology of otitis media during the first seven years of life in children in Greater Boston: A prospective cohort study. *Journal of Infectious Diseases* 160:83-94.

Teele, D.W., Klein, J.O., Chase, C., et al. 1990. Otitis media in infancy and intellectual ability, school achievement, speech, and language at age 7 years. *Journal of Infectious Diseases* 162:685-694.

Wald, E.R., Dashefsky, B., Byers, C., et al. 1988. Frequency and severity of infections in day care. *Journal of Pediatrics* 112:540-546.

Chapter 4

Special Issues Concerned with Screening for Middle Ear Disease in Children

Jerry L. Northern

INTRODUCTION

It is appropriate that this 1991 Symposium on Screening Children for Auditory Function is being held in Nashville, Tennessee, under the sponsorship of the Vanderbilt University School of Medicine and Bill Wilkerson Center. Fourteen years ago, during June of 1977, a major international symposium on immittance screening for middle ear disease in children was held in Nashville, also sponsored by Vanderbilt University Medical School and the Bill Wilkerson Center. This 1977 symposium holds a position of particular importance because the outcome of discussions held during the meeting resulted in the first set of recommended guidelines for immittance screening of children for middle ear disease. Since publication of these initial immittance screening guidelines, numerous other screening protocols have been developed and implemented, but in fact, none of the protocols have been universally accepted. What has become increasingly apparent is that screening children for middle ear disease varies by the demands and interests of health care systems, and as a function of the agreed purpose of the screening task: Are children to be screened and identified for medically treatable otologic problems, or is the concern to select out those children who are at risk for educational problems because of hearing loss related to a middle ear disorder?

In the United States, a considerable difference in attitude about screening for middle ear disorders is represented by pediatricians who are concerned about referral of children with serous otitis media for which there is no consensus regarding treatment (Paradise 1981) and audiologists who find immittance screening to be an important adjunct to hearing screening programs (Northern 1978). Roush (1990) recently pointed out that despite widespread and long-standing regard for the importance of middle ear screening in children, there is currently little standardization of hearing test or immittance procedures. According to Roush, the reasons for this unfortunate current state of affairs are due, in part, to our failure to produce clear-cut guidelines for achieving the optimal levels of predictive accuracy needed for screening, as well as our lack of critical scrutiny of existing practices and evaluation of various screening protocols.

Early Immittance Screening Protocols

The initial middle ear screening protocol developed at the 1977 Vanderbilt symposium (known thereafter as the Nashville Impedance Screening Guidelines) was not without controversy. In fact, a minority report was subsequently published (Feldman et al. 1978) that disagreed with the Nashville Task Force conclusion not to recommend the use of impedance measures for universal (mass) screening on a routine basis for the detection of middle ear disorders in children of any age group. The minority report charged that this statement was, in fact, "a blatant contradiction to the Nashville Task Force statement that early treatment of otitis media may be of advantage in preventing certain unfavorable long-term developmental consequences in some children." The minority report found fault with the Nashville Task Force recommendation that any child failing the initial screening should be retested in four to six weeks. The minority authors wanted *immediate* medical referral of children who were found with nonmobile (flat) tympanograms. It was charged that the Nashville guidelines were too conservative because of uncertainty about medical management of otitis media, and too focused on the overreferral problem associated with early research reports on immittance screening.

Within the next year, a second set of immittance screening guidelines was developed and published by the American Speech-Language-Hearing Association (1979). The ASHA 1979 guidelines were based on consideration of potential educational, social, and psychological sequelae of otitis media in children. The ASHA guidelines represented a proactive position that children screened who "failed" the middle ear screening (based on an abnormal tympanogram *and* an absent acoustic reflex) should be immediately referred for medical evaluation. Children classified to be "at risk," and therefore in need of rescreening, were to be retested within three to five weeks.

The opposing viewpoints of the Nashville and ASHA immittance guidelines led to a "debate" between Bess (1980) and Northern (1980). Bess felt that it was premature to mass screen children with immittance without additional research information about the natural history of otitis media. Northern advocated including tympanometry as an integral part of *all* hearing screening programs. Downs and Northern (in Bluestone et al. 1986) agreed that although much is yet to be learned about the natural sequence of otitis media, the potential educational sequelae associated with frequent occurrences of otitis media are sufficiently important that to wait for a definitive answer based on research put audiologists in an untenable position as advocates for optimal hearing children.

Actually the procedural considerations in both sets of recommendations, the Nashville guidelines and the ASHA guidelines, summarized in tables 1 and 2, are rather similar. Both standards are based on measurement of tympanometric peak pressure (TPP) and the presence or absence of the acoustic reflex (AR). The categorical description of what constitutes "pass" and "risk" classification of children screened with either of the protocols does not actually differ significantly. The "fail" classification, however, is different in the two guidelines in that a failure in the initial screen of the ASHA protocol results in an immediate medical referral, while the Nashville protocol recommends a retest in four to six weeks. Both sets of guidelines require interpretation of the presence or absence of the acoustic reflex in the "pass" and "fail" criteria. Subsequent research on inclusion of the acoustic reflex in the referral criteria indicates that absence of the acoustic reflex contributes substantially to the "failure" of many children when, in fact, referral to physicians reveals no middle ear disorder (Lucker 1980; Queen et al. 1981; Roush and Tait 1985).

Although data can be cited that support the use of immittance screening to detect middle ear disorders in school-age children, the extreme sensitivity of the procedures causes high false positive rates with less-than-adequate specificity rates in large-scale screening programs.

Table 1

Summary of 1977 Nashville Symposium Guidelines for Immittance Screening *

Classification	Initial Screen	Retest	Subject Outcome
1	Tympanogram: Normal ** and Acoustic reflex: Present***	Not required	Cleared
2	Tympanogram: Abnormal**** and/or Acoustic reflex: Absent***	Tympanogram: Abnormal**** and/or Acoustic reflex: Absent***	Referred
3	Tympanogram: Abnormal**** and/or Acoustic reflex: Absent***	Tympanogram: Normal** and Acoustic reflex: Present***	At risk Recheck at a later date

* From Harford, Bess, Bluestone, and Klein (1978). Reproduced with the permission of The Psychological Corporation.
** Clear peak between +50 and −200 daPa.
*** Contralateral or ipsilateral tone 1000 Hz at 105 dB HL.
**** Flat or rounded, or negative pressure equivalent beyond −200 daPa.

Table 2

Summary of 1979 ASHA Recommendations for Immittance Screening*

Classification	Retest	Subject Outcome
I. Pass	Tympanogram: Normal** or mildly positive/negative *** and Acoustic reflex: Present****	Clear, no return
II. At Risk	Tympanogram: Abnormal***** and Acoustic reflex: Present**** or Tympanogram: Normal** or mildly positive/negative*** Acoustic reflex: Absent****	Retest 3-5 weeks a) If results fall into class I, pass b) If results fall into class II, fail and refer
III. Fail	Tympanogram: Abnormal***** and Acoustic reflex: Absent****	Refer

* From ASHA 1979. Reprinted with the permission of the American Speech-Language-Hearing Association.

** Peak at ± 50 daPa.

*** +50 to +100 daPa or −50 to −200 daPa.

**** Contralateral tone 1000 Hz at 100 dB HL or ipsilateral tone at 105 dB HL.

***** Pressure peak more than +100 daPa or more negative than −200 daPa.

Table 3

Roeser–Northern 1988 Recommended Guidelines Combining Results from Hearing Screening and Immittance Measures*

Possible Outcome	Severity Type	Follow-up	Disposition after Follow-up
T[1]: Peak normal[4] 1 R[2]: Present[5] H[3]: Pass[6]	I	None–Pass	
T: Peak normal 2 R: Absent H: Pass	II	Retest[8]	A. Change to type I—pass B. No change or other type II—at risk—retest C. Type III—refer for audiologic testing D. Type IV—medical referral
T: Peak normal 3 R: Absent H: Fail	III	Retest	A. Change to type I—pass B. Change to type II—at risk—retest C. No change or other type III—refer for audiologic testing D. Change to type IV—medical referral
T: Peak normal 4 R: Present H: Fail	III	Retest	A. Change to type I—pass B. Change to type II—at risk—retest C. No change or other type III—refer for audiologic testing D. Change to type IV—medical referral
T: No peak or rounded 5 R: Present H: Pass	II	(Not a likely finding—check equipment) Retest if confirmed	A. Change to type I—pass B. No change or other type II—at risk—retest C. Change to type III—refer for audiologic testing D. Change to type IV—medical referral
T: No peak or rounded 6 R: Absent H: Pass	IV	Immediate medical referral	

	Type	Action
7 R: No peak or rounded R: Absent H: Fail	IV	Immediate medical referral
8 R: No peak or rounded R: Present H: Fail	IV	(Not a likely finding—check equipment) Immediate medical referral if confirmed
9 T: Abnormal peak[7] R: Present H: Pass	II	Retest A. Change to type I—pass B. No change or other type II—at risk—retest C. Change to type III—refer for audiologic testing D. Change to type IV—medical referral
10 T: Abnormal peak R: Absent H: Pass	II	Retest (Same as above)
11 T: Abnormal peak R: Absent H: Fail	III	Retest A. Change to type I—pass B. Change to type II—at risk—retest C. No change or other type III—refer for audiologic testing D. Change to type IV—medical referral
12 T: Abnormal peak R: Present H: Fail	III	Retest (Same as above)

(1) T=Tympanogram. (2) R=Reflex. (3) H=Hearing Screening. (4) +50 to −200 daPa. (5) 1000 Hz contralateral Tone at 100 dB HL. (6) Failure to respond to 1000 or 2000 Hz at 20 dB HL or 4000 Hz at 25 dB HL in either ear. (7) Greater than +50 daPa or more negative than −200 daPa. (8) Retest in 2-6 weeks.

* From Roeser, R., and Downs, M. (eds.) 1988. Reprinted with the permission of Thieme Medical Publishers.

These factors, combined with the lack of definitive research on specific referral criteria and the transient nature of middle ear disorders, have certainly affected the acceptance and use of immittance screening in school hearing screening programs.

An important project was undertaken in Denmark by Fiellau-Nikolajsen (1983) who attempted to elucidate certain diagnostic, epidemiologic, and therapeutic aspects of serous otitis media in more than 1,000 3-year-old children through more than 8,000 serial impedance tests. He concluded that impedance testing is an accurate, objective, and noninvasive tool for demonstrating middle ear pathology, is time efficient, and is therefore superior to alternative possibilities of diagnosing middle ear disease in young children. However, he expressed concern that the middle ear status in young children must be considered a link in an ever-changing, dynamic process, which thus *restricts the value of any single test*. He concluded "that case-finding by impedance testing of preschool children is technically practicable, but the results are difficult to interpret."

Roeser and Northern (1988) described a protocol for identifying middle ear disorders and hearing loss in school-age children that combines results from hearing screening with immittance measures. This procedure is an attempt to reach a compromise between the expense of unnecessary medical referral and the potentially important educational implications of delayed medical treatment. The Roeser-Northern protocol includes tympanometry, acoustic reflex measurement, and hearing screening. The results of the three tests are used to classify children into four management categories as shown in tables 3 and 4. Although the addition of hearing screening to the protocol does complicate interpretation matters somewhat, the plan is designed to reduce overreferrals and unwarranted treatment delays. This protocol, evaluated by Roush and Tait (1985) and compared to the ASHA and Nashville protocols in a group of 75 3- and 4-year-old children, produced the fewest number of children who needed retesting as well as no "over-referral" children. Roush and Tait concluded that the likelihood of overreferrals in preschoolers is high even when acoustic immittance rescreening is conducted. They also reported that pure-tone screening, by itself, is largely ineffective as a means of identifying preschool children with middle ear disorders.

Table 4
Characteristics of Severity Types Used with Roeser-Northern 1988 Recommended
Screening Procedures*

Severity Type	Characteristics	Follow-up
I	Normal	None-pass
II	Marginally abnormal immittance findings with pass on hearing screening	At risk-retest
III	Normal or marginally abnormal immittance findings with fail on hearing screening	Refer for audiometric threshold testing
IV	Grossly abnormal immittance findings and pass or fail hearing screening	Medical referral

* From Roeser, R.J., and Downs, M.P. 1988. Reprinted with the permission of Thieme Medical Publishers.

Haggard and Hughes (1988) comment that the screening of hearing in children, age 2 to 7 years, should on numerical grounds be mostly concerned with the accurate identification of otitis media. However, the fluctuation, persistence, and multiple-domain manifestations of otitis media with effusion entail that some of the traditional principles of screening cannot be applied to otitis media. Thus, the complexity of these circumstances leads to confusion about auditory screening objectives, optimal screening techniques to be used, the role of hearing assessment, and medical treatment of middle ear disorders.

REPORT OF THE FOURTH INTERNATIONAL SYMPOSIUM ON RECENT ADVANCES IN OTITIS MEDIA (1989)

Recognizing the controversy regarding mass immittance screening, the Fourth International Symposium on Otitis Media—Committee on Diagnosis and Screening took a somewhat different view of middle ear screening goals for children (Lim 1989). This report recommends that the goal of auditory screening should be the identification of the 10% of cases of otitis media that are truly chronic. Emphasis in screening should therefore be directed toward settings in which early recognition may forestall educational sequela, and in those groups of children that might otherwise not be screened (such as underserved populations). Key to the recommendations is the suggestion to only conduct hearing and middle ear screening during the initial year of school entry and during the following year. This strategy, it is suggested, will make screening more cost-effective and will survey children at the ages when they are most likely to have unrecognized middle ear effusion. It is also suggested that screening children, 7 years of age or older, is not likely to identify new cases of children with significant hearing loss.

The middle ear screening failure recommendation is based upon the finding of (1) middle ear pressure more negative than -200 mm H_2O and (2) low compliance of the tympanometric pattern. Acoustic reflex measurement, when conducted, is not to be considered as a pass-fail criterion. In addition, audiometric hearing screening is to accompany the middle ear screening protocol. The International Symposium on Otitis Media Report suggests that in young preschool-age children, hearing and middle ear screening should be done twice a year, preferably early in the school year and near the end of the school year. This is recommended for two reasons: (1) children with effusion early in the fall are more likely to have had chronic, persistent effusion over the preceding summer months, and (2) screening during the winter months is likely to identify cases associated with upper respiratory tract infections. Screening in the spring of the year should be reserved for children who were missed earlier or who failed the initial fall season screening.

The report states that the *bilateral* middle ear problem (as identified by pure-tone and immittance screening) is the key condition that should be sought in screening programs. Bilateral middle ear disorder is grounds for an immediate alerting letter to parents recommending assessment of the child by a physician at the earliest opportunity. A recommended rescreening in two months with pure tone and immittance should be scheduled for children who are found with bilateral middle ear and hearing problems to ensure resolution of the hearing difficulty. On the other hand, a child with a unilateral middle ear screening failure (by pure-tone and immittance screening) should be rescreened at the next routine screening session. Two consecutive unilateral failures in the same ear should result in an alerting letter to the parents recommending physician assessment at the child's next routine health examination or within one year. The report recommends that all children who fail the hearing or immittance screening protocol, whether unilaterally or bilaterally, should be rescreened at every routine biannual screening examination.

ASHA 1990 GUIDELINES FOR MIDDLE EAR SCREENING

The American-Speech-Language-Hearing Association published new Guidelines for Screening for Hearing Impairments and Middle Ear Disorders in 1990. Their published guidelines are taken nearly verbatim from an article published earlier by Margolis and Heller (1987). Margolis and Heller report results from an investigation of a prototype hand-held tympanometer that was used to collect normative values for static admittance (Peak Y), equivalent ear canal volume (V_{ec}), tympanometric peak pressure (TPP), and tympanogram gradient (TW) from 92 ears of 50 normal preschool children (mean age=4.7 years) and 87 ears from 48 adult subjects (mean age=30.5 years). From this limited set of normative data, a four-part protocol for medical referral of immittance screening failures was described. This four-part protocol was subsequently accepted and recommended by ASHA as national guidelines.

The 1990 ASHA immittance screening protocol incorporates standardized terminology for aural acoustic immittance measurements and acknowledges improved technologic advances in immittance meter instrumentation. The 1990 immittance guidelines are to be used in conjunction with the 1985 ASHA guidelines for hearing screening through identification audiometry. The goal of the 1990 immittance screening protocol is to identify potentially medically significant ear disorders that have been undetected or untreated.

The 1990 ASHA immittance guidelines were developed, in part, to decrease the excessive overreferral rates that characterized earlier recommended immittance guidelines. The 1990 guidelines include four sources of data for each child as shown in table 5: (1) history of recent occurrence of otalgia (ear pain) or otorrhea (ear discharge); (2) visual inspection for structural defects of the ear, head, and neck, ear canal or eardrum abnormalities; (3) pure-tone hearing screening; and (4) acoustic immittance measurements.

The referral criteria suggested for the acoustic immittance measurements include: (a) a flat tympanogram and equivalent ear canal volume (V_{ec}) outside normal range; (b) low static admittance (Peak Y) on two successive occurrences in a four- to six-week interval; or (c)

Table 5
Referral Criteria*

I.   History
     A. Otalgia
     B. Otorrhea
II. Visual inspection of the ear
     A. Structural defect of the ear, head, or neck
     B. Ear canal abnormalities
        1. Blood or effusion
        2. Occlusion
        3. Inflammation
        4. Excessive cerumen, tumor, foreign material
     C. Eardrum abnormalities
        1. Abnormal color
        2. Bulging eardrum
        3. Fluid line or bubbles
        4. Perforation
        5. Retraction
III. Identification audiometry - Fail air conduction screening at 20 dB HL at 1, 2,
     or 4 kHz in either ear (ASHA 1985; these criteria may require alteration for
     various clinical settings and populations)
IV. Tympanometry
     A. Flat tympanogram and equivalent ear canal volume (V_{ec}) outside normal
        range
     B. Low static admittance (Peak Y) on two successive occurrences in a 4-6
        week interval
     C. Abnormally wide tympanometric width (TW) on two successive
        occurrences in a 4-6 week interval

* From ASHA 1990. Reprinted with the permission of the American Speech-Language-Hearing Association.

abnormally wide tympanometric width (TW) on two successive occurrences in a four- to six-week interval. A schematic flowchart of the recommended management of a child in this screening protocol is shown in figure 1. The guidelines specifically exclude the traditional immittance screening data of tympanometric peak pressure (TPP) and the acoustic reflex (AR) because these measurements were indicated to contribute little to the overall sensitivity of the protocol—while, in fact, significantly lowering the specificity of the screening protocol.

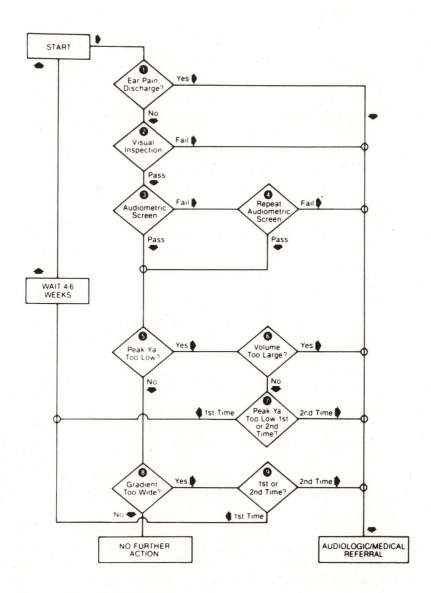

Figure 1. Flowchart for determination of the need for audiologic/medical referral incorporating case history, visual inspection, pure-tone audiometry, and tympanometry. Y_a = static admittance. From ASHA 1990. Reprinted with the permission of the American Speech-Language-Hearing Association.

The recommendations within the ASHA 1990 protocol introduce two areas of concern not routinely included in screening programs—history taking and visual inspection of the ear. Although the authors of the guidelines admit that it is beyond the scope of the screening program to obtain a complete history, recent occurrences of ear pain or ear discharge are cause for immediate medical referral. Except for obvious manifestations of these problems at the time of screening, our experience in hearing screening programs with young children suggests that the children are seldom able to provide accurate answers to medical history questions. Obviously, considerable effort will have to be expended to obtain this information from a responsible individual prior to or following the actual screening process.

The recommended visual ear inspection may raise even more problems in actual practice. The guidelines state that the visual inspection may be done with the unaided eye or an otoscope to identify obvious ear disease. It is further stated in the guidelines that because the skill and experience of the individual performing the otoscopic inspection will vary considerably, it is anticipated that subtle middle ear disorders will be detected in some screening programs and not in others. Clearly, the intent of the guidelines is that this visualization effort is only to identify the most obvious abnormalities of the ear canal and tympanic membrane, but nonetheless, this recommendation requires special skills not generally possessed by audiologists at this time. As a matter of fact, the skills of physicians and health professionals trained in otoscopy are often of question. A recent study of otoscopists' accuracy regarding the diagnosis of middle ear effusion in children during an "otoscopic validation" course found that 27 physicians and 3 pediatric nurse practitioners examining over 4,000 ears of children showed mean sensitivity and specificity for the group as a whole of only 87% and 74%, respectively (Kaleida and Stool 1991).

Otologic visual examination of the ear canal also brings forth questions concerning the audiologist's role in cerumen management since adequate observation of the ear canal and tympanic membrane depends on a clear, unobstructed view of the structures in question. Advocates have called for audiologists to accept responsibility for cerumen management and seek training in cerumen removal (Roeser and Crandell 1991a; 1991b). They support their position by citing the fact that few physicians actually perform cerumen removal but delegate the task to others. Roeser and Crandell recognize that cerumen management is associated with some risk of injury and infection to the external ear canal but indicate that when cerumen removal is performed judiciously, the risks are minimal. How active audiologists will become in otologic visual inspection and concomitant cerumen management tasks remains to be seen. However, it appears that to fully embrace the 1990 ASHA Guidelines for Screening for Hearing Impairments and Middle Ear Disorders, consideration will have to be given to these special issues of otoscopy and cerumen management. Further, it is likely that most children's hearing screening programs in the United States are conducted not by audiologists per se but by speech-language pathologists, school nurses, and nonprofessional volunteers who are likely not to have the necessary skills to fully abide with the 1990 ASHA four-part immittance screening protocol.

Few data are yet available regarding implementation of the 1990 ASHA guidelines. Roush et al. (1992) compared the 1978 and the 1990 ASHA acoustic immittance screening procedures on 204 3- and 4-year-old children from a rural area in eastern North Carolina. Some variance to the specific protocols was followed, i.e., during the 1978 ASHA protocol screening the immittance failures were not immediately referred for medical evaluation, and the 1990 guideline for visual inspection was conducted by a pediatric otolaryngologist coinvestigator. In general terms, this study found that the "traditional" protocol of 1978, which included tympanometric peak pressure and acoustic reflex measurement, was more successful in identifying ears needing medical attention than the newer 1990 ASHA protocol. These researchers conclude that use of the 1990 ASHA protocol should achieve a reasonable level of sensitivity and should increase the specificity above that obtained with the 1978 ASHA immittance screening procedure.

OTHER SCREENING TECHNOLOGIES

ACOUSTIC REFLECTOMETRY

A device known as the acoustic otoscope was initially described by Teele and Teele (1984) and was developed as a "by-product of the cold war and the arms race." The inventor (J.H. Teele), a radar engineer and military intelligence officer, undertook the challenge to produce a hand-held device that would detect middle ear effusion, independent of crying and cerumen, and not require pneumatic pressurization of the external ear canal (Teele et al. 1990).

The acoustic otoscope generates a 100-millisecond multifrequency sweep between 2000 Hz and 4500 Hz at a sound pressure of 80 dB (figure 2). The pickup microphone measures the amplitude of the reflected probe tone from the plane of the tympanic membrane. The instrument works on quarter-wavelength theory, so that the reflected wave completely cancels the principle wave in the external ear canal at a distance of one-quarter wavelength from the tympanic membrane. Thus, the reflected sound is inversely proportional to the total sound; a greater reflection produces a reduced amplitude suggestive of middle ear effusion. The examiner "aims" the speculum of the acoustic otoscope into the child's ear canal and presses the activator button. The instrument is quickly repositioned, and the activator button pressed again, until the highest level of reflectometry is noted on the LED vertical display. According to the manufacturer, reflectometry readings of 0 to 2 units represent normal middle ear findings; readings of 3 to 4 units suggest possible middle ear effusion; and readings of greater than 5 units suggest the presence of middle ear fluid.

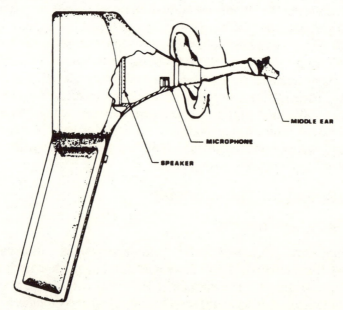

Figure 2. Cutaway view of the acoustic otoscope showing position at the ear as well as the relative position of the microphone and loudspeaker assemblies.

Early studies using the acoustic otoscope with children generally reported high sensitivity and specificity findings. Teele and Teele (1984) found sensitivity of 94% to 99% with specificity scores of 79% to 83%. Lampe et al. (1985) reported that the acoustic otoscope correctly identified 87% of ears in 75 children with middle ear effusion, and correctly identified 70% of ears without effusion. Schwartz and Schwartz (1987), from a cohort of 256 children seen in a private pediatric office, reported sensitivity of 88% and specificity of 83% using a cutoff criterion of 5 units on the LED display.

Recent research studies with the acoustic otoscope have verified its clinical utility in various study samples of children. Oyiborhoro et al. (1987) evaluated 200 children with the acoustic otoscope and verified their findings through otoscopy, tympanometry, pure-tone audiometry, and myringotomy. Using acoustic otoscope reflectivity greater than 4 to identify middle ear pathology, the sensitivity and specificity of the acoustic otoscope were reported to be 93% and 83%, respectively. Jehle (1989) reported use of the acoustic otoscope in an emergency room setting with 80 children. Using a reflectivity score of 5 or more units to signify otologic pathology, the sensitivity of the screening test was 82%, and specificity was 95%. After four years of clinical experience with the acoustic otoscope in emergency room applications, they found it to be an objective, reliable, and practical adjunct in the diagnosis of otitis media that is especially useful for evaluating hard-to-examine patients and for conducting quantitative repeat examinations on patients seen by multiple physicians. Particular value was reported for confirming the presence of a hemotympanum in patients with basilar skull fractures who showed reflectivity readings of 7 or more units.

Teele et al. (1990) examined the relationship between acoustic reflectomery and hearing loss, in ears with and without middle ear effusion, in 137 New Zealand children between the ages of 3 and 16 years. As expected, reflectometry was significantly associated with conductive hearing loss, and the three-frequency pure-tone averages were, in fact, associated with the degree of reflectivity. Using a reflectivity value of 6 or greater to detect a three-frequency pure-tone average hearing loss of 30 dB or greater, the sensitivity of the technique was 88% and the specificity was 44%. To be sure, the accuracy of the estimate of hearing loss from reflectivity readings permits only an estimate of the likelihood of significant (greater than 30 dB) conductive hearing loss, but the authors suggest that the procedure might be useful with very young children who pose difficult hearing test challenges.

HAND-HELD TYMPANOMETERS

The recent development of hand-held specific-purpose immittance screening tympanometers that are lightweight, cordless, and rechargeable will undoubtedly have major influence on immittance screening programs for children. This new instrumentation is currently available from two manufacturers (Welch Allyn, Inc., and Lucas GSI). These units are battery operated and include a storage base unit that contains a rechargeable battery system and a printer to record a hard copy of the data. These hand-held tympanometers are controlled by microelectronic computer systems comprised of speaker and microphone, mounted directly in the speculum of the hand-held unit, and a pressure transducer with a motor-driven pump in the handle of the device makes up the air-pressure system (Bak 1988).

As soon as a pneumatic seal is acoustically detected by the rubber tip on the speculum placed at the concha-meatal opening in the ear canal, the microcomputer starts the miniature pump that varies pressure to the ear from +200 daPa to −300 daPa in three seconds with a 226 Hz probe tone at 85 dB SPL. The unit comes with interchangeable tips of various sizes for use with children and adults. Test results obtained with these hand-held tympanometers are instantly shown on the LED display on the head of the device. Tympanometric data from two ears transfer immediately through the base unit to the printer, so the unit is instantly available for additional testing while the printer is printing results from the previous test.

Margolis and Heller (1987) used the Welch Allyn MicroTymp prototype hand-held tympanometer with normal preschool subjects to obtain the normative values of static admittance, equivalent ear canal volume, tympanometric peak pressure, and tympanogram gradient, which were subsequently used as the basis of the 1990 ASHA immittance screening guidelines. In a study of the diagnostic accuracy of the hand-held tympanometer, the Welch Allyn MicroTymp was compared with two other traditional immittance instruments on 152 patients by Wazen et al. (1988). From these patients, 99 tympanograms were obtained in the operating room just prior to a diagnostic myringotomy. This group included 50 children between the ages of 10 months and 15 years. Based on their operative findings at myringotomy, the authors concluded that the MicroTymp accurately measures static admittance and the tympanometric peak pressure.

Both of the new hand-held tympanometers record data consistent with the 1990 ASHA immittance screening guidelines. That is, the devices record static admittance (Peak Y) of the tympanogram, which is displayed against the normal variance parameters, as well as a visual display of the tympanometric width (TW). Both instruments also provide direct reading of the equivalent ear canal volume (V_{ec}). Availability and use of these tympanometers should contribute positively to the acceptance and utilization of the new ASHA immittance screening protocol.

SUMMARY

Immittance screening for middle ear disorders continues to be an important adjunct to children's hearing screening programs. A number of immittance screening protocols have been field evaluated, and sensitivity and specificity data are available. These studies have established that use of the acoustic reflex as a referral criterion lowers protocol specificity and is thus not recommended.

The 1990 ASHA Guidelines for Screening for Hearing Impairments and Middle Ear Disorders need additional field evaluation because little data are available regarding implementation. The guidelines call for "visual inspection" of the ear canal and tympanic membrane, which may require additional skills training for audiologists with otoscopy and cerumen removal. The ASHA guidelines are based on limited normative data, and additional information is needed on the protocol sensitivity, specificity, retest rate, and referral percentages.

New screening technologies, especially the lightweight, hand-held, cordless, rechargeable units, should facilitate the use of immittance measurements in children's hearing screening programs. These new devices incorporate the measurement variables recommended by the 1990 ASHA guidelines. However, additional field data are needed for evaluation of this new instrumentation.

REFERENCES

American Speech-Language-Hearing Association. 1979. Guidelines for acoustic immittance screening of middle ear function. *Asha* 21:283-288.

American Speech-Language-Hearing Association. 1990. Guidelines for screening for hearing impairments and middle ear disorders. *Asha* 32(Suppl. 2):17-24.

Bak, D.J. 1988. Microelectronics and a tiny pump make ear exams easy. *Design News.*

Bess, F.H. 1980. Impedance screening for children: A need for more research. *Annals of Otology, Rhinology and Laryngology* 89(3)(Suppl. 68):228-232.

Bluestone, C., Fria, T., Arjona, S., Casselbrant, M., Schwartz, D., Ruben, R., Gates, G., Downs, M., Northern, J., Jerger, J., Paradise, J., Bess, F., Kenworthy, O., and Rogers, K. 1986. Controversies in screening for middle ear disease and hearing loss in children. *Pediatrics* 77(1):57-70.

Feldman, A., Northern, J., Rosenberg, J., Wilber, L., and Howie, V.M. 1978. Communication to the editor re: Nashville symposium on impedance screening for children. *Annals of Otology, Rhinology and Laryngology* 87:738.

Fiellau-Nikolajsen, M. 1983. Tympanometry and secretory otitis media: Observations on diagnosis, epidemiology, treatment, and prevention in prospective cohort studies of three-year-old children. *Acta Otolaryngologica* Suppl. 394:1-73.

Haggard, M., and Hughes, E. 1988. *Objectives, values and methods of screening children's hearing—A review of the literature.* IHR Internal Reports, Series A, #4. Nottingham, England: Institute of Hearing Research.

Harford, E., Bess, F., Bluestone, C., and Klein, J. (eds.). 1978. *Impedance screening for middle ear disease in children.* New York: Grune and Stratton.

Jehle, D. 1989. Acoustic otoscopy in the diagnosis of otitis media. *Annals of Internal Medicine* 18(4):396-400.

Kaleida, P., and Stool, S. 1991. Assessment of otoscopists' accuracy regarding the diagnosis of middle-ear effusion in children ("otoscopic validation"). Abstract of the fifth International Symposium: Recent Advances in Otitis Media. Columbus, Ohio: The Ohio State University College of Medicine, Department of Otolaryngology, 31.

Lampe, R., Weir, M., Spier, J., and Rhodes, M. 1985. Acoustic reflectometry in the detection of middle ear effusion. *Pediatrics* 76:75-78.

Lim, D. (ed.). 1989. Diagnosis and screening. In *Recent advances in otitis media, report of the Fourth Research Conference. Annals of Otology, Rhinology and Laryngology* 98(4) part 2(Suppl. 139):39-41.

Lucker, J.R. 1980. Application of pass-fail criteria to middle ear screening results. *Asha* 22:839.

Margolis, R.H., and Heller, J.W. 1987. Screening tympanometry: Criteria for medical referral. *Audiology* 26:197-208.

Northern, J.L. 1978. Advanced techniques for measuring middle ear function. *Pediatrics* 61:761-768.

Northern, J.L. 1980. Impedance screening: An integral part of hearing screening. *Annals of Otology, Rhinology and Laryngology* 89(3)(Suppl. 68):233-235.

Oyiborhoro, J., Olaniyan, S., Newman, C., and Balakrishnan, S. 1987. Efficacy of acoustic otoscope in detecting middle ear effusion in children. *Laryngoscope* 97(4):495-498.

Paradise, J.L. 1981. Otitis media during early life: How hazardous to development? A critical review of the evidence. *Pediatrics* 68(8):869-873.

Queen, S., Moses, F., Wood, S., et al. 1981. The use of immittance screening by the Kansas City, MO, public school district. *Seminars in Speech Language and Hearing* 2:119-122.

Roeser, R., and Northern, J.L. 1988. Screening for hearing loss and middle ear disorders. In R. Roeser and M. Downs (eds.), *Auditory disorders in school children*. 2d ed. New York: Thieme Medical Publishers.

Roeser, R.J., and Crandell, C. 1991a. The audiologist's responsibility in cerumen management. *Asha* 33(1):51-53.

Roeser, R.J., and Crandell, C. 1991b. More on "The responsibility of audiologists in cerumen management." *Audiology Today* 3(3):20-21.

Roush, J. 1990. Identification of hearing loss and middle ear disease in preschool and school-age children. *Seminars in Hearing* 11(4):357-371.

Roush, J., and Tait, C. 1985. Pure-tone and acoustic immittance screening for preschool-aged children: An examination of referral criteria. *Ear and Hearing* 6(5):245-250.

Roush, J., Drake, A., and Sexton, J. 1992. Identification of middle ear dysfunction in young children: A comparison of tympanometric screening procedures. *Ear and Hearing* 13(2):63-69.

Schwartz, D., and Schwartz, R. 1987. Validity of acoustic reflectometry in detecting middle ear effusion. *Pediatrics* 29:739-742.

Teele, D., and Teele, J. 1984. Detection of middle ear effusion by acoustic reflectometry. *Journal of Pediatrics* 104:832-838.

Teele, D.W., Stewart, I.A., Teele, J.H., Smith, D.K., and Tregonning, S.J. 1990. Acoustic reflectometry for assessment of hearing loss in children with middle ear effusion. *Pediatric Infectious Disease Journal* 9(12):870-872.

Wazen, J.J., Ferraro, J.A., and Hughes, R. 1988. Clinical evaluation of a portable, cordless, hand-held middle ear analyzer. *Otolaryngology-Head and Neck Surgery* 99(3):348-350.

Chapter 5

Controversies in the Screening of Central Auditory Processing Disorders

Brad A. Stach

INTRODUCTION

Two fundamental assumptions underlying the screening of any disorder are, first, that the disorder is clearly defined, and, second, that it can be measured effectively. When tested in the context of central auditory processing disorder (CAPD), these assumptions face a rather stern challenge. For example, some individuals argue against the very existence of central auditory processing disorders. They view CAPD simply as the manifestation of poor control over linguistic and cognitive factors during behavioral testing. Others accept the concept but argue about the best way to measure it. If the definition of a disorder and the nature of its measurement are controversial, then the question of whether or not to screen for it surely must also be.

The purpose of this paper, then, is to ask the question, *Should mass screening of children for central auditory processing disorder be carried out?* In an effort to answer this question, the general definition of screening and how it relates to the CAPD are reviewed. In addition, public health questions related to mass screening are asked in relation to auditory processing disorder in an attempt to clarify whether or not it is a disorder for which screening programs should be implemented.

DEFINITION OF SCREENING

The definition of screening can be broken down into three parts. First, it is the application of rapid and simple tests to a large population.

Any technique designed to screen auditory processing disorder should involve tests that can be administered easily and rapidly to the population of children in general. Second, the population should consist of individuals who are undiagnosed and typically asymptomatic. Stated another way, if a disorder is symptomatic by nature, then there is no need to screen it with tests, since the symptoms provide all of the screening necessary. Third, the tests should identify those who require additional diagnostic procedures. Thus, the tests should not be the diagnostic measures themselves but screening tools to indicate the need for diagnostic measures. Implicit in this third aspect of the definition of screening is that the tests should also identify those who do *not* require additional diagnostic procedures.

Although there is nothing new in this definition of screening, when it is evaluated with auditory processing disorder in mind, it evokes some rather enlightening questions. Do we have screening tests of auditory processing disorder that can be easily and rapidly administered to the general population of children? Is auditory processing disorder asymptomatic and undiagnosed? Do screening tests of auditory processing disorder separate those children who require additional diagnostic procedures from those who do not?

PUBLIC HEALTH QUESTIONS

One way to approach the question of screening for CAPD is to cast it into an analysis of public health assumptions related to selection of disorders to screen. In 1974, Northern and Downs eloquently provided such an analysis of the assumptions related to mass screening of hearing in infants. They evaluated six public health assumptions related to hearing impairment and concluded that mass screening of hearing sensitivity was clearly appropriate from a public health perspective. While these six assumptions are appropriate for evaluating CAPD as a disorder to screen, they actually assume more about our knowledge of auditory processing disorder than most people would be willing to concede. Therefore, the six assumptions were expanded to eight assumptions in order to evaluate CAPD as a public health problem for which mass screening should be implemented.

The following eight questions are related to the assumptions underlying whether or not to screen for a particular disorder. The implication is that if most or all of these assumptions are met, then the disorder is one that is appropriate, from a public health viewpoint, to screen for in a large population.

Is the disorder to be screened a clearly defined disorder? That is, is auditory processing disorder an entity upon which there is general agreement? Probably in no other area in the fields of audiology and speech pathology is there more controversy than in defining CAPD. For example, Lasky and Katz (1983) contend that CAPD is part of a general category of language disorders in children. They believe that specific deficits characterizing CAPD affect all levels of linguistic development and that CAPD may have the most significant impact on development of phonemic structures of the language. Pinheiro and Musiek (1985), on the other hand, suggest that children with CAPD have difficulty listening to or comprehending auditory information. By this definition, a child must have a problem not necessarily in hearing but in listening or comprehending to have CAPD. Willeford and Burleigh (1985) suggest that children with CAPD have a problem in the perception of spoken language and other meaningful sounds in the environment. They contend that, in some children, difficulty may be due to a deficiency in basic linguistic capabilities, while in others, it may be due to a child's language skills.

By these definitions, then, CAPD may or may not be a language problem, may or may not be a listening deficit, and may or may not be a perceptual disorder. Jerger, Martin, and Jerger (1987) provided an interesting perspective when they evaluated CAPD in the context of two theoretical models of learning disability. One theoretical approach is termed the linguistic model. Individuals who ascribe to the linguistic model believe that CAPD is a conceptual problem, that the deficit is in representational or symbolic behavior, and that linguistic/cognitive factors are the primary problem involved in CAPD. Another theoretical approach is the auditory model. Individuals who ascribe to the auditory model contend that CAPD is a perceptual problem, that the deficit is in behaviors that are precursory to language, and that linguist/cognitive factors are secondary. They maintain that CAPD is an auditory perceptual problem, not a language disorder.

With regard to screening, it becomes readily apparent that if you were to consider CAPD a linguistic problem, you would develop a screening tool comprised of materials that represent a broad range of linguistic complexity so that children with language deficits would fail them. If, on the other hand, you were to view CAPD as a perceptual deficit, you would design a screening test that would hold language constant, or control for different levels of linguistic ability. In this way, perception could be specifically measured, and results of the test would not be influenced by different levels of linguistic competence in the children being tested.

Is the disorder well defined? No. There is simply not agreement as to whether this is a perceptual disorder, a language disorder, or some combination of disorders.

Does the disorder occur with sufficient frequency to warrant mass screening? The assumption underlying the question of frequency of occurrence of the disorder is that if the disorder is rare, then screening for it is probably not cost-effective. With regard to auditory processing disorder, the answer to this question is simply not known. To a large extent, this can be attributed to a lack of a clear definition. Because it is not a well-defined disorder, its incidence and prevalence have not been estimated in the childhood population.

Is the consequence of the disorder serious enough to warrant mass screening? Those individuals who evaluate and treat children with auditory processing disorder have reached a clear consensus on this issue. The consequences of all types of hearing disorders on speech and language development and on academic achievement are well documented. Because of the deleterious effects of these disorders on children's development, there is general agreement that auditory processing disorder may result in consequences serious enough to warrant screening.

Can the disorder be accurately diagnosed? The public health assumption underlying this question is that, once screening has occurred, the disorder can be accurately diagnosed with further testing. Can CAPD be accurately diagnosed? Because there is no biologic marker for CAPD, the disorder must be operationally defined on the basis of behavioral test results, which most often are speech audiometric measures. Unfortunately, interpretation of results of behavioral measures can be confounded by numerous nonauditory factors, such as deficits in language, cognition, and attention. Much of the controversy that surrounds diagnosis of CAPD results from the lack of a universally accepted clinical approach to controlling these confounding variables.

Evidence is emerging that well-controlled speech audiometric testing, in conjunction with auditory evoked potential measurements, may be powerful diagnostic tools for assessing CAPD. Nevertheless, the problem remaining in the diagnosis of CAPD is that there is no single gold standard against which to judge the effectiveness of any particular test. Although CAPD can be operationally defined on the basis of behavioral and electrophysiologic test results, and although nonauditory factors can be controlled to a certain extent, without a standard against which to compare the operational definition, agreement about the accuracy of CAPD diagnosis remains elusive.

Is the disorder amenable to treatment or prevention that will forestall or change the expected outcome? The public health assumption underlying this question is that if a disorder cannot be treated or prevented, then there is no reason to test for it, since the outcome for the individual patient would not vary, regardless of the test results. The answer to this question depends, fundamentally, on how CAPD is defined and diagnosed. If CAPD is thought of as an auditory disorder, the most important manifestation of which is difficulty understanding speech in background noise, and if treatment is focused on this manifestation, then, clearly, there are effective treatment strategies that will forestall or change the expected outcome related to the presence of CAPD.

Intervention strategies directed toward enhancement of signal-to-noise ratio (S/N) have proven to be effective in the treatment of children with CAPD (Stach 1990). There are at least two approaches to this type of intervention. The first approach is to alter the acoustic environment in order to enhance the S/N. Environmental alterations include such practical approaches as preferential seating in the classroom and manipulation of the home environment so that the child is placed in more favorable listening situations. It is not uncommon in children with CAPD for the diagnosis itself to serve as the treatment. That is, once parents and teachers become aware of the nature of the child's problem and that the solution is one of enhancement of S/N, they manipulate the environment in such a manner that the problem situations are eliminated, and the child's auditory processing difficulties become inconsequential.

In other cases, however, when severity of the auditory processing disorder is greater, the use of remote microphone technology may be indicated. Personal FM systems, which use remote microphones for S/N enhancement, have been used to assist these children in overcoming their deficit in understanding speech in background noise. In 1987, we summarized our experience at the Neurosensory Center of Houston with intervention in children with CAPD (Stach, Loiselle, and Jerger 1987). Of those children who were considered to have CAPD, 30 were successfully treated by enhancing the awareness of parents and teachers to the need for environmental alteration to reduce background noise. In 11 others, however, the more aggressive approach of personal FM-system use was taken. These were relatively young children whose average age was 7 years. Although some of the children had slight low- frequency hearing loss, all had pure-tone averages that were within normal limits. The majority (72%) also had a history of chronic otitis media. Evidence of improvement in 9 of the children using FM systems was gathered from interviews with parents and teachers. In 8 of the 9 children, improved grades and improved behavior were reported anecdotally by the teacher and parents. In addition, 2 of the children were reported to have improved speech and language abilities, 2 had improved attention, and in 2, there was a school placement change from a special education classroom to a regular classroom.

Given that CAPD is defined as an auditory problem and that its most important manifestation is difficulty understanding speech in background noise, treatment of the disorder can forestall or change the expected outcome, thus meeting the criteria for public health screening.

Are facilities for treatment and diagnosis readily available? The public health assumption underlying this question is that if treatment and diagnostic facilities are not available, then the outcome of screening will not be meaningful, since follow-up services will not be easily accessible. Are resources available throughout the country for accurate diagnosis and appropriate treatment of children with CAPD? This is very difficult to judge, and the answer remains unknown, primarily because of the difficulty that prevails in defining and diagnosing CAPD.

Are the costs of screening reasonably commensurate with benefits to the individual? In other words, what is the cost-benefit ratio to society of identifying an individual with a disorder? Most professionals involved with the provision of hearing health care are certain that the benefit to the individual patient is substantial. But that is not the entire question being asked here. The remainder of the question is whether or not this benefit can be accrued at a reasonable cost to society. The answer to this question is simply unknown because the cost of screening involves not only the cost of carrying out the actual screening test but also the cost of follow-up services to those who have failed the screening. While this cost is usually considered appropriate for those with the disorder, it can be elevated substantially by inaccurately identifying children as having a problem. If the number of false positive test results is large, then excessive resources will be spent on unnecessary follow-up testing. Since the test characteristics of the screening tools are unknown, the cost of identifying a child with the disorder cannot be estimated.

Are performance characteristics of the screening tools adequate? That is, do the tests that purport to screen for auditory processing disorder have adequate performance characteristics? Do they identify accurately those children who have the disorder? Do they identify accurately those children who do not have the disorder? What is the predictive value of a positive outcome? What is the predictive value of a negative outcome?

Although substantive data on performance characteristics of screening tests for CAPD do not exist, it is likely that currently available tests will be acceptable in terms of their sensitivity. That is, they will correctly identify those children who have the disorder. It is equally likely that these screening tests will be unacceptable in terms of their predictive value of a positive test. That is, too many children who do not have CAPD will fail the tests, thereby reducing the predictive value of a positive test. The percentage of all positive results that are true positives will be fairly low because many of the children who are identified probably do not have the disorder. This will result in a large number of false positive test results, which will burden the health care system with children who do not need further testing.

The main reason for conjecturing that screening tests of CAPD will have poor predictive values is that results can be influenced by the nonauditory factors of attention, cognition, and language skills. An excellent illustration of the problem was provided in 1986 by Gascon and colleagues (Gascon, Johnson, and Burd 1986). They evaluated a group of 9 children who were considered to be hyperactive and have attention deficit disorders. The children were evaluated with several tests of CAPD, including the Staggered Spondaic Word Test, the Competing Sentence Test, the Filtered Speech Test, and the Rapidly Alternating Speech Test. In addition, they were evaluated with several measures of attention, including motor impersistence, finger localization, face/hand extinction, visual tracking, and pointing span of objects in sequence. Both the CAPD test battery and the attention test battery were administered before and after the children were medicated with stimulants to control hyperactivity. Results showed that 79% of the children improved on the CAPD test battery following stimulants. In contrast, 50% of the children improved on the attention battery, and 53% showed improvement in their communication and attention behavior. What these results indicate, of course, is that the CAPD tests are very sensitive to the effects of attention. If this is true, then a poor test result is uninterpretable for CAPD because children who have attention disorders will perform poorly on the test even if they do not have auditory processing disorder. Therefore, the effects of auditory processing disorder cannot be separated from the effects that attention deficits have on a child's ability to carry out these particular test measures.

Similar problems with nonauditory influences on auditory test results have been reported on one of the most widely used CAPD screening tools, the SCAN: A Screening Test for Auditory Processing Disorders. For example, the test's author, Dr. Robert Keith, and his colleagues (Keith, Rudy, Donahue, and Katbamna 1989) reported that scores on the SCAN test were significantly correlated with scores on the Peabody Picture Vocabulary Test. These results can be interpreted in one of at least three ways: (1) children with CAPD are likely to have language deficits; (2) children with language deficits are likely to have CAPD; or (3) abnormal test results on the SCAN are uninterpretable for CAPD in children who have vocabulary deficits. A second finding, from the same study, showed that subjects with attention deficit disorders scored significantly worse on the SCAN than those who did not have attention disorders. Once again, this may mean that the two are correlated, so that children who are more likely to have one are more likely to have the other. Or it may mean that test results on the SCAN cannot be interpreted for CAPD because they are confounded by attention deficit disorders. Finally, Engineer and Keith (1991) showed that SCAN results improved significantly in hyperactive children when they were on stimulants, similar to the data from Gascon et al. (1986), indicating that the SCAN is sensitive to the effects of attention. What these studies suggest is that if children have a language deficit or an attention deficit,

Table 1

Questions Related to Public Health Assumptions Underlying the Appropriateness of Screening for Central Auditory Processing Disorder (CAPD). Should CAPD Be Screened?

	Yes	No	No Consensus
Clear definition?	○	●	○
Frequent occurrence?	○	○	●
Serious consequence?	●	○	○
Accurate diagnosis?	○	○	●
Amenable to treatment?	○	○	●
Available facilities?	○	○	●
Favorable cost-benefit?	○	○	●
Adequate screening tools?	○	○	●

then they are likely to fail this screening test for CAPD, regardless of their auditory processing ability. If the goal of the screening is to identify children with language deficits, attention deficits, and CAPD, then such a test might be appropriate. But if the goal is to screen exclusively for CAPD, then the influences of attention, cognition, and language skills must be controlled during the screening process.

Should auditory processing disorder be screened? Table 1 is a summary of the eight questions related to the assumptions underlying whether or not to screen for a particular disorder. Again, the implication is that if most or all of these assumptions are met, then the disorder is one that is appropriate, from a public health viewpoint, to screen in a large population. Is the disorder clearly defined? Clearly not. Is there a frequent occurrence of the disorder? The answer is simply not known. Does CAPD have a serious consequence? There seems to be a consensus that, yes, it does have a serious consequence. Can CAPD be accurately diagnosed? Yes, perhaps, although there are many who would disagree. Is it amenable to treatment? If it is defined as an auditory problem, it can be treated effectively. Are there available facilities? Maybe. What is the cost-benefit ratio? No one really knows. Are there adequate screening tools? There are certainly tools that have been developed or are under development. Only when the influence of nonauditory factors can be controlled will these tools be adequate for mass screening.

When the question of screening is viewed from a public health perspective, then, it becomes clear that, given our current level of understanding, it is inappropriate to carry out mass screening for CAPD. Consensus does not exist on a definition, operational or otherwise, of CAPD. There also is no gold standard against which to measure the effectiveness of diagnostic tools. Finally, there are not screening tools available that allow the differentiation of auditory problems from nonauditory problems.

Alternative Strategies

Although the foregoing summary paints a pessimistic picture of CAPD screening, it should not discourage us from trying to arrive at consensus about how to best identify and diagnose CAPD. Perhaps the most serious problem on which there is a lack of consensus is that of diagnosis of CAPD. Before screening can even be considered, general agreement needs to be reached on the appropriate strategies to use for diagnosis.

A PROPOSED APPROACH TO CAPD DIAGNOSIS

At the Neurosensory Center of Houston, the approach used to diagnose CAPD is based on the assumptions (1) that CAPD is a perceptual problem, not a language problem; (2) that it can be operationally defined on the basis of speech audiometric and electrophysiologic measures; and (3) that tests can be administered in a manner that limits the influences of attention, language, and cognition on interpretation of results. The test battery will be described briefly here to illustrate an approach to the diagnosis of CAPD that has proven successful clinically. While it is by no means the only strategy, it is successful because it controls the influences of cognition, attention, and language ability, thereby isolating auditory disorder from nonauditory influences on test interpretation. Such a strategy could readily be applied to any of a number of existing tests of CAPD.

Table 2
Test Battery for Assessing CAPD in Children

Speech Audiometry	Auditory Evoked Potentials
Younger Children Pediatric Speech Intelligibility Test	Auditory Brainstem Response Middle Latency Response Late Vertex Response
Older Children PB words in quiet Synthetic Sentence Identification Test Dichotic Sentence Identification Test	

The test battery for evaluating children with auditory processing disorder is summarized in table 2. It includes both speech audiometry and auditory evoked potential measurement. Speech audiometric measures vary depending on the child's language skills. For younger children, the Pediatric Speech Intelligibility (PSI) Test (Jerger, Lewis, Hawkins, and Jerger 1980) is used. Words and sentences, with both ipsilateral (ICM) and contralateral competing messages (CCM), are presented at various message-to-competition ratios (MCRs). For older children, adult speech audiometric materials are used. These include phonemically balanced (PB) words presented in quiet, the Synthetic Sentence Identification (SSI) Test (Jerger, Speaks, and Trammel 1968) with ipsilateral competing message, and the Dichotic Sentence Identification (DSI) Test (Fifer, Jerger, Berlin, Tobey, and Campbell 1983). Auditory evoked potential measurements include the auditory brainstem response (ABR), the middle latency response (MLR), and the late vertex response (LVR). CAPD is then operationally defined on the basis of patterns of speech audiometric scores and auditory evoked potential results.

The following cases illustrate the manner in which speech audiometric measures can be implemented to assess auditory processing ability while controlling the nonauditory effects of language, cognition, and attention. Audiometric data from a 4-year-6-month-old child who was diagnosed with CAPD are shown in figure 1. The child had a mild low-frequency conductive hearing loss bilaterally. In the right ear, speech understanding was normal for both PSI words and sentences. However,

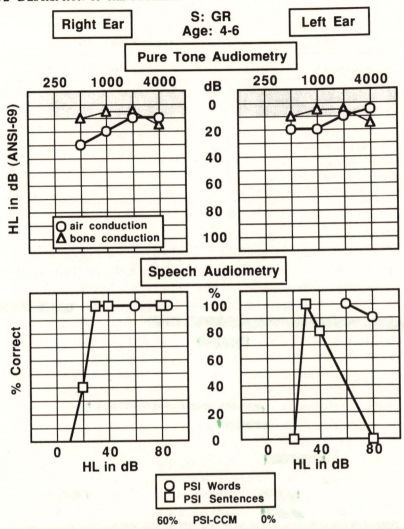

Figure 1. Pure-tone and speech audiometric results in a 4-year-6-month-old child with central auditory processing disorder.

in the left ear, there was a significant abnormality. While the PSI words were within normal limits, the performance-intensity function for PSI sentences showed substantial rollover, with very poor performance at high-intensity levels. In addition, performance on the PSI sentence task with contralateral competing message was abnormal for a child of this age, with 60% correct in the right ear and 0% in the left ear. This case illustrates how nonauditory effects can be controlled with appropriate testing strategies. If it were argued that CAPD does not exist in children and that these speech audiometric scores were simply the result of nonauditory factors affecting behavioral measures, some rather interesting explanations for the results would need to be invoked. For example, an argument would have to be made that explains ear asymmetry on the basis of a cognitive or language deficit. That is, can there be a left ear cognitive deficit? Can there be a left ear language deficit? Obviously, the likelihood of asymmetry resulting from a cognitive or language deficit is small. An argument would also have to be made to explain the rollover of the performance-intensity function. While the child performed well at a low-intensity level, he had difficulty understanding speech at a high-intensity level. Could it be that this child was somehow linguistically more impaired at higher intensity levels than at lower intensity levels? An intensity-level-specific language deficit would be very difficult to explain. Attention deficits could also be ruled out in this case. The child could obviously attend to the task, since performance in the right ear was excellent, and performance at various intensity levels in the left ear was also excellent. The child was cognitively capable of carrying out the task, linguistically capable of carrying out the task, and had the attention ability to carry out the task. The deficit, then, was in his auditory processing ability.

This point is illustrated further by the audiometric data of a 5-year-1-month-old child presented in figure 2. Although hearing sensitivity was within normal limits in both ears, speech audiometric results were strikingly abnormal. In the right ear, the performance-intensity functions for both words and sentences showed rollover. In addition, in the left ear, there was a substantial discrepancy between understanding of sentences and understanding of words. This was obviously not a language problem since, at 60 dB HL, the child understood all of the sentences correctly, and at an easier listening condition of +10 dB MCR, the child identified all of the words correctly. The child was clearly capable of doing the task linguistically and cognitively. Thus, use of performance-intensity functions, various MCRs, and word-versus-sentence comparisons permitted the assessment of auditory processing ability in a manner that reduced the likelihood of nonauditory factors influencing the interpretation of test results.

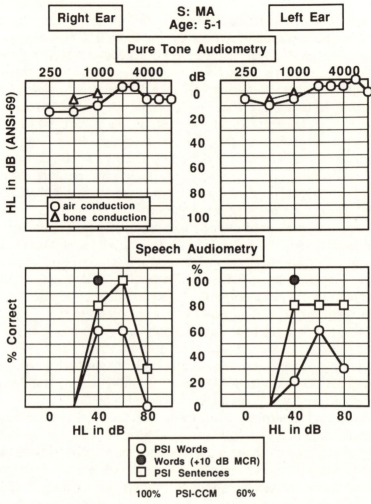

Figure 2. Pure-tone and speech audiometric results in a 5-year-1-month-old child with central auditory processing disorder.

Auditory evoked potential measurements are also included in the test battery in an effort to corroborate the results of speech audiometry. In 1988, we reported results from 44 children who were diagnosed as having CAPD, based on patterns of speech audiometric results (Stach, Loiselle, and Jerger 1988). Auditory evoked potentials were abnormal in 84% of the children tested. Of these 37 children, both the MLR and the

LVR were abnormal in 73%, the MLR was abnormal in isolation in 13.5%, and the LVR was abnormal in isolation in 13.5%.

Our clinical experience with this diagnostic strategy has been encouraging. In conjunction with thorough speech, language, and neuropsychological evaluations, the use of well-controlled speech audiometric measures and auditory evoked potentials has proven to be quite powerful in defining the presence or absence of an auditory processing disorder.

AN ALTERNATIVE APPROACH TO CAPD SCREENING

When consensus is reached on methods for diagnosing CAPD, the next challenge will be to identify those who are at risk for the disorder so that diagnostic testing can be implemented. As stated earlier, screening is usually carried out for problems that are asymptomatic. That is, if a child has the symptoms of a disorder, then there is no reason to screen. Instead, that child should receive diagnostic testing automatically. Since CAPD is, by its very nature, symptomatic, some would argue that it need not be screened but that the presence of its symptomatology be systematically investigated. Thus, one alternative to the use of a screening test is simply to assess the symptoms. Several efforts have been made to use checklists or performance scales, designed to be completed by teachers or parents, to evaluate the symptomatology of CAPD. For example, Fisher (1976) developed the Fisher Auditory Problems Checklist, and Smoski and his colleagues (Smoski, Brunt, and Tannahill in press) developed the Children's Auditory Processing Performance Scale for such a purpose. The underlying assumption of this approach is that there is no reason to screen for CAPD because it is symptomatic by its very nature. Therefore, the presence or absence of the symptoms need only to be evaluated and the child referred for diagnostic testing if symptoms are present. Although this alternative has been largely untested, it appears to have merit as a method for identifying those children who are at risk for CAPD.

SUMMARY

Should mass screening of children with CAPD be carried out? When tests of the assumptions underlying mass screening are applied to CAPD, the answer to this question becomes a rather clear no. Consensus has not been reached on a definition of the disorder, there is no universally accepted clinical approach to diagnosing it, and screening tools are not available that can differentiate auditory disorders from nonauditory disorders.

Although this conclusion may be discouraging, it should not fetter our search for models and strategies that can be used to better define and diagnose the disorder. If consensus can be reached on the nature of auditory processing disorder, and if operational definitions can be developed based on cogent diagnostic strategies, then many of the public health questions asked here can be answered. When this occurs, the questions of whether to screen and of how to screen will clearly be pertinent.

ACKNOWLEDGMENTS

I am grateful to Dr. James Jerger for his editorial insight and to Mary Lou Ginandt for her assistance in manuscript preparation.

REFERENCES

Engineer, P., and Keith, R.W. 1991. Effects of methylphenidate on auditory processing abilities of children with attention deficit-hyperactivity disorder. *Audiology Today* 3(2):44 (abstract).

Fifer, R.C., Jerger, J.F., Berlin, C.I., Tobey, E.A., and Campbell, J.C. 1983. Development of a dichotic sentence identification test for hearing-impaired adults. *Ear and Hearing* 4:300-305.

Fisher, L.I. 1976. *Fisher auditory problems checklist*. Cedar Rapids,Iowa: Grant Wood Area Educational Agency.

Gascon, G.G., Johnson, R., and Burd, L. 1986. Central auditory processing and attention deficit disorders. *Journal of Child Neurology* 1:27-33.

Jerger, J., Speaks, C., and Trammel, J. 1968. A new approach to speech audiometry. *Journal of Speech and Hearing Disorders* 33:318-327.

Jerger, S., Lewis, S., Hawkins, J., and Jerger, J. 1980. Pediatric speech intelligibility test. I. Generation of test materials. *International Journal of Pediatric Otorhinolaryngology* 2:217-230.

Jerger, S., Martin, R.C., and Jerger, J. 1987. Specific auditory perceptual dysfunction in a learning disabled child. *Ear and Hearing* 8:78-86.

Keith, R.W., Rudy, J., Donahue, P.A., and Katbamna, B. 1989. Comparison of SCAN results with other auditory and language measures in a clinical population. *Ear and Hearing* 10:382-386.

Lasky, E.Z, and Katz, J. 1983. Perspectives on central auditory processing. In E.Z. Lasky and J. Katz (eds.), *Central auditory processing disorders.* Baltimore: University Park Press.

Northern, J.L., and Downs, M.P. 1974. *Hearing in children.* Baltimore: Williams and Wilkins.

Pinheiro, M., and Musiek, F.E. (eds.). 1985. *Assessment of central auditory dysfunction: Foundations and clinical correlates.* Baltimore: Williams and Wilkins.

Smoski, W.J., Brunt, M.A., and Tannahill, J.C. In press. Listening characteristics of children with central auditory processing disorders. *Language, Speech, and Hearing Services in Schools.*

Stach, B.A. 1990. Hearing aid amplification and central processing disorders. In R.E. Sandlin (ed.), *Handbook of hearing aid amplification. Vol. 2: Clinical considerations and fitting practices.* Boston: College Hill Press.

Stach, B.A., Loiselle, L.H., and Jerger, J.F. 1987. FM system use by children with central auditory processing disorder. *Asha* 29(10):69 (abstract).

Stach, B.A., Loiselle, L.H., and Jerger, J.F. 1988. Auditory evoked potential abnormalities in children with central auditory disorder. *Asha* 30(10):133 (abstract).

Willeford, J.A., and Burleigh, J.M. 1985. *Handbook of central auditory processing disorders in children.* New York: Grune and Stratton.

Chapter 6

Prevalence Rates and Cost-Effectiveness of Risk Factors

Robert G. Turner and Barbara K. Cone-Wesson

INTRODUCTION

Risk factors are characteristics in the family or medical history of an infant that are thought to be associated with a disease or medical condition. Infants with the risk factor should have a higher prevalence of the medical problem than corresponding infants without the risk factor. Thus, infants who display a risk factor are considered at risk for the medical condition.

Certain risk factors are thought to be associated with hearing loss (table 1). The factors listed in table 1 are the ones most frequently discussed in the literature but not the only ones that have been considered. Most factors are self-explanatory; however, more detailed definitions are available (Gerkin 1986; Rossetti 1986).

Audiologists are interested in risk factors associated with hearing loss because these factors are the components used to construct a high-risk register (HRR). The HRR has been used for many years as a tool for early identification of hearing loss. In 1972, the Joint Committee on Infant Hearing (JCIH) recommended a five-factor high-risk register, the first five factors in table 1 (Gerkin 1986). They also recommended that infants who display one or more of these factors should be followed until accurate assessment of hearing was made. In 1982, the JCIH expanded the high-risk register to seven factors (see table 1). Infants displaying one or more factors should be screened by an audiologist, if possible, before

Table 1
Common Risk Factors for Hearing Loss

	1.	(FH)	Family history of childhood hearing loss
	2.	(TO)	Congenital infections, aka TORCH
	3.	(CA)	Craniofacial anomalies
	4.	(BW)	Birth weight < 1500 grams
1972	5.	(HB)	Hyperbilirubinemia requiring exchange
	6.	(BM)	Bacterial meningitis
1982	7.	(AX)	Asphyxia
		(AG)	Apgar score ≤ 3 at 5 minutes
	8.	(OX)	Ototoxic medication
	9.	(MV)	Mechanical ventilation ≥ 10 days
1990	10.	(SY)	Syndromes that include hearing loss
	11.	(GA)	Gestational age < 38 weeks
	12.	(IN)	Intubation
	13.	(MA)	Meconium aspiration
	14.	(RE)	Respiratory distress

The Joint Committee on Infant Hearing recommended a five-item high-risk register in 1972. These are the first five items listed. A seven-item register was recommended in 1982 and a ten-item register in 1990.

6 months of age (Joint Committee on Infant Hearing 1982). Again, in 1990, the JCIH expanded the HRR to ten factors (Joint Committee on Infant Hearing 1991). Neonates who manifest one or more factors should be screened with auditory brainstem response (ABR) prior to discharge from the nursery. If this is not possible, then the infant should be referred for ABR testing by 3 months but never later than 6 months.

We see that the HRR has been used for almost 20 years and continues to be recommended as an integral component in the early identification of hearing loss. If we are to continue to employ the HRR, we must address three fundamental questions.

1. How well do the individual risk factors predict hearing loss?
2. How do we combine these factors into a HRR?
3. How does the HRR compare to other hearing screening techniques?

This chapter will focus on what we currently know about these fundamental questions.

PREVALENCE DATA

How well do the individual risk factors predict hearing loss? Perhaps we can address this question by examining the clinical literature for some type of measure of the performance or accuracy of risk factors. We find a variety of statistics; the most common are what we will call prevalence data. To illustrate, assume a study found that 43 of 100 infants in the population had low birth weight. The prevalence of low birth weight in the infant population would be 43%. We could also say that 43% of the infants had low birth weight or that the probability of low birth weight in the population was 43%. All three descriptions are correct and equivalent. For consistency, we will consider these data as measures of prevalence.

To appropriately use the prevalence data in the literature, we must recognize that all of the data are not the same. There are three major classes of data based on the population of infants being studied. The first measure (PIP) is the prevalence of a risk factor in the initial population of infants, e.g., the well-baby nursery. The second measure (PAR) is the prevalence in the population of infants who have been identified as at risk by the risk factors. The third measure (PIL) is the prevalence in a population of infants who have hearing loss.

An example will demonstrate the difference between these measures. Assume there are 100 infants in an ICN. Twenty of those infants have low birth weight; PIP would be 20/100=20%. Several risk factors are used to screen the nursery. A total of 60 infants fail one or more factors. PAR for low birth weight would be 20/60=33%. Two of the 60 screening failures are found to have hearing loss; one of the two has low birth weight. PIL would be 1/2=50%. It should be clear that these three prevalence measures are quite distinct. A knowledge of one does not guarantee a knowledge of the others.

As a further complication, we must also consider the group of infants under study. The infants could come from the well-baby nursery (WBN), the intensive care nursery (ICN), or the general population (GP), which would contain infants from both the WBN and the ICN. We must consider each of these separately because the prevalence of a risk factor can be very different in each group. This is illustrated by data from Stein et al. (1983) for infants identified with hearing loss. The infants were separated into a WBN group and an ICN group. The prevalence of risk factors is quite different for the two groups (figure 1). For example, the prevalence of low birth weight is over 50% for the ICN infants but less than 10% for the WBN infants. Almost 50% of the WBN infants had no known risk factor, whereas all ICN infants could be associated with a risk factor. When we consider the three populations (initial, at risk, hearing loss) and the three groups (WBN, ICN, GP), we see that there are nine different prevalence statistics that can be reported in the literature. These nine measures are not equivalent and cannot be simply combined; they must be evaluated separately. Despite the limitations, these prevalence statistics are of some interest and can provide useful information. Results from several studies are summarized in tables 2 and 3. Comparison of different studies is difficult. The exact definition of a risk factor may vary as well as the criterion for determining if an infant meets a risk factor. Also, the group under study may be biased in some

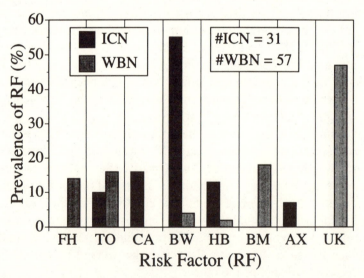

Figure 1. Comparison of risk-factor prevalence for intensive care and well-baby nurseries. All infants have hearing loss. See table 1 for definitions of risk-factor abbreviations. UK=no known risk factor. Data taken from Stein et al. 1983.

Table 2
Prevalence Statistics for Risk Factors as Calculated from Clinical Studies

RF	PIP (%)					PAR(%)				
	ICN			GP		ICN			GP	
	#1	#2	#3	#4	#5	#2	#6	#7	#4	#5
N	~2000	458	2192	17731	283298	234	168	137	~3600	25564
FH	1	2		5	6	3	5	1	22	62
TO	1	1	<1			3	1	7		
CA		3	1	<1		6	2		2	
BW	19	39	12	2	<1	76	25	57	8	9
HB		2	2	3		5	51	18	13	
BM		<1	0			<1		4		
AX		5	1			10				
AG			10	1	3				7	38
OX	17			<1				34	1	
MV										
SY										
GA	33									
IN										
MA										
RE	20									
NO	60	49		80	91	na	na	na	na	na

PIP: prevalence of risk factor in the initial population; PAR: prevalence of risk factor in the infants who fail one or more risk factors; RF: risk factor; N: number of infants in the study; ICN: intensive care nursery; GP: general population; NO: no risk factor could be identified; na: not applicable, by definition all infants in this group have some risk factors. The abbreviations for the risk factors are defined in Table 1. The numbers indicate the clinical studies that were evaluated. #1 Halpern et al. 1987; #2 Shimizu et al. 1990; #3: Barton 1991; #4 Feinmesser and Tell 1976; #5: Mahoney and Eichwald 1987; #6: Shannon et al. 1984; #7: Swigonski et al. 1987.

Table 3

Prevalence Statistics for Risk Factors as Calculated from Clinical Studies

PIL(%)

RF	ICN			WBN		GP					
	#1	#8	#9	#9	#4	#10	#11	#12	#13	#14	#15
N	50	23	33	55	25	262	2355	2897	69	179	117
FH	0	13	0	14	40	28	50	11	32	55	33
TO	10	26	10	16		23	6	16	4	5	16
CA	8	9	16	0		12	2		1	13	2
BW	31		55	4			9		1		
HB	14	70	13	2	8	2	3	4	6		
BM	0	4	0	18				6		7	3
AX	24		7								
AG	12	57			4			4	1		
OX	45	78				<1		1			2
MV	33					10					
SY		78				3					4
GA	63										
IN	90										
MA	20										
RE	37	57									
NO		4	0	47	28	20		45	49	83	27

PIL: prevalence of risk factor in infants with hearing loss; RF: risk factor; N: number of infants in the study; ICN: intensive care nursery; WBN: well-baby nursery; GP: general population; NO: no risk factor could be identified. The abbreviations for the risk-factors are defined in Table 1. The numbers indicate the clinical studies that were evaluated. #1: Halpern et al. 1987; #4: Feinmesser and Tell 1976; #8: Simmons et al. 1979; #9: Stein et al. 1983; #10: Northern and Downs 1974; #11: Fraser 1976; #12: Martin 1981; #13: Feinmesser et al. 1982; #14: Kankkunen 1982; #15: Parving 1983.

way, as discussed in more detail later in this paper. Finally, some judgment and interpretation were necessary by the authors to create these tables. The data reveal some general characteristics about the risk factors; more quantitative conclusions are questionable.

The most obvious conclusion from the data is that we have little information on the WBN, at least for the studies we found in the literature. This reflects a tendency of researchers to concentrate on the ICN or retrospectively on the general population. The prevalence statistics for the ICN differ significantly from those for the GP. Obviously, the factors relating to prenatal or perinatal problems are going to be more common in the ICN because these problems will place the infant in the ICN. For infants with hearing loss, family history is a major factor in the GP but relatively minor in the ICN. Also, a high percentage in the GP have no evident risk factor; this percentage is low in the ICN. Medical conditions that are major factors in the ICN have low prevalence in the GP. These results are not surprising. The GP consists primarily of infants from the WBN, not the ICN. If we had sufficient information on the WBN, we would probably see the results for the GP parallel statistics for the WBN.

EVALUATING RISK FACTORS

Can the prevalence data be used to evaluate the accuracy and utility of the risk factors? In general, the answer is no. Consider the first measure, PIP. This indicates the percentage of infants in an initial population who fail a particular risk factor. What this statistic does not tell us is how many normal hearing and hearing-impaired infants fail the risk factor. All we know is the total number of failures. Without information as to hearing status, we cannot evaluate the risk factors.

The second measure, PAR, tells us the prevalence of a risk factor in the infants who have failed one or more risk factors. Although this is a popular statistic to report, it is actually a meaningless measure. If the infant were screened with only one risk factor, then PAR for that factor would be 100%. If many factors were used, then PAR for that same factor could be very small. We see that the value of PAR will depend upon how many risk factors were used. This tells us little about the performance of the risk factor. In addition, like PIP, PAR does not distinguish between normal hearing and hearing-impaired infants.

The third measure, PIL, tells us the prevalence of a risk factor in infants with hearing loss. In most studies, only infants who fail the risk-factor screening are followed and evaluated for hearing loss. Thus, PIL is calculated for infants who have hearing loss *and* have failed one or more risk factors. Hearing-impaired infants who have passed the screening are not followed or evaluated. In this situation, PIL does not give us a valid measure of the accuracy of a risk factor because we do not know the number of hearing-impaired infants who have passed the risk factor.

The prevalence data provide useful and interesting information, but they are not adequate for evaluating the risk factors. With PIP we can never know exactly how many normal hearing or hearing-impaired infants failed the risk factor. PAR is a useless measure, and PIL frequently does not reflect the total number of hearing-impaired infants.

Is there any way to evaluate the risk factors? Yes, if we treat each risk factor as an individual screening test. When we do this, we can use all of the measures of performance and cost that have been developed for diagnostic and screening tests. While a number of measures are available, the most basic measures of test performance are hit rate (HT) and false alarm rate (FA). These can be applied to risk factors, even though that is seldom done. Hit rate of a risk factor (HTr) is the percentage of hearing-impaired infants in the initial infant group (WBN, ICN, or GP) who fail the risk factor. False alarm rate of a risk factor (FAr) is the percentage of normal hearing infants in the initial group who fail the risk factor. Unlike the prevalence data, HTr and FAr are measures that tell us exactly how normal hearing and hearing-impaired infants are evaluated by a risk factor.

Calculating HTr and FAr requires an appropriately designed experiment. We must know the exact number of hearing-impaired infants in the population who fail the risk-factor screening and the number who pass the screening. All infants must be followed and evaluated for hearing loss, not just those who fail the screening. Typically, studies that we reviewed did not adhere to this experimental design. This means that HTr and FAr cannot be calculated.

Is there any way to estimate these measures from the prevalence data usually provided? Under some conditions, the prevalence data can be used to derive an estimate of HTr and FAr. PIP can provide a reasonable approximation to FAr. This is best illustrated with an example. Assume that 500 infants in an ICN are screened with a multiple risk-factor HRR and that 300 infants fail the screen. Of these 300, 150 have low birth weight. In this case, PIP equals 150/500=30% for low birth weight. The prevalence of hearing loss in the ICN is usually small, 2% to 4%. If we assume 3%, then there would be 15 hearing-impaired infants in the ICN. Even if all 15 had low birth weight, at least 135 of the 150 low birth weight failures would be false alarms, and the false alarm rate would be 135/485=28%. In general, FAr will be a few percent smaller than PIP in the ICN. In the WBN and GP where prevalence is much smaller, there would be even less difference between FAr and PIP. Thus, PIP can provide an estimate of risk-factor false alarm rate.

In some studies (e.g., Stein et al. 1983), hearing-impaired children are retrospectively evaluated for risk factors. This approach avoids the normal problem when calculating PIL in that the infants are not restricted to those who have failed an initial screening. If these children are a representative sample of hearing-impaired children in their corresponding group (WBN, ICN, or GP), then PIL is an estimate of HTr for that group. Of course, there really is never any way to know that the children are an appropriate sample.

Even though HTr and FAr are good measures of performance, we still need some measure of cost to adequately evaluate the risk factors. A useful measure is the financial cost per hearing-impaired infant identified (CPHL), a measure of cost-effectiveness. By our definition, the

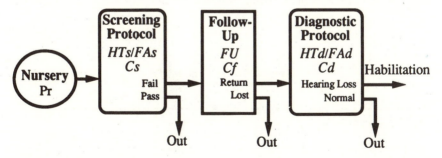

Figure 2. Basic model of early identification protocol. The following parameters must be specified for the model. Pr: prevalence of hearing loss in nursery; HTs: hit rate of screening protocol; FAs: false alarm rate of screening protocol; Cs: cost per infant of screening; FU: follow-up success; Cf: cost per infant for follow-up; HTd: hit rate of diagnostic protocol; FAd: false alarm rate of diagnostic protocol; Cd: per infant cost of diagnostic evaluation. "Out" means that an infant is no longer tested or followed by the protocol. Model adapted from figure 1 in Turner 1991a.

greater the CPHL, the poorer the cost-effectiveness. We can determine CPHL using a model of the early identification process that has been developed to evaluate different hearing screening strategies (Turner 1991a). The basic model is shown in figure 2. Infants come from either a well-baby nursery or an intensive care nursery. In general, infants in the nursery are referred to a screening protocol. The outcome of screening is either pass or fail; the screening is not diagnostic. Infants who fail are referred for diagnostic testing; infants who pass are not followed. Some infants will be lost from follow-up and will not receive additional testing. The final component in the early identification process is the diagnostic protocol. Infants who demonstrate hearing loss would return for additional audiologic testing and evaluation by other professionals.

To use the model, we must specify a number of parameters such as prevalence of hearing loss and cost of testing. For everything except the screening protocol, we will use the parameters suggested by Turner (1991a), which are based on the clinical literature (table 4). The screening protocol in the model would correspond to each individual risk factor or, as a control, no screening tests (figure 3a,b). In the latter case, all infants are referred for follow-up and diagnostic testing. For the screening protocol, we must specify a hit rate (HTs), a false alarm rate (FAs), and the cost per infant of the screening. HTs is the percentage of hearing-impaired infants in the nursery who fail the screening. FAs is the percentage of normal hearing infants in the nursery who fail the

Table 4
Parameters Used with Model

	ICN	WBN	$/Test
Prevalence (%)	3.0	0.1	
Follow-Up Success (%)	50	50	13
Diagnostic Protocol			160
Hit rate (%)	100	100	
False alarm rate (%)	0	0	
Test Correlation	Zero	Zero	

ICN: intensive care nursery; WBN: well-baby nursery. Values taken from Turner 1991a.

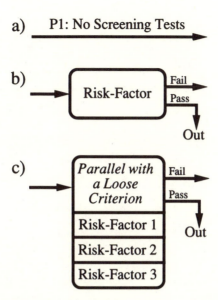

Figure 3. Screening protocols using risk factors. a) Protocol 1(P1): This protocol uses no screening tests and serves as a comparison for other screening protocols. All infants in nursery are referred for follow-up and diagnostic evaluations. b) Each risk factor constitutes a different screening protocol. c) Risk factors are combined in parallel with a loose criterion to form screening protocols. This means that an infant is evaluated with each risk factor in a protocol; if the infant fails at least one factor, then the infant fails the screening. Risk factor 1 is the most cost-effective risk factor. Risk factor 2 is the second most cost-effective, and so forth. Risk factor 1 is the first screening protocol. Risk factor 1 plus risk factor 2 make up the second protocol. Risk factor 1 plus risk factor 2 plus risk factor 3 constitute the third. This process is continued until there is an 11-factor screening protocol.

screening. When an individual risk factor is the screening protocol, HTs equals HTr, and FAs equals FAr. The cost of screening would equal the cost of administering a one-factor HRR. We assume a per infant expense of $1 for each risk factor. When there is direct referral to follow-up (P1), HTs equals 100%, and FAs equals 100%. This is because all infants have effectively "failed" screening. In this case, the cost of screening is $0.

EXAMPLE

Once all parameters are specified, we can use the model to calculate CPHL. This measure combined with HTr is sufficient for a basic

Table 5
Performance and Cost of Risk Factors

RF	HTr (%)	FAr (%)	CPHL ($)
TO	9.8	0.5	1170
CA	7.8	0.4	1350
MA	19.6	5.4	2180
OX	45.1	16.5	2530
GA	62.7	33.9	3540
RE	37.3	19.7	3540
BW	31.4	18.5	3940
AX	23.5	13.6	4950
MV	33.3	21.4	4250
AG	11.8	8.4	5030
IN	90.2	86.4	6020
HB	13.7	13.6	6640
P1	100.0	100.0	6200

RF: risk factor; HTr: hit rate of risk factor; FAr: false alarm of risk factor; CPHL: cost per hearing-impaired infant identified. Abbreviations for risk-factors are defined in table 1. Risk factors are arranged in increasing CPHL. Calculations of HTr and FAr are based upon data in Halpern et al. 1987. CPHL was calculated using the model described in the text. P1: protocol 1, no screening tests.

evaluation of the risk factors. To illustrate the concept, we will use data from Halpern et al. (1987). This study is one of the most comprehensive in terms of number of risk factors and infants (over 800); all infants were from the ICN. The results are presented in such a way that hit rate and false alarm rate can be calculated. The authors provide the number of normal hearing and hearing-impaired infants who pass and fail each risk factor in this population of 800 infants. Unfortunately, the 800 infants were selected from an initial population of 2,000 because they failed a screening with a small subset of risk factors. In addition, the infants who passed were not evaluated for hearing loss. Thus, the experimental results are corrupted by the experimental design, but for this example, we will pretend that the 800 infants constitute an unbiased sample of ICN infants. We used this study because it came the closest to meeting all of the requirements for this example.

HTr and FAr are calculated in the following way. From the results of Halpern et al., we see in their table 3 that 16 hearing-impaired infants had low birth weight whereas 35 did not. HTr for low birth weight would equal 16 divided by 51, the total number of hearing-impaired infants. There were 360 normal hearing infants with low birth weight and 405 with normal weight. FAr would equal 360 divided by 765, the total number of normal hearing infants. A list of risk factors with corresponding HTr and FAr is shown in table 5.

The model was used to calculate CPHL for each risk factor as well as for the no-screen control (P1). The techniques for making these calculations are described in detail by Turner (1991a) and will not be repeated here. We can easily compare the risk factors by plotting CPHL (cost-effectiveness) as a function of HTr (performance) (figure 4). The location of each abbreviation in the figure indicates the HTr and CPHL for that risk factor.

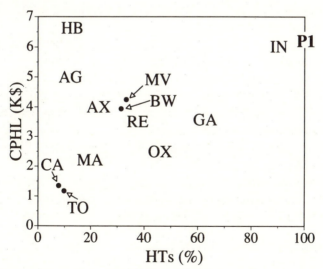

Figure 4. Comparison of cost and performance of individual risk factors. CPHL: cost per hearing-impaired infant identified; HTs: hit rate of screening protocol, which is, in this case, the hit rate of the individual risk factor. See table 1 for definitions of abbreviations for risk factors. Location of abbreviation indicates datum point. P1: protocol 1, no screening tests.

Note that CPHL is the cost per hearing-impaired infant identified. The higher the CPHL, the lower the cost-effectiveness. Therefore, we want risk factors to have high HTr and low CPHL. This corresponds to the lower right area of the plot. Unfortunately, no risk factor occupies that region. The upper right area corresponds to high hit rate and low cost-effectiveness. Intubation (IN) occupies this region and is near P1, which corresponds to failing all infants in the ICN. This means that most infants are intubated, but the percentage with hearing loss is about the same as the general ICN population. Intubation is not a good predictor of hearing loss.

The upper left region means low hit rate and poor cost-effectiveness. Hyperbilirubinemia (HB) and low Apgar score (AG) occupy this area. Few infants have these factors, and the percentage of hearing loss in those who do is about the same as the general ICN population. Factors in this region are the least desirable to use. The lower left corresponds to low hit rate but cost-effectiveness. Few infants have factors in this region, producing the low hit rate, but a high percentage of those with these factors have hearing loss, producing the low CPHL. These factors are desirable to use, although no one factor would identify many hearing-impaired infants. The factors in the middle of the plot represent moderate hit rate and cost-effectiveness.

This approach provides a simple way to compare objectively risk factors in terms of performance and cost. For example, ototoxic medication (OX) is clearly superior to low birth weight (BW) because it is below and to the right in figure 4. This means that OX has both higher hit rate and lower cost than BW. In addition, these data permit a rank ordering of risk factors by performance or cost, which is important if we want to combine risk factors into a HRR. The purpose of this example is to illustrate the technique; the results do not provide a valid comparison of the risk factors. As stated previously, the data presented by Halpern et al. are biased by the experimental design and do not really permit an accurate calculation of HTr or FAr.

COMBINING RISK FACTORS

How do we combine these factors into a HRR? It is evident from figure 4 that a number of risk factors offer cost-effectiveness better than P1 (no tests), but none of these have a hit rate greater than 65%. This is a problem because a general strategy when screening is to maximize hit rate, even at the expense of a higher false alarm rate and reduced cost-effectiveness. The reason is that false alarms are usually preferable to misses. An infant who is missed by screening will not be followed and may not be identified for years. A false alarm will be followed and correctly identified by the diagnostic procedure.

Is there any way to combine risk factors to increase hit rate? Yes, we can combine them in parallel with a loose criterion (Turner et al. 1984). The infant is screened with all factors, and if the infant fails at least one, the infant fails the screen. This typical strategy has been used when constructing a HRR from individual risk factors. The only problem is that combining risk factors in this way will also increase false alarm rate, decreasing cost-effectiveness.

The individual risk factors evaluated in figure 4 can be combined in parallel to form a HRR (figure 3c). This serves as the screening protocol in the model. If we can estimate a hit rate and false alarm rate for the combined risk factors, we can calculate CPHL. Thus, we can determine if a combination of risk factors will provide better performance and cost than any individual factor.

The risk factors were combined in the following way. They were rank ordered from lowest to highest CPHL (table 5). We began with the factor with the lowest CPHL, congenital infections (TO). This is the most cost-effective single factor and serves as a comparison for the combinations. The factor with the second lowest CPHL, craniofacial anomalies (CA), was combined with TO to produce a 2-factor HRR. The factor with the next lowest CPHL, meconium aspiration (MA), was combined with TO and CA to produce a 3-factor HRR. The process was repeated up to an 11-factor HRR consisting of the 11 most cost-effective factors. Thus, we have 11 HRRs to evaluate ranging from a 1- to an 11-factor screening protocol. Intubation (IN) was not included because it functions essentially the same as no screening tests.

The hit rate and false alarm rate of the 11 screening protocols were calculated using equations provided by Turner et al. (1984). To use these equations, we must specify the hit rate and false alarm rate of the individual risk factors, how the factors are combined, and the test correlation. The hit rates and false alarm rates have already been calculated (table 5). As stated above, the risk-factors are combined in parallel with a loose criterion. Test correlation is the tendency of tests to identify the same patients the same way. There are little clinical data on correlation between risk factors. For this example, we will specify zero test correlation; that is, the tests are uncorrelated.

Cost of a screening protocol was determined using $1 per risk factor per infant and $2 per risk factor per infant. Two values were used to represent a reasonable range of clinical expense, since there is little information in the published literature on the cost of administering a HRR. Thus, a four-factor screening protocol would cost either $4 or $8 per infant. CPHL was calculated for each screening protocol using both costs (figure 5). As each factor is added, the hit rate of the screening protocol increases, but so does the CPHL. For comparison, the value for the no screen control (P1) is shown. The first several factors that are added significantly increase hit rate with a modest increase in CPHL. The five-factor HRR has a hit rate of about 85% at two-thirds the cost of P1. This is an improvement in performance over any individual risk factor, plus cost-effectiveness is much better than for P1. Some would consider a hit rate of 85% a little low for screening. One out of every six

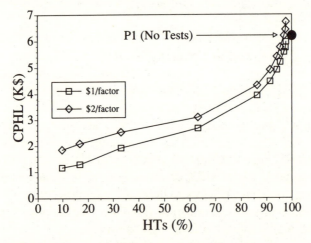

Figure 5. Cost and performance of high-risk registers formed by combining risk factors. The two curves correspond to two different estimates of cost for administering the high-risk register: $1/factor/infant and $2/factor/infant. Left-most pair of symbols correspond to the single most cost-effective risk factor. Moving right, the second pair represent a high-risk register formed by the 2 most cost-effective factors. The third pair are the 3 most cost-effective factors. This continues until the right-most pair, which are for the high-risk register consisting of the 11 most cost-effective risk factors. The solid circle is the datum for protocol 1 (P1), which uses no screening tests. CPHL: cost per hearing-impaired infant identified; HTs: hit rate of screening protocol, which is, in this case, the hit rate of the risk factors when combined in parallel with a loose criterion.

hearing-impaired infants would be missed. As more risk factors are added to increase hit rate above 85%, CPHL increases rapidly. When a high hit rate is achieved, the HRR offers little advantage over using no screening tests.

EVALUATING THE HIGH-RISK REGISTER

How does the HRR compare to other hearing screening techniques? Both the JCIH (1991) and the American Speech-Language-Hearing Association (ASHA) Committee on Infant Hearing (1989) have recommended that every infant be tested with the HRR. Is this the best possible strategy? If we are to continue using the HRR for the early identification of hearing loss, we need some measure of its utility, particularly compared to other hearing screening protocols.

The HRR can be evaluated in much the same way as the individual risk factors if we recognize that the HRR is a hearing screening test (Turner 1990). Some have argued that the HRR is not a screening test but a procedure that identifies infants at risk (ASHA Committee on Infant Hearing 1990). Which concept is correct? That really depends on how one defines a hearing screening test. We offer the following, which we feel is reasonable:

A hearing screening test is a procedure that identifies a subpopulation of individuals that has a higher prevalence of hearing loss than the original population.

There are several points to note. The definition says nothing about how good or cost-effective the test is. One procedure may be a better screening test than another, but they both are screening tests if they both perform better than chance. The definition says nothing about the mechanics of the test. It is the performance of the test that is important, not how it is conducted. If the subpopulation has a prevalence greater than the initial population, then the infants in the subpopulation are at risk. We see that a hearing screening test, by definition, identifies infants at risk for hearing loss.

Using our definition, the HRR is a hearing screening test even though it involves no physical contact with the infant. Auditory brainstem response (ABR) testing in the nursery is a hearing screening test even though it does not measure hearing. And the mere presence of an

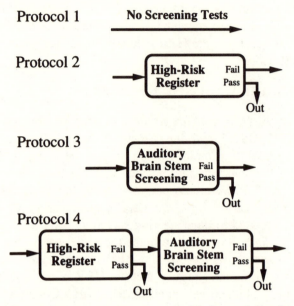

Figure 6. Four screening protocols that are evaluated. Protocols are described in text. Adapted from figure 2 in Turner 1991b.

infant in an ICN can be a hearing screening test because the prevalence of hearing loss in the ICN is greater than the general newborn population.

We can evaluate the HRR against other screening strategies using the model presented earlier. Most of the work presented below is from Turner (1991b in press). We will consider four screening protocols, two of which will use the HRR (figure 6).

Protocol 1 (P1): This protocol consists of no screening tests. All infants are scheduled for diagnostic testing. This protocol was considered previously when we evaluated the individual risk factors.

Protocol 2 (P2): This protocol consists of the HRR. Infants who fail the HRR are scheduled for diagnostic testing. Infants who pass are no longer followed.

Protocol 3 (P3): This protocol consists of ABR screening. Infants who fail are scheduled for diagnostic testing.

Protocol 4 (P4): This protocol consists of the HRR combined in series-positive with the ABR. Infants who fail the HRR receive ABR

Table 6
Parameters for Screening Protocols

	ICN	WBN	$/Test
High-Risk Register		13	
Hit rate (%)	95	60	
False alarm rate (%)	65	10	
Auditory Brainstem Response Screening			60
Hit rate (%)	95	95	
False alarm rate (%)	15	10	
Protocol 1 (No Tests)			0
Hit rate (%)	100	100	
False alarm rate (%)	0	0	
Protocol 2 (HRR)			13
Hit rate (%)	95	60	
False alarm rate (%)	65	15	
Protocol 3 (ABR)			60
Hit rate (%)	95	95	
False alarm rate (%)	15	10	
Protocol 4 (HRR+ABR)			73
Hit rate (%)	90	57	
False alarm rate (%)	10	1	

ICN: intensive care nursery; WBN: well-baby nursery; HRR: high-risk register; ABR: auditory brainstem response. Values taken from Turner 1991a; 1991b.

testing. Those who fail the ABR screening are scheduled for diagnostic testing. This is similar to the screening protocol recommended by the ASHA Committee on Infant Hearing (1989).

The parameters for the screening protocols are given in table 6. The values for the HRR were derived from the clinical literature. We did not use the values calculated previously from the individual risk factors. It is necessary to evaluate the ICN and WBN separately because the prevalence of hearing loss is very different, as well as the performance of the HRR. In the ICN, we have assumed HT/FA=95/65% based on Simmons et al. (1979). This is one of the few articles that provide performance information on the HRR in the ICN. In the WBN, it is well

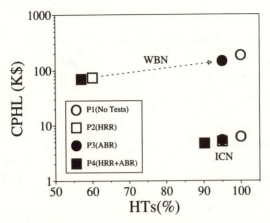

Figure 7. Comparison of four screening protocols. The protocols are evaluated separately for the intensive care nursery and the well-baby nursery. CPHL: cost per hearing-impaired infant identified; HTs: hit rate of screening protocol. Adapted from figure 5 in Turner 1991b.

documented that the hit rate of the HRR can be as low as 50%. We have used HT/FA=60/10%.

We can compare the four protocols by plotting CPHL versus HTs (figure 7). In the ICN, all four screening protocols group fairly close together, although there is some tradeoff between performance and cost. The most expensive protocol (P1) is only 1.3 times as expensive as the least expensive (P4). Any of the four seems reasonable for use in the ICN. The decision could be based on more subjective factors. In the WBN, the screening protocols form two groups. The two with the HRR (P2 and P4) have lower cost but relative poor hit rate (<60%). The two without the HRR (P1 and P3) have high hit rate, but the CPHL is 2 to 2.5 times as great as that for P2 or P4. In the WBN, we are forced to choose between high cost or poor performance.

DISCUSSION

Many studies have attempted to evaluate risk factors. We would like to collapse the results of these studies to provide "average" statistics that can be used in a model, like that presented in this paper, to evaluate the performance of the different risk factors. Unfortunately, these studies have produced a variety of statistics that are not equivalent and cannot be easily combined. In addition, many of these studies provide questionable data because of an inappropriate experimental design. In some, the risk factors were evaluated using a subset of infants from the nursery population. This subset was identified by using a small number of the risk factors. Obviously, the prevalence statistics were biased toward the factors that selected the infants for study. Either all infants in the nursery should have been evaluated, or the subset of infants should have been randomly selected.

Another common problem has been mentioned earlier in this paper. In many studies, the only infants followed and evaluated for hearing loss were those who failed the HRR. In this situation, it is impossible to know how many hearing-impaired infants in the nursery failed the risk factors. Thus, calculations of hit rate for the risk factor may be in error. This was the case in the paper by Halpern et al. (1987). All infants should be followed, or the subgroup followed should be randomly selected, not selected by the risk factors.

A number of papers we examined demonstrated a variety of problems with the experimental design. Given the described difficulties with the clinical data, it is probably impossible to accurately evaluate the usefulness of the individual risk factors at this time. There are not enough studies with adequate experimental design to provide meaningful "averaged" measures for the risk factors.

We have examined the HRR in two ways. We have combined individual risk factors into HRRs and compared them to the individual factors and to a no screening control (figure 5). In addition, we have compared two screening protocols using the HRR to other screening strategies (figure 7). In both cases, the arguments for the use of the HRR are not compelling. In the ICN, once a sufficient number of risk factors had been combined to produce a hit rate greater than 90%, the resulting HRR is no more cost-effective than using no screening tests. The comparison of four screening protocols demonstrated that there was little difference in the ICN between protocols that do and do not use the HRR.

There are other potential problems using the HRR in the ICN. The reported failure rate in the ICN for the HRR varies from 20% to 90%. When the failure rate is very high (>70%), it can actually cost more to screen with the HRR (Turner 1991c in press). P4 (HRR+ABR) becomes less cost-effective than P3 (ABR) and P2 (HRR) becomes less than P1 (No Tests). While failure rate is low, we must also be concerned. The few studies that provide data on hit rate in the ICN indicate a high value, but in these studies the failure rate was also high. It is possible that a low failure rate also means a low hit rate. We simply do not know enough about the performance of the HRR to be comfortable about its use in all situations.

At the moment, the HRR is the only cost-effective way to screen in the WBN. To forgo screening or to screen with just ABR would be extremely expensive. The problem is the poor hit rate; up to one-half of the hearing-impaired infants may be missed. This is particularly disturbing considering that as many as two-thirds of all hearing-impaired infants may pass through the WBN (Stein et al. 1983; Elssmann et al. 1987; Stein et al. 1990). Of course, screening with the HRR is significantly better than no early identification program in the WBN.

What needs to be done? Do we need more studies of the risk factors? If we really want to use the risk factors effectively, then more information is required. Additional investigations must be tightly controlled. This is necessary to ensure that the experimental design is error-free and that the appropriate statistics are calculated. Then, results from different facilities could be combined to provide average prevalence data that would permit a reliable evaluation of the factors.

Evaluation of risk factors in the ICN would be feasible. Assuming a prevalence of 3% in the ICN, it would only be necessary to screen about 3,000 infants to generate 100 infants with hearing loss. This seems like a reasonable number to evaluate the risk factors. There are a number of ICN-based screening programs in existence. A multicenter project could be organized and could screen 3,000 infants within a reasonable time.

The situation in the WBN is quite different. We need a good alternative to what is now available. One strategy would be to improve the hit rate of the HRR. As discussed previously, the JCIH has recently expanded the HRR from seven to ten factors. This should improve hit rate, although it is difficult to predict how much. This will also increase false alarm rate resulting in reduced cost-effectiveness. Again, the amount of change is unclear. Another alternative is to better evaluate the risk factors using either the approach presented in this paper or more complex statistical analysis as illustrated by Halpern et al. (1987). In either case better clinical data are required, which may be a problem. If we assume a prevalence of 1 per 1,000, then it would be necessary to screen 100,000 newborns to generate 100 infants with hearing loss. A multicenter project would require far more centers or a much longer project duration than the same study in the ICN. In addition, there are far fewer existing WBN screening programs to incorporate into such a study. The final alternative is a new screening test, possibly otoacoustic emissions, that has the appropriate cost and performance characteristics. For a variety of reasons, evaluating a test like otoacoustic emissions for use in the WBN may be fundamentally easier than evaluating risk factors.

SUMMARY

The audiologist is interested in risk factors because they are used to construct a high-risk register, a tool that has been used for many years for early identification of hearing loss. In 1972, the Joint Committee on Infant Hearing recommended a five-factor high-risk register. In 1982, the Joint Committee expanded the high-risk register to seven factors. Again, in 1990, the high-risk register was expanded to ten factors in hopes of improving its performance.

The high-risk register has been used for almost 20 years and continues to be recommended as an integral component in the early identification of hearing loss. If we are to continue to employ the high-risk register, we must address three fundamental questions.

1. How well do the individual risk factors predict hearing loss?
2. How do we combine these factors into a high-risk register?
3. How does the high-risk register compare to other hearing screening techniques?

A variety of measures have been used to evaluate risk factors. These measures are not equivalent and cannot be easily combined to provide "average" measures of performance. In addition, many studies have flawed experimental design, diminishing even further the value of clinical data on risk-factor performance. At this time, there is insufficient data to adequately evaluate the individual risk factors.

Given adequate clinical data, good techniques exist for evaluating the performance and cost-effectiveness of the risk factors. Hit rate and false alarm rate, while seldom applied to risk factors, are excellent measures of performance, far superior to most of the measures that have been used. The cost-effectiveness of the risk factors can be calculated using a simple model of the early identification process.

Designing a high-risk register from risk factors is a fairly complex problem. We really do not know enough about the relation of risk factors to hearing loss to evaluate their individual value to a high-risk register. Also, we do not know enough to predict the performance of a high-risk register based upon its specific risk factors. We can always return to the nursery to collect more information, but do we want to bother? There is less need to use the high-risk register in the ICN because good alternatives are available for screening. Plus, there are other potential problems using the high-risk register. Today, the high-risk register is the only cost-effective way to screen in the WBN. Unfortunately, the high-risk register may miss up to half of the hearing-impaired infants. If we can develop a reasonable alternative for the WBN, then the high-risk register may appropriately become an historical footnote.

ACKNOWLEDGMENT

The authors would like to thank Dr. Lorraine Barton, Department of Pediatrics, Neonatal Division, University of Southern California, for the LAC-USC hospital ICN statistics.

REFERENCES

American Speech-Language-Hearing Association. 1989. Guidelines for audiologic screening of newborn infants who are at risk for hearing impairment. *Asha* 31(3):89-92.

American Speech-Language-Hearing Association. 1990. Guidelines for infant hearing screening—Response to Robert G. Turner's analysis. *Asha* 32(9):63-66.

Barton, L. 1991. Statistics for 1990, Los Angeles County-University of Southern California Hospital. Personal communication.

Elssmann, S., Matkin, N., and Sabo M. 1987. Early identification of congenital sensorineural hearing impairment. *The Hearing Journal* 40:13-17.

Feinmesser, M.D., and Tell, L.T. 1976. Neonatal screening for the detection of deafness. *Archives of Otolaryngology* 102:297-299.

Feinmesser, M., Tell, L., and Levi, H. 1982. Follow-up of 4000 infants screened for hearing defect. *Audiology* 21:197-203.

Fraser, G.R. 1976. *The causes of profound deafness in childhood*. Baltimore: Johns Hopkins University Press.

Gerkin, K.P. 1986. The development and outcome of the high-risk register. In E.T. Swigart (ed.), *Neonatal hearing screening*. San Diego: College Hill Press.

Halpern, J., Hosford-Dunn, H., and Malachowski, N. 1987. Four factors that accurately predict hearing loss in "high risk" neonates. *Ear and Hearing* 8(1):21-25.

Joint Committee on Infant Hearing. 1982. Position statement. *Asha* 24(12):1017-1018.

Joint Committee on Infant Hearing. 1991. 1990 position statement. *Audiology Today* 3(4):14-17.

Kankkunen, A. 1982. Pre-school children with impaired hearing in Goteborg, 1964-1980. *Acta Otolaryngologica* Suppl. 391.

Mahoney, T.M., and Eichwald, J.G. 1987. The ups and "downs" of high-risk screening: The Utah statewide program. *Seminars in Hearing* 8(2):155-163.

Martin, J.A.M., Bentzen, O., Colley, J.R.T., et al. 1981. Childhood deafness in the European Community. *Scandinavian Audiology* 10:165-174.

Northern, J.L., and Downs, M.P. 1974. *Hearing in children*. Baltimore: Williams and Wilkins.

Parving, A. 1983. Epidemiology of hearing loss and etiological diagnosis. *International Journal of Pediatric Otorhinolaryngology* 5:151-165.

Rossetti, L.M. 1986. *High risk infants: Identification, assessment, and intervention*. Boston: Little, Brown and Company.

Shannon, D.A., Felix, J.K., Krumholz, A., Goldstein, P.J., and Harris, K.C. 1984. Hearing screening of high-risk newborns with brainstem auditory evoked potentials: A follow-up study. *Pediatrics* 73:22-26.

Shimizu, H., Walters, R.J., Proctor, L.R., Kennedy, D.W., Allen, M.C., and Markowitz, R.K. 1990. Identification of hearing impairment in the neonatal intensive care unit population: Outcome of a five-year project at the Johns Hopkins hospital. *Seminars in Hearing* 11(2):151-166.

Simmons, F., McFarland, W., and Jones, F. 1979. An automated hearing screening technique for newborns. *Acta Otolaryngologica* 87:1-8.

Stein, L., Clark, S., and Kraus, N. 1983. The hearing-impaired infant: Patterns of identification and habilitation. *Ear and Hearing* 3:232-236.

Stein L., Jabaley, T., Spitz, R., Stoakley, D., and McGee, T. 1990. The hearing-impaired infant: Patterns of identification and habilitation revisited. *Ear and Hearing* 11:128-133.

Swigonski, N., Shallop, J., Bull, M., and Lemons, J. 1987. Hearing screening of high risk newborns. *Ear and Hearing* 8:26-30.

Turner, R.G. 1990. Analysis of recommended guidelines for infant hearing screening. *Asha* 32(9):57-61.

Turner, R.G. 1991a. Modeling the cost and performance of early identification protocols. *Journal of the American Academy of Audiology* 2(4):195-205.

Turner, R.G. 1991b in press. Comparison of four hearing screening protocols. *Journal of the American Academy of Audiology*.

Turner, R.G. 1991c in press. Factors that determine the cost and performance of early identification protocols. *Journal of the American Academy of Audiology*.

Turner, R.G., Shepard, N.T., and Frazer, G.J. 1984. Formulating and evaluating audiological test protocols. *Ear and Hearing* 9:177-189.

Chapter 7

Newborn Hearing Screening—
Education of the Medical Profession

Stephen Epstein

INTRODUCTION

A newborn and infant hearing screening program cannot be successful without the support and participation of the medical profession.[1] The physicians that are primarily involved in the early identification of hearing loss include neonatologists, pediatricians, family practitioners, public health physicians, and the otolaryngologists-head and neck surgeons.

Physician support is essential for the campaign to establish mandated statewide hearing screening programs. In those states where newborn and infant hearing screening already exists, physician participation is necessary for public and patient education as well as the actual implementation of the hearing screening process within the participating hospitals. Neonatologists, pediatricians, and family practitioners either supervise or participate in the process of completing the high-risk questionnaire for hearing loss in all newborns in those areas where the

---

[1] The Advocacy Committee for Early Identification of Hearing Loss shall endorse and promote whatever the most reliable, practical, and cost-effective method for screening newborn and infant hearing is universally accepted. At the time of this presentation, screening all newborns by means of the high-risk register followed by an ABR screening test on those newborns at risk for having a hearing loss was the most accepted protocol.

questionnaire is utilized as part of the screening process. These physicians are also responsible for recommending that those newborns who are at risk for hearing loss by having one or more risk factors have an auditory brainstem response (ABR) test, preferably *prior* to that newborn leaving the hospital. If the ABR test cannot be performed prior to hospital discharge, these same physicians are responsible for seeing that the high-risk newborns and infants have their hearing evaluated within three months after hospital discharge. The public health physician is responsible for those newborns and infants who do not have a private physician and are followed through the public health system.

Description of the Problem

A major problem is that once a high-risk infant leaves the hospital without any hearing evaluation prior to discharge, an average of about 50% of these infants are lost to follow-up. An effective solution to solve the problem of poor follow-up would be to have greater and more effective physician participation in assuming the responsibility to see that all high-risk newborns and infants have appropriate hearing evaluations.

With the publication of the 1990 Position Statement of the Joint Committee on Infant Hearing (see Appendix 1), which establishes a more effective list of risk criteria for hearing loss, physician participation is even more essential. In the 1990 Position Statement, the risk criteria for hearing loss are now divided into two age groups: *neonates* (birth to 28 days) and *infants* (29 days to 2 years). The risk criteria for neonates can still be checked for in all newborns while still in the hospital using an updated high-risk questionnaire. The new risk criteria for infants will have to be checked for by the physicians who care for the child once he or she is discharged from the hospital.

Unfortunately, at the present time, complete cooperation and participation of the medical profession does not exist for several reasons. There is a general lack of knowledge and concern among many physicians about the effects of hearing impairment in children and the necessity for *early* diagnosis and early intervention in the management of hearing loss in children. Many physicians are generally not aware that children's hearing can be tested *at any age* starting shortly after birth. They are also not aware that management of hearing loss must be implemented *as early as possible* to prevent delay of speech, language, and educational development. Even today, when confronted with parental concern that a child is not hearing or the speech and language are not developing like other children of the same age, physicians generally ignore or minimize parental concerns. To solve this problem and educate physicians about newborn and infant screening as well as inform them about the management of hearing loss in children, efforts are now being undertaken on both the national and the statewide levels, which will be discussed in this presentation.

POSSIBLE SOLUTIONS

On the national level, in March 1989, the American Academy of Otolaryngology-Head and Neck Surgery joined forces with the Alexander Graham Bell Association for the Deaf to create what is now called the Advocacy Committee for Early Identification of Hearing Loss (formerly called the Joint Committee on Early Identification of Hearing Loss in Children). One of the main purposes of this joint venture is to educate the medical profession about the importance of *early* identification and *early* intervention in the management of hearing loss in children. The Advocacy Committee is in the process of establishing working relationships with the American Academy of Neonatology, the American Academy of Pediatrics, the American Academy of Family Practice, the American Academy of Public Health Physicians, and the American Academy of Otolaryngology-Head and Neck Surgery. The plan is to encourage these organizations to incorporate into their residency training programs the principles and protocols involved with early identification of hearing loss in children. This information is also expected to be incorporated in postgraduate continuing medical education programs for physicians past their residency programs. Plans are being undertaken to investigate the incorporation of this same information into the medical school curriculum so that future physicians will become aware of the importance of early diagnosis and early management of hearing loss in children during the formative years of their medical career.

An example of how education of the medical profession can be undertaken on the statewide level is illustrated by the State of Maryland Program to Identify Hearing Impaired Infants. Incorporated into law by the Maryland legislature in 1985 and implemented statewide in 1988, this mandated program clearly illustrates the effectiveness of education of physicians, which resulted in their participating in the initial high-risk hearing screening phase as well as assuming responsibility for encouraging follow-up hearing evaluations.

The Advisory Council for Hearing Impaired Infants, the organization that administers the statewide hearing screening program in Maryland, played an active role in physician education and recruitment. The Advisory Council created a leaflet entitled "Program Information for Primary Care Physicians," which was distributed to all physicians involved with the care of newborns, infants, and children. The leaflet educated the physicians about the statewide hearing screening program, the importance of early identification and early intervention, and the necessity of their role in the program. In another capacity, members of the Advisory Council were divided into teams that went to all 36 participating hospitals within the state and to the regional public health facilities. These teams provided in-service education programs for the physicians and staff members, assisted them with the actual implementation of the in-hospital screening protocol, and further educated them about newborn and infant hearing screening. A considerable effort is now being made within the state to encourage all participating hospitals to have facilities available to perform ABR testing on all high-risk newborns prior to their hospital discharge.

To solve the problem of follow-up of high-risk infants once they leave the hospital, letters are sent to the physicians of these infants. This letter includes a questionnaire requesting the current status and address of the infant and inquiring if his or her hearing has been tested. Based on the physician's response, the state program can then maintain a follow-up on the status of this particular high-risk infant by means of a computerized tracking system.

The statewide hearing screening program has already begun to make changes and adaptations to comply with the 1990 Position Statement of the Joint Committee on Infant Hearing (see Appendix 1). Until the Advisory Council receives legislative approval or authority to change the present high-risk questionnaire, it has sent out notification to all statewide participating hospitals to voluntarily incorporate the changes within the present questionnaire to comply with the new neonatal risk criteria. A letter is being prepared that will be distributed to all physicians involved with the care of children to implement routinely the infant risk criteria as part of their routine examination. The letter will also recommend a hearing evaluation for all infants at risk who have one or more risk criteria present, including the crucial parental or caregiver concern about a child's hearing or speech and language development.

SUMMARY

If we are to reduce the average age of identification of hearing loss in children in the United States to below 1 year of age by the year 2000 (U.S. Department of Health and Human Services 1990), effective statewide newborn and infant hearing screening programs must be implemented throughout the country. In order for these statewide programs to become established and fully implemented, physician support and participation are essential. It is the role of the Advocacy Committee for Early Identification of Hearing Loss on a national level and established statewide hearing screening programs such as the State of Maryland Program to Identify Hearing Impaired Infants to educate the medical profession and to enlist their participation.

REFERENCES

U.S. Department of Health and Human Services, Public Health Service. 1990. *Healthy people 2000: National health promotion and disease prevention objectives*. Washington, D.C.: U.S. Government Printing Office.

For copies of:

The Advocacy Committee for Early Identification of Hearing Loss flyer, the State of Maryland Program to Identify Hearing Impaired Infants leaflet (Program Information for Primary Care Physicians) or the 1990 Position Statement of the Joint Committee on Infant Hearing, please write to:

> Stephen Epstein, M.D.
> Director
> The Ear Center
> Wheaton Plaza-South Annex
> 11160 Veirs Mill Road
> Wheaton, Maryland 20902

Chapter 8

Policy Formulation: A Real World View

Alfred A. Baumeister

INTRODUCTION

Perhaps we can all accept the proposition that systematic policy analysis is important. As professionals vitally interested in promoting health and welfare of children, we should understand that unless we impact public policy we are unlikely to exert great practical influence on decisions to provide early and comprehensive services and programs designed to avert serious and crippling disabilities. Many early impairments, such as hearing loss, can have adverse long-term consequences on the child's quality of life and ultimately on society. Humanitarian, social, and economic considerations all converge upon the conclusion that prevention and prompt remediation of children's impairments should be taken as a given to secure the future, as reflected in public policy. Certainly, this is a mandate that the angels should decree, and we are on the side of the angels, are we not? It is in this context that public policy initiatives are absolutely critical.

Indeed, the specialization of policy analysis in various disciplines, such as economics, education, medicine, and public planning, has become a major academic growth industry over the past two decades. Practically every major university now boasts a policy research institute or center. Vast sums of federal money have fueled this process, resulting in countless position papers, reports, dissertations, new journals, newspaper articles, conferences, and fancy and expensive social gatherings that, perhaps, attest to the importance of the academic search for a new and more realistic social policy relevance.

Policy Analysis

A fundamental question is whether national resolve, as reflected in current public policy, is adequate to the investment necessary to secure the futures of children given the unremitting demands of the present (Baumeister 1981). Research and the professional technology it spawns do not drive public policy, although scientific analysis is often employed to bolster a policy decision and to provide validation of preexisting ideas. This is a fact of life too often ignored by professionals who would attempt to influence policy, whether it derives from legislative, administrative, or judicial sources. Moreover, public declarations about health policies are not always closely related to what actually happens. Effective influence, rooted in policy analysis, is contingent on a precise understanding of how programs are actually implemented, a levelheaded understanding of barriers to the implementation of formally declared policy, and a clear statement of objectives and how these objectives will serve the purposes of policy makers.

Much of the activity of policy analysis has been rooted in important classical intellectual and philosophical traditions, with an emphasis on value neutrality, rationality, efficiency, and the unassailable scientific method. It should be emphasized that formal policy inquiry has largely focused on improving means of policy making, i.e., focus on the process rather than on ends, a point that is central to the arguments advanced here. The emphasis on ends obviously requires a different understanding of means.

The weaknesses of policy analysis as a detached and intellectual analytical pursuit are increasingly apparent. The major consumers of policy analysis—politicians, administrators, and managers at every level—have come to express doubts about the relevance of policy research findings. Recently, the head of a governmental agency commented that while everybody seems to be for policy analysis, few who have responsibility for broad decision making have come to expect much of it. Various studies bear out this assertion (Fischer and Forester 1987). There are numerous reasons for this inability to connect the analysis and the decision makers.

My conclusions about the nature of policy formulation and implementation do not come so much by way of the formal traditions and commitment to the theories of some philosophers long dead but not entirely forgotten. Instead, my recommendations relative to policy influence derive from quite another, more mundane, direction—as one who has attempted to influence legislation, testifying before congressional committees, providing information directly to political candidates, and serving on and advising government committees.

The basic premise advanced here is that the focus should be on ends, ends to be pursued aggressively by whatever means are available, within reason. Some will recognize this assertion derives from the Aristotelian or Machiavellian traditions of practical political thought. Through this experience one comes to understand something about how policy is formed in the political trenches, so to speak, and a little of how to influence the process while learning to accept many failures in exchange for the occasional accomplishment. This is not a system to be disdained, although many academics find it aversive to become involved in a world that seems to operate at a more visceral, meaner, unpredictable, and primitive level than the purer academic pursuit of knowledge. Nevertheless that is not the truth at all—the world of policy formulation operates in a lawful sense, with its rules, values, and rationality, susceptible to understanding and change. But I readily acknowledge that it is an activity not for everyone, especially those who have an aversion to walking through cow fields or, even worse, mine fields.

THE POLITICS

Now, the specific focus here bears on the question of how to ensure that every child is screened early to identify significant hearing impairments and, further, how to provide systematically and comprehensively the services that prevent or minimize the varied disabilities that accompany undetected and uncorrected auditory deficits. Many share these concerns. For instance, specific goals that bear upon these and related child health issues are contained in the comprehensive *Healthy People 2000* report recently published by the Department of Health and Human Services. They are also included in a fairly detailed report we recently prepared for the president through the President's Committee on Mental Retardation (Baumeister, Kupstas, Klindworth, and Woodley-Zanthos 1990). This planning *Guide* contains dozens of recommendations designed to articulate a national policy to prevent health and behavior handicaps among children, especially those at elevated risk owing to a myriad of social, economic, and biologic circumstances. The report connects the *Healthy People 2000* objectives. Even so, the *Guide* had to undergo political and administrative scrutiny (i.e., "technical clearance"), an integral aspect of policy formulation. This is where our science connects with politics.

Space does not permit any detailed account concerning the background, rationale, compromises, data, and methods that guided us through these difficult processes of attempting to balance scientific, health, economic, and political realities. Nor is this the proper context in which to describe the partisan sensitivities that are inevitably aroused. But I should like to share some general observations that have conditioned the approach taken in our efforts to impact public health, social, and educational policy.

I shall, in this respect, conclude with a few practical recommendations that might be of some value to those who wish to influence policy with regard to early screening for hearing impairments. It is first worthwhile to examine a bit of the background regarding the nature of the politics of policy formulation. The term politics is used here not to incite to riot but to convey the sense of real-life issues that inevitably must be confronted if professionals wish to have direct impact in the policy area. Decision criteria are always certainly political in nature (Fischer and Forester 1987).

Each of the occasions I have testified before the Senate and House Appropriations Committees has been memorable in some aspect—because it can be an intimidating experience, but also because of some of the interesting and enlightening verbal exchanges that have taken place. Two of these are worth recounting because they place into stark reality the crux of the issues before us: namely, power, money, and choices.

After hearing me describe the health plight of poor and minority children, then Senator Weicker observed: "Dr. Baumeister, you have made a very compelling statement. The situation for many groups of children is, no doubt, becoming worse. But the problem you face is that children do not vote."

A little over a year ago, this time on the House side, after I had concluded my statement, a representative remarked: "You have provided this committee with important information. But please understand that we are laymen and that others, like you, have given us equally compelling arguments. How are we to choose among the problems that should be addressed because the needs, as critical as they are, exceed our ability to manage them within a finite and shrinking resource base?"

Of course, both of these gentlemen are correct. Public statements on the record, scientific articles in learned journals, and good intentions may be necessary, but they are insufficient. It is the background work together with a thorough appreciation of the process that really counts. Our pursuit of public analysis must address the fundamental clashes of values that raise basic questions about quality of societal life and who, therefore, should be accorded special consideration in the ultimate interests of society. For instance, should we reinforce the strong and the bright at the expense of the weak of body and/or mind? If we continue to rely mainly on the criterion of cost-effectiveness of a particular policy initiative, we shall have not addressed the main questions, yet alone provided any meaningful answers.

THE FORMULATION OF SERVICE POLICY

Human service policies do not evolve in a regular developmental sequence; rather, the process follows a wavelike more than a linear course. We often lurch from one position or fad to the next depending on prevailing political and economic climates. Good current professional information, such as that presented at this conference, does have a role in the process. But the tie is neither direct, certain, nor decisive. Even in those areas where there are solid data suggesting effective courses of intervention—such as screening for sensory disorders, reduction of exposure to toxic substances, provision of adequate prenatal care, immunizations to prevent infectious diseases—systematic and comprehensive public policy often has been excruciatingly slow to evolve.

This causes no little consternation among researchers and other professionals who generally believe that public policy would be better served if decisions were based on our own definitions of rationality. It naturally follows from this reasoning that health policy should be derived from the best professional knowledge available. Thus, policy surely will be sounder, wiser, and fairer. Scientists and health care professionals are all versed in the science method. Because we believe that science is the most rational of systems, it follows that public policy, in this case the delivery of health services to children at risk for auditory impairments, should always be grounded in empirical and professional understanding.

Not only does that proposition contain a certain logic, it recognizes the professional's centrality in the natural order of things and, not incidentally, validates one's career choice. In short, the view commonly held by professionals is that public policy requires science. On reflection, this proposition is audacious because it is not only false, but its converse is true. Research and professional services are the products of public policy, which, in turn, are derived from normative assumptions or value judgments. The contingencies that control the behavior of researchers are not the same as those that control the behavior of policy makers. Furthermore, there is no greater truth in one than the other, for truth is ultimately a moral test. These circumstances lead to a vast and sometimes unbreachable communications barrier in which the two interests operate at fundamentally different levels of discourse, frequently accompanied by a distrust of each other's intentions.

In addition, professionals are not any more likely to agree with each other as to what is important than are politicians. But when it comes to policy, we play in another ballpark, according to political rules. Disagreements among researchers cost credibility in this game. Moreover, we are inclined, when it comes to suggesting public action, to make enormous and sometimes fragile intellectual leaps from our professional base. As Mark Twain once observed: "There is something fascinating about science. One gets such wholesale returns of conjecture out of such trifling investment of fact."

Relevance is more a political concept than scientific. It is not only futile but counterproductive for us, as professionals, to lecture policy makers as to the meaning of relevance. Observing how driven we in the sciences are by shifting paradigmatic considerations, I am persuaded that it is undesirable to fashion public policy entirely on the basis of prevailing scientific considerations. Today's grand theory often becomes tomorrow's nonsense. Certainly to replace our decision-making system, as awful as it sometimes might seem, with a technology orientation is an unattainable and precarious position. I remain persuaded that it is undesirable to fashion health policy entirely on the basis of scientific professional considerations. Policy should reflect the expression and competition of personal and social values or normative foundations. There are those who will argue that we are increasingly a technologic culture and that we should exploit technology to provide a more rational basis for social decision making. But that is only one form of rationality, one that may even be in conflict with other normative assumptions, like returning to a simpler life or empowering the individual. Technology does not free us from our dependency on the world around us; it merely changes the nature of that dependency. Moreover, ends preexist in means, and means are dependent on one another.

Therefore, when we are talking about policy, we are necessarily addressing tradeoffs—costs balanced against benefits. Professionals may tell policy makers about how to design programs and how to minimize costs. But professionals cannot say how much cost is acceptable—that is a value judgment. Actually, cost-benefit analysis is not value neutral but is an administrative instrument to rationalize a decision (Byrne 1987). That is to say, cost-benefit analyses are themselves conditional on a number of normative assumptions, the political nature of which drastically affect the calculus against which the tradeoff is assessed. A screening program for hearing disorders may make good economic sense, but whether it is socially imperative may be a more important benefit.

There is nothing at all wrong with articulation of a value or normative argument that says we should set policies that enhance the health of all children. But in making the case we often mistakenly disguise personal values under a scientific veil, usually in language that does not communicate. One cannot argue the case for a scientific conclusion before decision makers as we might before a peer review group. Truly, this is easier said than done because empirically based arguments seek value neutrality. But policy analysis demands an integration of professional and normative concerns.

I should like to describe briefly the process of formation of public policy. There is substantial and informative literature on the subject, although sometimes rather abstract. Again, it is difficult to improve on the lessons of experience in attempting to influence policy and, therefore, to identify the points at which we can exert influence. Formation of public policy is not an event but a dynamic process with identifiable components. First, there must be public awareness of a problem and, consequently, a significant sentiment by powerful agents toward rectifying the problem. Second, laws and measures must be formulated specifically for dealing with some important aspects of the problem. Third, programs must be designed, funded, and implemented. Finally, accountability through continuing systematic evaluation, including a wide array of criteria, needs to be an integral feature of the process.

These are not events that occur spontaneously or incidentally. In each of these components there is the opportunity to apply scientific and professional knowledge, but this is a fragile dynamic. As one observer (Rein 1976) put it, "The link is neither consensual, graceful nor self-evident." Indeed, it can be demonstrated that funds for research and service are typically allocated and legitimized after the policy decision. Perhaps there is no better example than our national Head Start program. As one examines, in retrospect, the empirical knowledge base at the time Head Start was initiated as national policy, one must conclude that the program was conceived, planned, and implemented primarily on the basis of political and social considerations. Of course, research on early intervention did enter the picture in a significant way but largely after the fact. Even then research has been used to justify selectively the basic policy decision or, in the case of opponents, to select data to show that the policy is flawed.

As another example, the current pediatric HIV/AIDS epidemic represents one of the greatest threats to children we have confronted. A great deal of funding support for research on the problem of AIDS has been forthcoming, although the vast bulk of the money is not directed at these children. In any event, the most salient aspects of the national epidemic are expressed in debates over rights, values, and discrimination. We do have the technology and the capabilities to slow down the rate of pediatric AIDS, but the application of these interventions will require tradeoffs that we, as a society, appear unwilling to make at the present. In sum, studies of information transfer indicate that research has only a modest effect on policy decisions.

The frustration and occasional feelings of ingratitude that professionals sometimes experience when policy makers fail to wear a path to our doors may be self-inflicted. A major problem is that we fail, too often, to understand the needs, attitudes, and problems of policy makers, especially those who are in a position to implement the service systems that we know would be good for society, if they could just be shown the scientific facts. But these facts, as important and integral to the process as they are, constitute only a portion of the process.

OBSTACLES

While it is clearly important to explain clearly and precisely the virtues of a particular health objective, such as screening for sensory impairments, it is equally important to appreciate the obstacles to a broad and concerted public effort. These obstacles, rooted in the social, economic, and political vectors that drive public attitudes, include: (*a*) disorganization among the constituencies that would elevate the issue to a priority in the national agenda; (*b*) a disease-oriented and piecemeal health care system that, while one of the most expensive in the world as reflected in percent of GPN, fails too often to connect reliably with those in particular need of a service; (*c*) fragmented and uncoordinated service and support systems at the local, state, and federal levels; (*d*) the lack of a current comprehensive and integrated national data base from which to fashion and justify policy recommendations; (*e*) lack of documentation regarding epidemiologic factors, assessment of outcomes, and evaluation of effectiveness, both in terms of costs and satisfaction; (*f*) inconsistency of eligibility requirements for entitlement programs for services between and even within states; (*g*) budgetary constraints (or better, choices) that have resulted in continuing cutbacks of needed programs; (*h*) belief systems and ethical issues that often set conditions for delivery of services; and (*i*) competition for resources among important social programs.

These basic concerns threaten the overall national effort to promote prevention and intervention services. Some of these, such as the need to create an ongoing data base, will elicit little disagreement, except perhaps with respect to costs. Others, such as restructuring the nation's health care system to include those who are at the margins, are, by their nature, politically volatile.

ORDINARY KNOWLEDGE

We have consistently and collectively made the mistake that we can supply authoritative knowledge to the pursuit of social policy if only we were asked. All too often we wait to be asked. As important as our professional knowledge is, it does not equate with what Lindblom and Cohen (1979) have called "ordinary knowledge." This is not to imply that ordinary knowledge is trivial, unimportant, or necessarily wrong. It is derived from common sense, intuition, experience, speculation, understanding of values, appreciation of political contingencies and fiscal exigencies, and personal desires. Scientific knowledge becomes ordinary knowledge when it filters into the public consciousness. This is the reason that journalists are more directly effective in influencing public policy than are professionals—they touch the public chords by stressing, in ordinary language, the immediacy and importance of a problem. While we may prefer to argue the case at an intellectual level, the affective dimensions may represent the more important element in policy formulation.

Therein lies another of our problems of understanding. Policy makers, especially elected politicians and those who serve them, require immediate information and feedback. They are unlikely to invest in an uncertain future. Research, in particular, tends to be future oriented, and that has little appeal to those who play and must win on the political stage. We must appreciate better the role of ordinary knowledge in the complex constellation of factors that bring about policy, for it represents a more veridical view of societal values than scientific knowledge.

We also need to understand how policy is formed. There are formal and informal intersecting avenues. Who makes policy? The obvious answer is "we the people." But in this regard, we are not all equally created. Presidential campaign rhetoric notwithstanding, there is no single authoritative source of policy. With respect to broad social and health issues, power is diffused among interest groups at all levels, from the communities to the federal establishment. Even within a single major governmental entity such as the Department of Health and Human Services, power is fragmented into numerous agencies, branches, and offices. At any level, each unit is naturally concerned with protecting its identity and turf. The participants in this process have different interests, constituencies, and perspectives. They also, therefore, have different solutions. Administrators exercise great discretion in translating legislative and judicial mandates into policy. A bureaucrat sitting in a secluded office often has the ability to change policy by altering administrative directives, i.e., by the simple word change from *may* to *will*. Unless we understand these dynamics, until we know the players and their roles, and when we can offer them something in return for support, as a professional constituency, we shall have buried our signal under a mountain of noise.

SOME RECOMMENDATIONS

Against this very sketchy background I should like to offer some suggestions for the ways in which we can have some impact on public policy—in this case serving children who are at risk for auditory dysfunction.

1. Develop a clear and unambiguous consensus about what must be done, by whom, when, and where. Be specific and give good reasons for your decisions. To be sure, professional debate and argument are an integral aspect of the scientific enterprise. Confrontation in this sphere does promote progress. But in the public domain of policy and politics, discordancy will be interpreted as indecisiveness. In this regard, it is necessary to have a broad conception of prevailing public purposes.
2. Identify two or three well-respected individuals who have the interest, time, and energy to study and understand in detail the political environment, the major players, and the obstacles to implementation. Be informed by the contemporary political philosophy. It is also helpful to include people from states represented by powerful senators and congressmen. At the state and local levels, the representation should include those who have or can cultivate the proper connections.
3. Generate a plan of action that calls for continuous lobbying efforts, coordination among the various professional organizations and disciplines, and constant updating of scientific information.
4. Enlist the involvement of advocacy groups who share the common cause. A number of congressmen have indicated by word and vote that they are far more impressed by what the public has to say than bureaucrats and special interest professional groups.
5. Identify those members of Congress and in state legislatures as well as agency officials who, by reason of personal circumstances, can be expected to be sympathetic to your interests and agenda. We can serve the needs of policy makers by improving our knowledge of their perceptions, their values, and the ways in which they operate.
6. Cultivate and exploit the power of the press through high visibility events, statements by prominent figures, and release of information with high news value. Actually, reporters can be very nice and helpful people. Policy makers use information gleaned from the media to ensure that their awareness is in touch with contemporary attitudes (Davis and Salasin 1978).

7. Work together politically, rather than competitively, with other organizations also interested in affecting public policy—for example, those concerned with vision defects, Down syndrome, etc.
8. Because public policy formulation is primarily a vertical rather than a lateral transmission of information, speak English, not jargon. Ordinary language enables the opportunity for public policy debate.
9. Policy makers are more impressed by information obtained from real-life observation than from controlled experiments. It is rare that policy is determined from an explicit analysis of empirically grounded data (Caplan, Morrison, and Stambaugh 1975). The lesson is that our scientific data, especially data derived from basic research, need to be presented in the context of lives of children, not as nameless faces identified as numbers.
10. Set realistic annual targets that represent an incremental approach to the ultimate goal—but always request somewhat more than you know you will achieve at that moment.
11. Accept the need for compromise, given that other needs and interests must also be addressed within a system that is longer on demands than the resources can accommodate. Moreover, political activity inevitably involves deep-rooted ethical dilemmas, and any effort to affect the policy without appropriate cognizance of these ethical conflicts will likely fail.
12. Put into place an ongoing system of information exchange within your own professional groups and those with parallel interests, lobbying efforts, and review.
13. As an advocacy group, be prepared to pay for the effort because rarely can we expect to find an individual or a group with the resources to handle this sort of lobbying effort alone.
14. Don't be discouraged, because there will be setbacks and tradeoffs.

These are but a few general suggestions, among many others, that one could offer. Obviously, the specific strategy to be employed depends on the issue to be joined and the values to be expressed. One such value, well worth the investment, is to enhance the quality of life of children. Children are too often the hapless and helpless victims of a system that responds to many other vested and powerful interests. The challenge to society is to generate new knowledge to serve the common cause. A far greater challenge is to ensure that all children share equally in this wisdom, to achieve a fair start and a fair chance to succeed. If children have not us, what hope have they? They are the future, and it is to our societal benefit to invest in that future. This is a value expressed so well by Hubert Humphrey: "The measure of a nation is how it treats people in the twilight of life, people in the dawn of life, and people in the shadows of life."

REFERENCES

Baumeister, A.A. 1981. Mental retardation policy and research: The unfilled promise. *American Journal of Mental Deficiency* 5:449-456.

Baumeister, A.A., Kupstas, F.D., Klindworth, L.M., and Woodley-Zanthos, P. 1990. *Guide to state planning for the prevention of mental retardation and related disabilities associated with socioeconomic conditions.* Washington, D.C.: President's Committee on Mental Retardation.

Byrne, J. 1987. Policy science and the administrative state: The political economy of cost-benefit analysis. In F. Fischer and J. Forester (eds.), *Confronting values in policy analysis: The politics of criteria.* New York: Sage.

Caplan, N., Morrison, A., and Stambaugh, R.J. 1975. *The case of social science knowledge in policy decisions at the national level.* Ann Arbor: University of Michigan, Institute for Social Research.

Davis, H.R., and Salasin, S.E. 1978. Strengthening the contribution of social research and development to policy making. In L.E. Lynn, Jr. (ed.), *Knowledge and policy: The uncertain connection.* Washington, D.C.: National Academy of Sciences.

Fischer, F., and Forester, J. (eds.). 1987. *Confronting values in policy analysis: The politics of criteria.* New York: Sage.

Lindblom, C.E., and Cohen, D.K. 1979. *Usable knowledge.* New Haven: Yale University Press.

Rein, M. 1976. *Social science and social policy.* New York: Penguin.

PART II.

Screening Newborns for Auditory Function

Chapter 9

Auditory Brainstem Response (ABR) in Infants: Screening and Diagnostic Applications

Deborah Hayes

INTRODUCTION

Auditory brainstem response (ABR) is an important component in evaluation of infants at risk for hearing impairment. Both the American Speech-Language-Hearing Association (ASHA) and the Joint Committee on Infant Hearing, a multidisciplinary body of representatives from audiology and speech-language pathology, pediatrics, otolaryngology, and deaf education, recommend that, prior to hospital discharge, newborn infants at risk for hearing loss receive hearing screening by ABR (ASHA 1989; Joint Committee on Infant Hearing 1991). In many neonatal intensive care units (NICU), ABR is routinely used to screen hearing of infants (Stein, Clark, and Kraus 1983; Galambos, Hicks, and Wilson 1984; Gorga et al. 1987).

For newborn hearing programs, the ABR is typically applied as a screening procedure (Stein, Ozdamar, Kraus, and Paton 1983; Jacobson and Morehouse 1984; Galambos, Hicks, and Wilson 1984; Committee on Hearing, Bioacoustics, and Biomechanics 1987; Delano et al. 1987; ASHA 1989). That is, the infant either "passes" or "fails" the hearing screen based on presence of an electrophysiologic response to click stimuli at a predefined intensity criteria, usually 30 or 40 dB nHL. The advantages of this approach are (1) it is a relatively rapid procedure, and (2) volunteers or technicians can be trained to carry out the procedure because no on-line decision making is required (Amochaev 1987). Recently, an automated instrument has been introduced that not only performs the test but also determines presence of the response (Kileny 1987).

For most infants in the NICU, this screening approach is adequate and results in a "pass" on the initial test. In many reported studies, approximately 80% to 90% of infants "pass" initial ABR screen (Jacobson and Morehouse 1984; Galambos, Hicks, and Wilson 1984; Hyde et al. 1984; Worthington et al. 1985; Delano et al. 1987). For infants who "fail" ABR screen, however, information available from the single intensity level test may not be adequate to predict degree of sensitivity loss or site of dysfunction (Stein, Clark, and Kraus 1983; Kileny 1987). This information is important not only for appropriate otologic and medical management of the infant but also for development of effective follow-up strategies. Immediate application of the ABR as a diagnostic procedure with responses evaluated for threshold, and latency measures obtained at a number of intensity levels, can provide information relevant to both predicted degree of loss and probable site of dysfunction. In addition, threshold and latency measures permit validation of test accuracy and differentiation of hearing disorder from neurologic abnormality (Despland and Galambos 1980; Stein, Ozdamar, Kraus, and Paton 1983).

When we initiated an ABR program in our NICU in 1985, we were specifically concerned about providing complete audiologic information for management and follow-up. Because many infants we test are transported to our facility from communities in a seven-state region, we do not have the opportunity to follow all infants who fail the initial test. For this reason, we chose to develop a program that would provide relevant audiologic information to professionals in the infant's home community. We designed our ABR NICU program on a diagnostic model that included evaluation of response threshold, latency, and morphology for each infant tested. This chapter summarizes results of that experience.

METHOD

SUBJECTS

From January 1985 through May 1991, we evaluated 1,281 infants in our newborn ABR program. Most infants were referred from The

Children's Hospital neonatal intensive care nurseries, but some babies were referred as outpatients from community physicians. In the NICU, infants were identified at risk by their primary care nurse based on the seven-point criteria recommended by the Joint Committee on Infant Hearing (1982), 1982 position statement. Infants considered to have significant birth defects (i.e., neural tube defects) or a significant neonatal course (i.e., persistent pulmonary hypertension of the newborn, or extracorporeal membrane oxygenation treatment, etc.) were also referred for evaluation. In some instances, infants were referred due to parental concern. Average age at test was 40 weeks postconception and ranged from 33 weeks to 6 months corrected age. Seven hundred fourteen infants were male; 567 infants were female.

TEST PROCEDURE

Infants were tested in their bassinet in the nursery or in a quiet room in the Audiology Service. In general, noise level at the test site did not exceed 60 dB A. Whenever possible, electronic monitoring and treatment equipment surrounding the infant was disconnected to reduce electrical artifact. Infants were tested in natural sleep. In general, NICU infants were evaluated within one to three days prior to hospital transfer or discharge.

ABRs were recorded on standard clinical evoked potential instrumentation (Nicolet CA1000; Nicolet Compact Auditory) or ABR screening instrumentation (Grason Stadler Instruments 55). Electroencephalographic (EEG) disk electrodes were attached to the forehead at hairline (positive, or noninverting input) ipsilateral earlobe (negative, or inverting input) and contralateral earlobe (neutral, or ground). Responses were filtered (150 or 220 Hz to 2000 or 3000 Hz) and amplified (x100,000 or more).

Acoustic stimuli were alternating polarity clicks (100 microseconds duration) presented routinely at 20 or 31.1 clicks/second. Although most infants were tested at one of these two click rates, other click rates (i.e., 11.1 clicks/second) were used when slower rates were considered necessary to improve response detectability. Clicks were presented either through TDH 39P earphones mounted in MX-41 cushions hand-held to the infant's ear (Nicolet CA1000 and Compact Auditory) or through infant insert eartips (Grason Stadler Instruments 55). For some infants, clicks were also delivered via bone conduction with the bone vibrator held firmly against the infant's forehead. Bone conduction testing was attempted whenever response threshold to air conduction clicks was elevated (i.e., thresholds were greater than 35 to 40 dB nHL). Responses to either 1,024 or 1,500 clicks were averaged, and each average was replicated to determine reproducibility of test results. Responses were averaged over a 12 or 20 millisecond time base.

ABR was recorded to clicks presented at a minimum of two intensity levels, 30 or 40 dB nHL and 60 dB nHL (re: behavioral threshold for clicks of normally hearing adult listeners as measured in a quiet room). For infants who failed to demonstrate a response at these click intensities, or whose response latency or morphology was abnormal, ABR threshold to clicks was determined for each ear by adjusting click intensity in 5 or 10 dB steps until the lowest click intensity yielding a response was identified. For all infants, latency of wave I and wave V was measured and compared to normative data from control infants of equivalent age.

DEVELOPMENT OF NORMATIVE LATENCY-INTENSITY FUNCTIONS

Normative data were collected from an additional 71 infants in the NICU. Definition of what constitutes "normal" responses from preterm infants is necessarily arbitrary. We attempted to account for the effects of maturation, middle ear dysfunction, and peripheral hearing sensitivity loss in our control infants.

To account for effects of maturation, we developed separate latency-intensity functions for infants (1) less than age 36 weeks postconception, (2) age 36 through 37 weeks postconception, (3) age 38 through 42 weeks postconception, (4) age 43 weeks postconception through 2 months corrected, and (5) age 2 through 6 months corrected. Figure 1a shows a representative latency-intensity function for infants less than 36 weeks postconception; figure 1b shows a representative latency-intensity function for infants age 38 to 42 weeks postconception. To control for middle ear effects, we limited acceptable latency of wave I of the response to 3.2 milliseconds (msec) or less at 60 dB nHL (Worthington et al. 1985). To control for peripheral hearing sensitivity loss, we required control infants to demonstrate a well-defined response to clicks presented at 40 dB nHL or less. Responses from only one ear of each control infant were included in the normative data set. Number of infants in normative control groups varied from as few as 8 infants in age group

Auditory Brainstem Response (ABR) Report Form

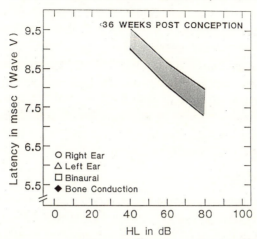

Figure 1a. Normative latency-intensity function form for infants less than 36 weeks postconception. The area within the lines encompasses the normal range of wave V latency by intensity.

Auditory Brainstem Response (ABR) Report Form

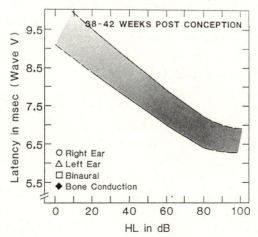

Figure 1b. Normative latency-intensity function form for infants age 38 to 42 weeks postconception. The area within the lines encompasses the normal range of wave V latency by intensity.

less than 36 weeks to 29 infants in age group 38 through 42 weeks. All other age groups contained at least 10 infants. Responses from infants in the normative groups were not included in further data analysis. (When new instrumentation was introduced to the clinical procedure [i.e., Nicolet Compact Auditory and Grason Stadler 55], responses of at least 10 apparently normally hearing infants in each age category were evaluated relative to these established norms. No significant difference in response latencies related to instrumentation was found. Thus, the normative latency-intensity functions established at program initiation in 1985 were used throughout the study.)

RESPONSE ANALYSIS

Test infants were categorized in two ways based on results of ABR evaluation. The two-way categorization scheme was developed to permit prediction of both degree of peripheral sensitivity loss and probable site of dysfunction.

To predict degree of peripheral sensitivity loss, all infants were subgrouped based on lowest click intensity yielding a repeatable ABR. Infants who exhibited ABR threshold differences between their two ears were subgrouped based on responses from the better hearing ear. The following criteria were developed for predicting degree of sensitivity loss:

Subgroup A—Presence of a response to clicks presented at 30 to 40 dB nHL in at least one ear. Subgroup A represented infants whose ABR predicted either normal sensitivity or no more than a very mild (i.e., less than a 30 dB HL) sensitivity loss in some portion of the 1k to 4k Hz region of the pure-tone audiogram (results are discussed as predicting hearing sensitivity in "at least some portion of the 1k to 4k Hz region of the pure-tone audiogram" because of the nonfrequency specific nature of the click stimulus). We initially selected 40 dB nHL as the "pass" criteria to limit failures due to test environment (Hyde et al. 1984). In June 1989, we reduced "pass" criteria to a more stringent 30 dB nHL without subsequent increase in ABR failures.

Subgroup B—Responses to clicks presented at 45 to 55 dB nHL (or 35 to 55 dB nHL after June 1989) and no response to clicks presented at lower click intensities. Subgroup B consisted of infants whose ABR predicted at least a mild (i.e., 30 to 45 dB HL) sensitivity loss in some portion of the frequency region 1k to 4k Hz of the pure-tone audiogram.

Subgroup C—Responses to clicks presented at 60 to 75 dB nHL and no response to clicks presented at lower click intensities. Subgroup C consisted of infants whose ABR predicted at least a moderate (i.e., 50 to 65 dB HL) sensitivity loss in some portion of the frequency region 1k to 4k Hz of the pure-tone audiogram.

Subgroup D—Either no response to clicks presented at highest click intensities tested (in general, 80 dB nHL, or for infants with aural atresia, 95 dB nHL) or responses at 80 to 95 dB nHL only. No responses were observed to clicks presented at lower click intensities. Subgroup D consisted of infants whose ABR predicted at least a severe (i.e., greater than 70 dB HL) sensitivity loss in some portion of the 1k to 4k Hz region of the pure-tone audiogram.

To predict probable site of auditory dysfunction, responses of infants with apparent hearing sensitivity losses (subgroups B, C, and D) were categorized on characteristics of response latency and morphology. For this categorization scheme, absolute latency of wave I and wave V, the wave I to wave V interwave interval, and response morphology were evaluated. Absolute latency of wave I and wave V was considered normal if responses fell within the range of results obtained from control infants of equivalent age. Wave I to wave V interwave interval was considered normal if it fell within two standard deviations of the mean of control infants of equivalent age. Finally, response morphology was considered abnormal if wave I was present and later waves III and V could not be identified, or if only a repeatable, rounded response without distinct, peaked morphology could be distinguished. Three categories were formed:

Category I—Wave I and wave V absolute latency within normal limits, wave I to wave V interwave interval within normal limits, and normal response morphology. Responses in this category were considered consistent with a sensorineural dysfunction affecting hearing sensitivity in the 1k to 4k Hz region of the pure-tone audiogram, and normal brainstem auditory pathway function. Infants were placed in this category based on responses from the better hearing ear if there was a difference in ABR thresholds between ears.

Category II—Wave I and/or wave V prolonged, wave I to wave V interwave interval normal, and normal response morphology. If wave I to wave V interwave interval could not be measured due to absence of wave I, threshold to bone-conducted clicks at lower intensity levels than thresholds to air-conducted clicks also resulted in placement in this category. Responses in this category were considered consistent with conductive (middle ear) dysfunction affecting hearing sensitivity in the 1k to 4k Hz region of the pure-tone audiogram, and normal brainstem auditory pathway function. Infants were placed in this category based on responses from the better hearing ear if there was a difference in ABR thresholds between ears.

Category III—Wave I within the normal range and wave V prolonged relative to the normal range resulting in a prolonged wave I to wave V interwave interval, or abnormal response morphology. Responses in this category were considered consistent with brainstem pathway dysfunction. Infants were placed in this category only if responses from both ears met these criteria.

RESULTS

Table 1 shows results of ABR evaluation based on lowest click intensity yielding a response in the 1,281 infants tested (subgroups A, B, C, and D). The overwhelming majority of infants tested "passed" the initial ABR with responses to clicks at 40 dB nHL or lower (subgroup A, 1,162 infants, or 90.7%). These results indicate either normal peripheral hearing sensitivity or no more than a very mild (i.e., less than 30 dB HL) sensitivity loss. Sixty-six infants (5.1%) were placed in subgroup B based on response thresholds of 45 to 55 dB nHL (or 35 to 55 dB nHL after June 1989). Responses of these infants predicted mild (i.e., 30 to 45 dB HL) peripheral sensitivity loss. There were 38 infants (3.0%) in subgroup C, with click ABR thresholds of 60 to 75 dB nHL.

Table 1

Results of auditory brainstem response (ABR) evaluation in 1,281 infants. Responses of infants were subgrouped on the basis of the lowest click intensity yielding a replicable response in at least one ear.

	Subgroup A (Normal)	Subgroup B (Mild Loss)	Subgroup C (Moderate Loss)	Subgroup D (Severe Loss)
N	1,162	66	38	15
% of total	90.7	5.1	3.0	1.2

Table 2

Distribution of predicted site of dysfunction in 66 infants whose initial ABR threshold was consistent with mild sensitivity loss (subgroup B).

	Category I (Sensorineural)	Category II (Conductive)	Category III (Brainstem Pathway)
N	16	50	0
% of total	24.2	75.8	0.0

Responses of these infants predicted moderate (i.e., 50 to 65 dB HL) sensitivity loss. Finally, 15 infants (1.2%) were placed in subgroup D with responses predicting at least a severe sensitivity loss (either responses to clicks presented at 80 to 95 dB nHL or no response to clicks presented at any intensity level).

Table 2 shows distribution of predicted site of dysfunction in 66 infants whose ABR threshold of 35 to 55 dB nHL was consistent with mild sensitivity loss. Most infants (50 of 66, or 75.8%) demonstrated response latency and morphology characteristics that suggested conductive (middle ear) dysfunction (category II). The remaining 16 infants (24.2%) showed response characteristics consistent with sensorineural dysfunction (category I). No infants with predicted mild sensitivity loss demonstrated abnormality of response latency or morphology consistent with brainstem auditory pathway dysfunction (category III).

Table 3 shows distribution of predicted site of dysfunction in 38 infants whose ABR threshold of 60 to 75 dB nHL was consistent with moderate sensitivity loss. Once again, most infants (34 of 38, or 89.5%)

Table 3

Distribution of predicted site of dysfunction in 38 infants whose initial ABR threshold was consistent with moderate sensitivity loss (subgroup C).

	Category I (Sensorineural)	Category II (Conductive)	Category III (Brainstem Pathway)
N	1	34	3
% of total	2.6	89.5	7.9

demonstrated characteristics of response latency and morphology consistent with conductive (middle ear) dysfunction (category II). Only 1 infant (2.6%) demonstrated response characteristics consistent with sensorineural dysfunction (category I), and 3 infants (7.9%) showed response latency and morphology abnormalities suggesting brainstem auditory pathway dysfunction (category III). One of these infants, with a medical history of birth asphyxia, profound hypoglycemia, and seizures, demonstrated normal ABR thresholds, latency, and morphology upon follow-up evaluation. The other 2 infants expired before follow-up evaluation could be completed.

Of 15 infants whose ABR threshold was consistent with at least a severe sensitivity loss (subgroup D), 4 infants demonstrated no response to clicks presented by either air conduction or bone conduction. Response characteristics for these infants could not be subcategorized. Medical diagnoses of these infants included bilateral atresia (1 child), bacterial meningitis (2 children), and Down syndrome (1 child). Hearing loss has been confirmed in all 4 of these infants through additional evoked potential and behavioral assessment, and medical evaluation. All 4 infants are receiving auditory habilitation services.

Categorization of predicted site of dysfunction for the remaining 11 infants with predicted severe sensitivity loss is shown in table 4. Four of these 11 infants (36.4%) demonstrated characteristics of response latency and morphology consistent with conductive (middle ear) dysfunction (category II). Three of these infants had craniofacial or syndromal anomalies affecting external and/or middle ear structures. Three of the 11 infants (27.3%) had response characteristics consistent with

Table 4

Distribution of predicted site of dysfunction in 11 infants whose initial ABR threshold was consistent with severe sensitivity loss (subgroup D). (An additional 4 infants in this subgroup were not included in this analysis because they exhibited no response to ABR clicks.)

	Category I (Sensorineural)	Category II (Conductive)	Category III (Brainstem Pathway)
N	3	4	4
% of total	27.3	36.4	36.4

sensorineural dysfunction (category I). Medical diagnosis of these children included Down syndrome and cleft palate (1 child), bacterial meningitis (1 child), and congenital heart disease (1 child). Finally, 4 infants in subgroup D (36.4%) had ABR characteristics consistent with brainstem auditory pathway dysfunction (category III). All of these infants demonstrated medical or radiographic evidence of central nervous system dysfunction.

DISCUSSION

An NICU ABR program should result in (1) accurate identification of infants with probable hearing impairment and (2) appropriate follow-up recommendations. Based on our experience, we believe that accurate identification can be enhanced when the ABR is applied as a diagnostic procedure to those infants who fail its administration as a screening test. For those infants, immediate diagnostic application permits prediction of both degree of sensitivity loss and probable site of dysfunction. This information is important to the managing physician who must make treatment decisions based on test results and physical examination, and to the managing audiologist who must develop audiologic follow-up strategies.

Our data highlight three important aspects of NICU ABR testing. First, in our sample, a "pass" criteria of 30 or 40 dB nHL in one or both ears resulted in an initial pass of more than 90% of 1,281 infants tested, even in less than ideal acoustic test conditions. Average age of infants tested in our program was 40 weeks postconception. Clinical studies in which the average age at test was less than approximately 38 weeks postconception report a lower initial pass rate (and consequently a higher initial failure rate) than the present study (Roberts et al. 1982; Swigonski et al. 1987). Higher failure rate in younger infants may be related to neuromaturational factors rather than to peripheral hearing sensitivity loss (Salamy 1984; Lary et al. 1985). Age at test, therefore, must be considered when evaluating infants in the NICU. As recommended by others, we believe that infants should be tested prior to discharge and as close to full term (38 to 42 weeks) as possible (Committee on Hearing, Bioacoustics, and Biomechanics 1987; ASHA 1989). For infants who must be tested at an earlier age because of discharge or transfer considerations, we recommend testing strategies that will enhance response detection (i.e., slower click rate, longer response window). It is important to recognize the nontransitive nature of presence versus absence of a response at threshold criterion in very young premature infants. Presence of a response at 30 or 40 dB nHL in these babies effectively rules out significant peripheral sensitivity loss; absence of a response at these levels does not preclude the possibility of normal hearing sensitivity.

Second, most infants who failed the "pass" criteria of 30 or 40 dB nHL demonstrated responses to clicks at levels suggesting mild sensitivity loss (subgroup B, N = 66, 5.1% of all infants tested). Only 38 infants (subgroup C, 3.0% of all infants tested) had response thresholds suggesting moderate sensitivity loss, and only 15 infants (subgroup D, 1.2% of all infants tested) had no response or response thresholds consistent with severe to profound sensitivity loss. These results suggest that, in graduates of the NICU, there are more infants with mild and moderate sensitivity loss than with severe to profound sensitivity loss. Follow-up studies of NICU graduates confirm this finding (Hosford-Dunn et al. 1987). The importance of this finding is related to the definition of "significant" hearing loss in infants and the goal of NICU hearing screening programs. There is little debate that even mild hearing impairment can have important effects on speech-language development, social-emotional adjustment, and academic achievement in preschool- and school-age children (Bess 1985). There has been considerable debate, however, about the value of detecting mild sensitivity loss in infants (Simmons 1982; Galambos, Hicks, and Wilson 1982).

We would argue that in the NICU, a setting of high-risk newborns, identification of hearing impairment of any degree sufficient to affect speech and language development is possible and should be the screening goal. We are especially concerned about infants with mild hearing loss. In the absence of systematic identification programs, there is an inverse relationship between age of identification and degree of hearing loss (Elssmann, Matkin, and Sabo 1987). A screening program that passes infants with mild sensitivity loss may actually contribute to delayed identification because parents may equate "pass" on a screening test with normal hearing. At a minimum, we believe that an infant hearing screening program should identify hearing losses of approximately 30 dB HL and greater. Inevitably, some will argue that it is not cost-effective to identify infants with this degree of hearing loss, especially when the hearing loss may be transient in most cases. Even accounting for false positives related to transient hearing disorders, ABR remains the most sensitive and cost-effective screening approach (Durieux-Smith et al. 1985; Prager, Stone, and Rose 1987). It also meets the 30 dB HL goal.

Finally, these data illustrate the ease of predicting both degree of sensitivity loss and site of dysfunction at initial test. This information is useful for developing follow-up strategies specific to the predicted hearing disorder. For example, for infants with predicted mild conductive hearing loss, an appropriate follow-up strategy might be medical/otologic evaluation and management, and audiologic reevaluation by behavioral audiometry and acoustic immittance measures at age 6 months. For infants with predicted moderate sensorineural loss, however, it would be important to obtain medical/otologic evaluation and ABR reevaluation within one to two months to ensure rapid confirmation of permanent hearing loss and to initiate habilitation. Although fitting of amplification may be postponed pending completion of behavioral and acoustic immittance measures, parental information, education, and support can initiate the habilitative program.

Unfortunately, we have found, as have other investigators, that follow-up of screening failures is less than ideal, regardless of the screening technique (Stein, Clark, and Kraus 1983; Galambos, Hicks, and Wilson 1984; Delano et al. 1987; Mahoney and Eichwald 1987; Kramer, Vertes, and Condon 1989; Stein et al. 1990). Factors that contribute to failure to follow up include financial, medical, social, emotional, and transportation issues (Stein et al. 1983; Hayes 1987). These issues are not easily resolved. By reducing the number of infants needing follow-up through a predischarge ABR screening/diagnostic program, more aggressive follow-up and management strategies can be developed for a fewer number of babies. For those infants who are discharged to communities with limited pediatric audiology services, information provided by the diagnostic component of the NICU ABR program can be invaluable to the managing physician.

The following components are necessary for an NICU ABR screening/diagnostic program. First, each program must develop appropriate normative data. Although normative ABR latency data for preterm infants have been published (Gorga et al. 1987), each program should develop its own norms related to test site (NICU versus sound-treated enclosure), stimulus conditions, and recording parameters.

Specific recommendations have been made regarding these test conditions (Murray, Javel, and Watson 1985; Committee on Hearing, Bioacoustics, and Biomechanics 1987).

Second, responses should be analyzed on-line to determine what changes in stimulus or recording parameters are necessary. The audiologist should evaluate not only presence of a response to each stimulus condition but also response latency and morphology. Evaluation of these components of each response permits prediction of both degree of sensitivity loss and probable site of dysfunction.

Finally, the test technique must allow flexibility in stimulus conditions and recording parameters. The audiologist should be able to change a variety of stimulus and recording conditions to enhance response detection and evaluation. We routinely change stimulus intensity, click rate, and response window to search for responses. In addition, we change stimulus transducer, preamplifier filter settings, and stimulus characteristics to obtain more complete diagnostic information. This flexibility is necessary for maximum diagnostic efficiency.

SUMMARY

Application of the ABR as a "screening" procedure is adequate to "pass" most NICU infants. For babies who do not pass the initial screen, however, immediate application of a diagnostic ABR is both cost-effective and time efficient, and permits better management and follow-up of infants.

In this study of more than 1,200 infants, 90% "passed" initial ABR evaluation with electrophysiologic response to clicks at 30 to 40 dB nHL. Of those infants who did not pass, most demonstrated responses consistent with mild hearing sensitivity loss (66 infants or 5.1% of the total sample). Only 15 infants (1.2% of the sample) demonstrated results suggesting severe hearing sensitivity loss. These results highlight the importance of screening infants at risk for hearing loss for mild degree (i.e., loss of 30 dB HL and greater) of hearing loss, and the utility of ABR evaluation with analysis of response threshold, latency, and morphology for this purpose.

We encourage expanded use of ABR evaluation in newborn hearing screening programs to provide information relevant to probable degree of peripheral hearing sensitivity loss and predicted site of dysfunction to assist in management and follow-up of infants who fail initial evaluation.

REFERENCES

American Speech-Language-Hearing Association. Committee on Infant Hearing. 1989. Audiologic screening of newborn infants who are at risk for hearing impairment. *Asha* 30:61-64.

Amochaev, A. 1987. The infant hearing foundation—a unique approach to hearing screening of newborns. In K. Gerkin and A. Amochaev (eds.), *Seminars in Hearing* 8:165-168.

Bess, F. 1985. The minimally hearing-impaired child. *Ear and Hearing* 6:43-47.

Committee on Hearing, Bioacoustics, and Biomechanics. Working group on brainstem audiometry of prelanguage groups. 1987. Brainstem audiometry in infants. *Asha* 29:47-55.

Delano, S., Carrigan, V., Sabo, D., and Nozza, R. 1987. Confirmation and management of hearing-impairment following ABR screening. Paper read at annual convention of the American Speech-Language-Hearing Association, November 1987, New Orleans.

Despland, P., and Galambos, R. 1980. The auditory brainstem response (ABR) is a useful diagnostic tool in the intensive care nursery. *Pediatric Research* 14:154-158.

Durieux-Smith, A., Picton, T., Edwards, C., Goodman, J., and MacMurray, B. 1985. The Crib-O-Gram in the NICU: An evaluation based on brain stem electric response audiometry. *Ear and Hearing* 6:20-24.

Elssmann, S., Matkin, N., and Sabo, M. 1987. Early identification of congenital sensorineural hearing impairment. *The Hearing Journal* 40:13-17.

Galambos, R., Hicks, G., and Wilson, M. 1982. Identification audiometry in neonates: Reply to Simmons. *Ear and Hearing* 3:189-190.

Galambos, R., Hicks, G., and Wilson, M. 1984. The auditory brain stem response reliably predicts hearing loss in graduates of a tertiary intensive care nursery. *Ear and Hearing* 5:254-260.

Gorga, M., Reiland, J., Worthington, D., and Jesteadt, W. 1987. Auditory brainstem responses from graduates of an intensive care nursery: Normal patterns of response. *Journal of Speech and Hearing Research* 30:311-318.

Hayes, D. 1987. Problems in habilitation of hearing-impaired infants. In K. Gerkin and A. Amochaev (eds.), *Seminars in Hearing* 8:181-185.

Hosford-Dunn, H., Johnson, S., Simmons, F., Malachowski, M., and Low, K. 1987. Infant hearing screening: Program implementation and validation. *Ear and Hearing* 8:12-20.

Hyde, M., Riko, K., Corbin, H., Moroso, M., and Alberti, P. 1984. A neonatal hearing screening research program using brainstem electric response audiometry. *Journal of Otolaryngology* 13:49-54.

Jacobson, J., and Morehouse, C. 1984. A comparison of auditory brainstem response and behavioral screening of high risk and normal newborn infants. *Ear and Hearing* 5:247-253.

Joint Committee on Infant Hearing. 1982. Position statement. *Asha* 24(12):1017-1018.

Joint Committee on Infant Hearing. 1991. 1990 position statement. *Asha* 33(Suppl. 5):3-6.

Kileny, P. 1987. ALGO-1 automated infant hearing screener: Preliminary results. In K. Gerkin and A. Amochaev (eds.), *Seminars in Hearing* 8:125-131.

Kramer, S., Vertes, D., and Condon, M. 1989. Auditory brainstem responses and clinical follow-up of high-risk infants. *Pediatrics* 83:385-392.

Lary, W., Briassoulis, G., deVries, L., Dubowitz, L., and Dubowitz, V. 1985. Hearing threshold in preterm and term infants by auditory brainstem response. *Journal of Pediatrics* 107:593-599.

Mahoney, T., and Eichwald, J. 1987. The ups and "downs" of high risk hearing screening: The Utah statewide program. In K. Gerkin and A. Amochaev (eds.), *Seminars in Hearing* 8:155-163.

Murray, A., Javel, E., and Watson, C. 1985. Prognostic validity of auditory brainstem evoked response screening in newborn infants. *American Journal of Otolaryngology* 6:120-131.

Prager, D., Stone, D., and Rose, D. 1987. Hearing loss screening in the neonatal intensive care unit: Auditory brainstem response versus Crib-O-Gram: A cost effectiveness analysis. *Ear and Hearing* 8:213-216.

Roberts, J., Davis, H., Phon, G., Reichert, T., Sturtevant, E., and Marshall, R. 1982. Auditory brainstem responses in preterm neonates: Maturation and follow-up. *Journal of Pediatrics* 101:257-263.

Salamy, A. 1984. Maturation of the auditory brainstem response from birth through early childhood. *Journal of Clinical Neurophysiology* 1:293-329.

Simmons, F. 1982. Comment on "Hearing loss in graduates of a tertiary intensive care nursery." *Ear and Hearing* 3:188.

Stein, L., Clark, S., and Kraus, N. 1983. The hearing-impaired infant: Patterns of identification and habilitation. *Ear and Hearing* 4:232-236.

Stein, L., Ozdamar, O., Kraus, N., and Paton, N. 1983. Follow-up of infants screened by auditory brainstem response in the neonatal intensive care unit. *Journal of Pediatrics* 103:447-453.

Stein, L., Jabaley, T., Spitz, R., Stoakley, D., and McGee, T. 1990. The hearing-impaired infant: Patterns of identification and habilitation revisited. *Ear and Hearing* 11:201-205.

Swigonski, N., Shallop, J., Bull, M., and Lemons, J. 1987. Hearing screening of high risk newborns. *Ear and Hearing* 8:26-30.

Worthington, D., Gorga, M., Reiland, J., and Beauchaine, K. 1985. Evaluating ICN graduates II: Abnormal ABR patterns. Paper read at annual convention of the American Speech-Language-Hearing Association, November 1985, Washington, D.C.

Chapter 10

Newborn Hearing Screening with Auditory Brainstem Response (ABR): Experience with 1982 Versus 1990 Joint Committee Risk Criteria

James W. Hall III and Charlotte H. Prentice

INTRODUCTION

The Joint Committee on Infant Hearing is a national multidisciplinary group composed of representatives from audiology, otolaryngology, pediatrics, and speech pathology. The Committee was established first in 1969. The current official statement of Joint Committee recommendations, a revision and expansion of earlier position papers, was developed in 1990 (Joint Committee 1991). The 1990 Joint Committee Position Statement, including a listing of risk criteria, is reproduced in Appendix 1. Until now, newborn hearing screening programs have typically relied on the 1982 Joint Committee risk criteria for identification of infants to be screened (Joint Committee 1982). Now that the 1990 Joint Committee risk criteria are available and have been disseminated, most screening programs will presumably adhere to these most recent guidelines.

When newborn hearing screening was introduced at the Vanderbilt University Hospital in October 1988, infants were identified as at risk for hearing impairment according to criteria recommended by the 1982 Joint Committee on Infant Hearing (Joint Committee 1982). Since October 1990, however, infant chart review protocol has followed recommendations by the 1990 Joint Committee. In this paper, we compare our experiences with the 1982 versus 1990 Joint Committee recommendations, including some clinical challenges encountered in making the transition to the new risk criteria for hearing impairment.

DESCRIPTION OF JOINT COMMITTEE RISK CRITERIA

INTRODUCTION

A thorough discussion of each Joint Committee risk criterion is beyond the scope of this review. The pediatric, audiologic, and otolaryngologic literature contains papers on the relation between various risk factors and infant hearing impairment. There are also review papers on the topic (Gerkin 1984; Hall 1992). The 1982 Joint Committee listed seven risk criteria for neonatal hearing impairment. Three additional neonatal risk criteria were added by the 1990 Joint Committee. In addition, the 1990 Joint Committee Position Statement includes one set of risk criteria for neonates, defined by the Committee as from birth to 28 days, and another set for infants, which the Committee defines as between 29 days and 2 years. Each neonatal risk criterion for hearing impairment will now be explained briefly.

1982 RISK CRITERIA

Family history. A family history of hearing impairment is perhaps the most obvious risk factor, yet the one in practice that is most difficult to document with certainty, especially by review of an infant's medical chart. Information on family history in the medical chart is typically sparse, at best. Halpern, Hosford-Dunn, and Malachowski (1987), for example, reported that family history was not indicated as a risk factor in medical charts of any of 975 intensive care nursery infants.

Congenital infections. Perinatal infections are often listed according to the TORCH complex. The letters in this acronym refer to Toxoplasmosis, Other (an example of an infection in this category is syphilis), Rubella, Cytomegalovirus (CMV), which is the most common infection in the TORCH complex, and Herpes simplex virus. These perinatal infections, and their relation to hearing impairment, were recently reviewed by Hall (1992).

Craniofacial anomalies. One of the most apparent risk factors upon physical examination is anatomic malformation involving the head or neck. This may range from complete and bilateral aural microtia or atresia (absence or severe malformation of the external and often middle ear) to relatively subtle aberrations of the pinna (e.g., low set or posteriorly rotated ears) to absent philtrum or a low hairline. Anatomic malformations may occur in isolation or as part of a syndrome along with heart, kidney, genital, or skeletal defects (e.g., Treacher Collins syndrome).

Low birth weight. The Joint Committee defines low birth weight (LBW) as less than 1500 grams. Since 1000 grams (1 kilogram) is equivalent to 2.2 pounds, the cutoff for low birth weight is approximately 3.3 pounds. There is, in fact, no direct correlation between low birth weight and hearing impairment in newborn infants. There is a definite tendency for low birth weight among infants born prematurely, although low birth weight does not necessarily imply or equate with prematurity. Prematurity is, therefore, more closely related to possible hearing impairment than low birth weight. A brief definition of several terms used in describing infant age would perhaps be appropriate at this point. *Gestational age* (GA) is defined as the time interval from the last menstrual period up to the time of delivery. Gestational age is also described in terms of infant development, in comparison to the normal standard (normative data for infants born after a full-term pregnancy). *Conceptional age* is calculated from the date of conception versus the date of the last menstrual period. Thus, conceptional age is 2 weeks less than gestational age. Gestational age for a complete, full-term pregnancy is between 37 and 42 weeks (40 weeks on the average). Although reference to *gestational age* does not continue beyond birth, the term *conceptional age* may be used to describe an infant's gestational age (at birth), plus chronological age (after birth).

Hyperbilirubinemia. Hyperbilirubinemia is defined as bilirubin concentration in the blood in excess of 6 to 8 mg/dl. At that level, jaundice (characterized by yellowish skin) becomes apparent. Hyperbilirubinemia is a very complex metabolic disorder, which may result from too much production of bilirubin or too little clearance of bilirubin from the blood by the liver. Approximately 5% to 10% of all newborns have bilirubin concentrations above 13 mg/dl. To be considered a risk factor according to the Joint Committee recommendations, hyperbilirubinemia must be at a level that requires exchange transfusion.

Bacterial meningitis. The meninges are thin membranes that surround the brain and enclose a plasmalike fluid. Meninges form a barrier between the brain and the skull. Bacterial infection reaches the meninges from the bloodstream. Meningitis occurs more often in premature than term neonates. In large series of high-risk infants, meningitis is relatively infrequent.

Asphyxia (severe depression). Asphyxia is a disruption of oxygen to the body, including the brain. It can result from extrinsic causes, such as strangulation, crushing injury to the chest, or drowning, or from intrinsic causes, such as a foreign body in the trachea (windpipe), lung disease, or heart deficiency. In neonates, the two mechanisms for asphyxia are interruption of placental or maternal blood flow before delivery or blockage of the infant's airway at delivery. In either case, the amount of oxygen available to the infant is reduced (and the amount of carbon dioxide is increased), and hypoxia or ischemia develops. Asphyxia can effect the cochlea and the auditory regions of the brain. The Apgar score is a common tool for definition of the asphyxia risk criterion. Named after the person who developed it, the Apgar score consists of five criteria: (1) heart rate, (2) respiratory effort, (3) muscle tone, (4) response to stimulation, and (5) color. The highest score is 10. The Apgar score is determined at 1 minute and 5 minutes after birth. Asphyxia is more likely for infants with low Apgar scores. The 1990 Joint Committee defines severe depression as Apgar scores of 0 to 3 at 5 minutes, or failure to initiate spontaneous respiration by 10 minutes, or hypotonia persisting for 2 hours after birth.

ADDITIONAL 1990 JOINT COMMITTEE RISK CRITERIA

Ototoxic medications. This 1990 Joint Committee criterion is defined as "ototoxic medications including but not limited to the aminoglycosides used for more than five days (e.g. gentamicin, tobramycin, kanamycin, streptomycin) and loop diuretics used in combination with aminoglycosides" (Joint Committee 1991). There is general agreement in the literature that these widely used drugs, and others such as cis-platinum, are potentially ototoxic in adult populations (see Griffin 1988 for a review). Also, serious sensorineural hearing loss has been reported for over 20% of young severely burned children treated with one or more of these medications (Hall et al. 1986; 1987). Whether these clinical experiences can be generalized to newborn infants, however, is less clear. For example, Colding, Andersen, Prytz, Wulffsberg, and Andersen (1989) reported that continuous intravenous infusion of gentamicin during neonatal intensive care failed to cause hearing impairment. In addition, Hall, Brown, and Hargadine (1985) found no evidence of hearing impairment in an infant with advanced renal disease who inadvertently received ten times the acceptable dosage of vancomycin (an antibiotic that is not in the aminoglycoside class). There are other similar reports (McCracken 1986). One major methodological problem inherent in such clinical studies of at-risk infants is parceling out the ototoxic factor from the other potential causes of hearing impairment, including the risk factors just reviewed and confounding variables such as infection, prolonged respiratory care, acute central nervous system insults, and high levels of noise in the NICU environment. It is probable that synergistic effects among several of these drugs, particularly an aminoglycoside in combination with the loop diuretic furosemide (lasix), will prove most ototoxic in the neonatal population.

Prolonged mechanical ventilation. A second additional 1990 Joint Committee risk criterion is prolonged mechanical ventilation, for a duration of ten or more days. This disorder occurs most often in relatively large infants (greater than 2500 grams) who are born close to term and is usually associated with persistent pulmonary hypertension (PPH). In most cases, these infants would not be identified as at risk for hearing impairment by 1982 Joint Committee recommendations.

Stigmata of syndrome. Infants with signs or other findings of a syndrome that may be associated with a sensorineural hearing loss, such as Waardenburg's or Usher's syndrome, are at risk for hearing impairment according to the 1990 Joint Committee.

EXPERIENCE WITH 1982 VERSUS 1990 RISK CRITERIA

VANDERBILT UNIVERSITY HOSPITAL NEWBORN HEARING SCREENING PROGRAM

Vanderbilt University Hospital (VUH) is a 650-bed tertiary care facility in Nashville, Tennessee. It is the primary teaching hospital of the Vanderbilt University School of Medicine. The Hospital was one of the first to introduce intensive care of neonates in the early 1960s. VUH serves as a regional perinatal referral center for the Middle Tennessee region, southern Kentucky, and northern Alabama. Infants requiring level four intensive care nursery services are transported to VUH via ground, in specially designed ambulances, or via Life Flight helicopter.

In spring of 1988, the first author assumed responsibility as Director of Audiology at VUH. A newborn hearing screening program was proposed to the Division of Neonatology, and in October of that year, the program was implemented. Details of the newborn screening program are described in Appendix 3. Briefly, infants are identified as at risk for hearing impairment by Joint Committee criteria. Medical charts of all infants admitted to the NICU or intermediate nursery are reviewed, usually within one or two days after admission, by audiology staff or trained audiology graduate students. Those infants meeting one or more risk criteria undergo hearing screening by ABR at bedside within the final days before discharge from the hospital. An automated ABR device (ALGO-1)[1] is used for most hearing screenings. The remainder are conducted with a conventional ABR system. ABR screening protocol is summarized in Appendix 3. Screening is scheduled with the help of a discharge nurse or the infant's primary care nurse. We attempt to recall, for comprehensive follow-up audiologic assessment within 3 to 6 months of age (chronological age after 40 weeks gestational age), all infants who fail the hearing screening on either ear or bilaterally, and infants at risk for progressive hearing loss. This assessment always includes behavioral audiometry and tympanometry. A full ABR assessment (with latency-intensity functions, and tone burst and bone conduction stimulation, as indicated) is carried out whenever behavioral audiometry is inconclusive or incomplete. Infants with confirmed hearing impairment, and without audiologic or otologic evidence of medically or surgically treatable disease, are referred to the Bill Wilkerson Center for long-term audiologic and educational management and parent-infant stimulation.

GENERAL HEARING SCREENING STATISTICS

We reviewed a total of 2,093 infant medical records from October 1988 through May 1991 (table 1). An additional 107 infants admitted to the VUH nurseries died before chart review was completed. Of the 2,093 infants, 769 (37%) met one or more of the Joint Committee risk criteria. This proportion is considerably lower than we anticipated, based on experiences reported by other newborn hearing screening programs. In our initial proposal to Neonatology, we had requested a standing order to screen all nursery admissions with the expectation that over 85%

---

[1]ALGO-1™ Natus Medical Incorporated, Forest City, California.

Table 1
General Statistics for Vanderbilt University Hospital Newborn Hearing
Screening Program (October 1988 to May 1991)

Medical charts reviewed	2,093
Infants deceased	
before chart review	107
before hearing screening	44
Infants at risk by chart review	769 (37%)
Infants screened	441
unconditional pass outcome	296 (67%)
unconditional fail outcome	65 (15%)
pass but at risk for progressive loss	30 (7%)
fail but at risk for progressive loss	2 (.004%)
could not complete screening	48 (11%)
Did not screen *	271

* Infants discharged to home or back transported to another hospital before screening
could be completed (see table 2 for details).

would be at risk according to Joint Committee criteria. The request was
denied. We predicted that routine screening of all infants would reduce
the demand for chart review. At our Hospital, however, by screening all
NICU admissions we would, in fact, create three times the demand for
screenings. Based on this experience, we advise those proposing a
hearing screening program based on Joint Committee recommendations
to first review medical charts on a trial basis to estimate the proportion
of infants admitted to the NICU who are at risk by Joint Committee
criteria. This information will also be valuable in determining staffing
and equipment needs for the screening program.

Among the 441 infants screened, 67% passed unconditionally. That
is, there was an ABR within the acceptable latency region bilaterally.
And since ototoxicity was included among risk criteria in October 1990,
this group of infants presented no risk criterion for a progressive hearing
loss. Most previous newborn hearing screening studies report a "pass"
rate of over 85% to 90% (see Hall 1992 for review). Our unconditional
failure rate of 15% is consistent with these reports. However, we also
found that 7% of our population passed the screening but were at risk for

progressive hearing loss. Other reasons for the relatively low proportion of pass outcomes will be discussed below. For 11% of the infants, screening was attempted but could not be completed for both ears. In some cases, the infant passed on one ear and then became excessively restless. Other reasons for the aborted screening included excessive electrical artifact, excessive ambient noise, or excessive test time (e.g., more than 45 minutes to an hour). Conditions are often suboptimal because we must conduct the screenings in the NICU or intermediate nursery. Finally, in the time period of this study 271 infants were discharged prior to hearing screening.

VUH is the major regional referral center for newborn intensive medical care. Infants are commonly transported from outlying hospitals soon after birth and, after appropriate medical and/or surgical management, returned to this hospital (back transported) for follow-up care before discharge to home. In fact, the majority of infants at risk for hearing impairment at VUH are back transported (table 2), whereas only one-third are discharged to home. The high proportion of back transported infants presents at least four practical hearing screening problems. First, at the time of screening, they are in an NICU environment, which can be hostile relative to ABR measurement. That is, there are numerous sources of electrical artifacts and excessive ambient noise. Second, they are often preterm (less than 40 weeks gestational age) at the time of discharge. This results in a higher hearing screening failure rate (Hall 1992). Third, most infants remain in an isolette, rather than a bassinet, up until VUH discharge. Technically, it is more difficult to carry out hearing screening with the infant in an isolette versus an open bed. In addition, many of these infants are on oxygen support during testing. Finally, infants are often back transported

Table 2
Infant Discharge Statistics for Vanderbilt University Hospital Newborn
Hearing Screening Program (October 1988 to May 1991)

Total number discharged	722
Back transported to another hospital	424 (59%)
Directly to home	237 (33%)
Deceased before discharge	47 (6%)
Unknown disposition	14 (2%)

Table 3
Comparison of 1988 Versus 1990 Hearing Screening Statistics for
Vanderbilt University Hospital

	Since October 1988	Since October 1990
Medical charts reviewed	2,093	563
Infants at risk by chart review	769 (37%)	216 (38%)
Screening completed	393 (51%)	148 (68%)
Could not complete screening	48 (6%)	6 (3%)
Did not screen *	271 (35%)	62 (29%)

* Infants discharged to home or back transported to another hospital before screening could be completed.

with little warning. The decision may be based not on a generally predictable criterion of health status, such as weight gain or independence from oxygen support, but on unpredictable factors (e.g., overcrowding of the NICU or availability of a bed at the receiving hospital). The clinician planning a hearing screening program at a major hospital with an NICU is advised to first estimate the volume of back transported infants, and then to develop a strategy for ensuring that these are screened before discharge and, also, that an adequate follow-up system is in place.

During the first two years of the hearing screening program, we realized that screening was not completed for an unacceptable number of infants. We identified various reasons for the problem, ranging from inconsistent communication with the discharge nurse to inadequate audiology staffing. When these problems were addressed, the proportion of infants screened increased (table 3). Most of the infants in the "did not screen" category were back transported to another hospital before their health status permitted successful testing. These infants are, of course, still at risk and are placed on our follow-up list.

SCREENING FOLLOW-UP STATISTICS

Follow-up was required for 25% of the infants with completed hearing screening (table 4). These infants could be subdivided rather equally into three groups; slightly over one-third failed the screening bilaterally, and slightly under one-third either failed unilaterally or passed but were at risk for progressive hearing impairment. Most

Table 4
Hearing Screening Outcome for Vanderbilt University Hospital
(October 1988 to May 1991)

Pass bilaterally	296 (75%)
Follow-up required	97 (25%)
fail bilaterally	34 (35%)
fail unilaterally	31 (32%)
right ear	19
left ear	12
fail and at risk for progressive loss	2 (2%)
pass but at risk for progressive loss	30 (31%)

published newborn ABR hearing screening reports cite follow-up rates of 8% to 12%. There are at least two reasons why the proportion of infants requiring follow-up in our program is two times greater than that reported by other investigators. First, according to our protocol each ear must be tested separately. If we are unable to complete the screening for each ear, the infant is classified as "could not test" and followed on an outpatient basis, even if one ear passes the screening. Clearly, follow-up rates will be lower for screening programs without ear specific stimulation (e.g., Crib-O-Gram technique) or programs that define a pass outcome on the basis of results for only one ear. That approximately one-third of our screening failures were unilateral argues strongly for a protocol requiring monaural stimulation of each ear. A second factor contributing to the greater demand for infant follow-up with our program has to do with potentially progressive hearing loss. Close monitoring of the auditory status of infants at risk for progressive hearing loss is essential to minimize the likelihood of a long-term "false negative" outcome; that is, infants who pass a hearing screening at birth yet develop permanent hearing loss. The requirement for infant follow-up is substantially greater for the 1990 versus 1982 Joint Committee recommendations, as detailed below. Thus, our higher follow-up rate may, in fact, reflect sensitivity in the hearing screening program.

Follow-up statistics for the VUH hearing screening program are summarized in table 5. During the past year, we have routinely attempted to perform behavioral audiometry for NICU graduates who return for a six-month pediatric assessment at the low-birth-weight (LBW) clinic, whether they passed or failed hearing screening in the

Table 5
Follow-Up Statistics for Vanderbilt University Hospital Hearing Screening Program
(October 1988 to May 1991)

Passed screening and followed in LBW* clinic	36 out of 296 (12%)
Follow-up of failures	
fail bilaterally	18 out of 34 (53%)
fail right ear	11 out of 19 (58%)
fail left ear	6 out of 12 (50%)
screening not completed	15 out of 48 (31%)
discharged before screening	59 out of 271 (22%)
pass but at risk for progressive loss	4 out of 30 (13%)

* LBW=low birth weight.

NICU. As a result of the effort, 12% of this population have undergone audiologic follow-up. Slightly over one-half of the infants failing hearing screening return for the recommended follow-up audiologic assessment. This proportion is similar for bilateral and unilateral screening failures. Unfortunately, among the infants who were not successfully screened in the hospital or who were discharged before screening was scheduled, less than one-third returned for the follow-up audiologic assessment. Finally, the poorest follow-up rate was found for infants passing the screening yet at risk for progressive hearing impairment. The implications of this statistic will become clear in the following review of our experiences with the 1990 Joint Committee risk criteria.

EXPERIENCE WITH 1990 JOINT COMMITTEE RISK CRITERIA

DISTRIBUTION OF AT-RISK INFANTS

The distribution of infants at risk for hearing impairment according to the original seven 1982 Joint Committee criteria, plus the three additional 1990 Joint Committee criteria, is displayed in table 6. Recall that these 769 infants were identified by chart review from an NICU and intermediate nursery population of over 2,000 infants. The total of percentages listed in the table exceeds 100% since some infants met more than one criterion. As expected (e.g., Hall 1992; Halpern et al. 1987), the most common risk criterion was LBW (birth weight less than 1500 grams or about 3.3 pounds). Since such data were collected, the second most common criterion was ototoxicity, as defined by the 1990 Joint

Table 6

Distribution of Infants At Risk for Hearing Impairment According to 1990 Joint Committee Criteria by Chart Review at Vanderbilt University Hospital (October 1990 to May 1991) (N=769)

Criterion	N	%*
Family history	3	1
Perinatal infection	6	3
Craniofacial anomalies	13	6
Low birth weight	129	60
Hyperbilirubinemia	2	1
Meningitis	1	0.5
Asphyxia		
Apgar <6 at 5 minutes	32	15
Apgar <4 at 5 minutes	16	7
Ototoxicity	49	23
Syndrome	5	2
Prolonged ventilation (PPH)**	NA	3 (estimated)
Physician order	25	12

* Percentage exceeds 100 because some infants met more than one criterion.
** PPH =persistent pulmonary hypertension.
NA =data not available.

Committee. Relatively few infants met the other eight risk criteria. In fact, less than one-third of the infants met any of these criteria. It is important to keep in mind that these data reflect the 1990 Joint Committee recommendations only for neonates (birth to 28 days), not infants (29 days to 2 years). One would expect that the proportion of infants meeting certain criteria, such as meningitis, would be substantially higher in the older age grouping.

Two of the 1990 Joint Committee criteria accounted for a very small proportion of the at-risk infants. For three of the five infants with evidence of a syndrome, this was the only risk factor. VATER association was cited most often among this group. VATER is an acronym for Vertebral defects, Anal atresia, Tracheal-esophageal fistula with esophageal atresia, and Renal dysplasia (Temtamy and Miller 1974). Ear defects are sometimes a component of VATER association. None of the infants with prolonged ventilation (persistent pulmonary hypertension) would have been identified with the other risk criteria. Two additional risk criteria listed in table 6 need further explanation. Asphyxia is categorized according to two sets of criterion. For the first two years of our screening program, asphyxia was defined by an Apgar score of 5 or less at 5 minutes, without regard to the timing of initiation of spontaneous respiration or hypotonia. Since October 1990, however, we have also applied the specific definition of asphyxia recommended by the 1990 Joint Committee (stated earlier in this chapter). Clearly, by lowering the acceptable Apgar cutoff at 5 minutes from 5 to 3, the number of infants meeting this criterion will be reduced by approximately 50%. The last criterion listed in table 6 (physician order) is not recommended by either Joint Committee. Various reasons account for a physician order for hearing screening of these 25 infants who were not at risk for hearing impairment by Joint Committee criteria, including evidence of neurologic insult (e.g., grade IV intraventricular hemorrhage and seizure disorder), ototoxicity not detected by chart review, extracorporeal membrane oxygenation (ECMO), and "general sickness."

The 1990 Joint Committee recommendations regarding ototoxicity will have the most pronounced impact on newborn hearing screening programs in terms of screening and follow-up demands. For example, almost one-fourth of the infants in our series met this risk criterion for hearing impairment. Furthermore, for approximately 50% of these infants, ototoxicity was the only risk criterion (3% of the total number of at-risk infants). Details on specific ototoxic drugs administered to infants meeting this criterion are shown in table 7. Data were available for 25 of the 49 neonates who received one or more of the ototoxic

Table 7

Distribution of Infants Meeting 1990 Joint Committee Ototoxicity Risk Criterion for Hearing Impairment at Vanderbilt University Hospital (October 1990 to May 1991)**

Ototoxic Drug(s)	N	%*
Gentamicin only	17	68
Gentamicin + vancomycin + lasix	6	24
Gentamicin + vancomycin	1	4
Vancomycin + lasix	1	4

* Calculated from N of 25.

** A total of 49 infants met the ototoxicity risk criterion (23% of series). Among these 49 infants, 24 (49%) met no other 1990 Joint Committee risk criteria. However, data on the specific ototoxic drug(s) were available for only 25 infants.

drugs. Gentamicin is commonly administered in the NICU setting as a prophylaxis for infection. Within the ototoxicity category, most infants were receiving gentamicin (for more than five days). The six infants receiving a combination of gentamicin, lasix, and vancomycin, however, are more likely to have hearing impairment due to the synergistic effects of the drugs. Inclusion of the 1990 Joint Committee ototoxicity criterion, in summary, increases the number of infants who require screening and whose hearing should be monitored after hospital discharge, regardless of the screening outcome (pass or fail). Unfortunately, in our experience follow-up rates are lowest for this group.

CONFIRMED HEARING IMPAIRMENT AMONG AT-RISK INFANTS

Most at-risk infants do not actually have hearing impairment. Still, if it is not feasible to screen all infants, then risk factors are useful in making decisions as to which infants should be screened. The two best predictors of hearing impairment in NICU graduates, length of stay in the unit and gestational age (Halpern, Hosford-Dunn, and Malachowski 1987), are not included in Joint Committee recommendations. The two Joint Committee criteria with the highest predictive value for hearing impairment are craniofacial anomalies and TORCH infections (Hall 1992; Halpern, Hosford-Dunn, and Malachowski 1987). Statistical correlation between other risk factors, such as LBW, and hearing impairment is lacking.

We have analyzed risk factors for 18 infants with audiologically confirmed hearing impairment, unilateral and bilateral and of varying degrees (table 8). Our experiences are in general agreement with Halpern et al. (1987). LBW was the most common risk factor (occurring in one-half of the group), yet for all but two infants it was in combination with ototoxicity, asphyxia, and/or a craniofacial anomaly. One was an infant with an extended stay in the NICU or intermediate nursery (over one year) who later expired. Perinatal infection was a risk criterion for just six of our series of 769 at-risk infants (3%). Three of these infants, however, had profound hearing impairment (two unilateral and one bilateral). The infectious disease for each was cytomegalovirus (CMV). Fifty percent of this group of hearing-impaired infants were at risk for progressive hearing loss, due to either ototoxicity or CMV infection, and thus continued to require audiologic monitoring.

Table 8

Summary of Characteristics for 18 Infants at Vanderbilt University Hospital Who Were At Risk by Joint Committee Criteria (these infants failed a hearing screening and had hearing impairment confirmed at follow-up audiologic assessment)

Infant	Risk Criterion*	Hearing Status**
1	LBW; asphyxia; ototoxicity	bilateral, mild-severe, high frequency SNHL
2	asphyxia	bilateral, mild-moderate, SNHL
3	not at risk	unilateral, SNHL
4	family history; syndrome	bilateral, profound, SNHL
5	perinatal infection (CMV)	unilateral, profound, SNHL
6	perinatal infection (CMV)	unilateral, profound, SNHL
7	LBW	bilateral, mild, SNHL***
8	LBW; asphyxia; ototoxicity	bilateral, mild-moderate, SNHL
9	perinatal infection (CMV)	bilateral, profound, SNHL
10	LBW; ototoxicity	bilateral, mild-moderate, SNHL
11	not at risk (physician's order)	unilateral, profound, SNHL
12	LBW; anatomic malformation; syndrome	bilateral, mild, SNHL
13	LBW; ototoxicity	bilateral, mild, high frequency, SNHL
14	hyperbilirubinemia	auditory brainstem dysfunction
15	hyperbilirubinemia	bilateral, SNHL
16	LBW; ototoxicity; IVH	unilateral, moderate, SNHL
17	LBW; ototoxicity; IVH	unilateral, moderate, SNHL
18	LBW	bilateral, moderate, SNHL***

*   LBW = low birth weight; CMV = cytomegalovirus; IVH = intraventricular hemorrhage Grade IV.

**   SNHL = sensorineural hearing loss.

***   Infant expired.

1990 JOINT COMMITTEE CRITERIA — CLINICAL CHALLENGES

Adherence to 1990 versus 1982 Joint Committee recommendations presents two major clinical challenges. The first involves the chart review process. During the initial chart review, more time is required to verify whether or not an infant meets the asphyxia (severe depression) risk criterion. Whereas notations on Apgar scores at 1 and 5 minutes are usually quite prominent in the medical record, information on spontaneous respiration and hypotonia may not be readily apparent. Then, during the baby's hospital stay, charts must be repeatedly monitored for documentation of prolonged ventilation, a syndrome, or ototoxicity. Such information will not, of course, appear in the admission note or in progress notes for the first week of the infant's hospital stay. The increased chart review time puts an additional demand on hearing screening personnel, increases dependence on NICU staff, and heightens the need for physician and nurse education. This problem is compounded at our Hospital since the majority of at-risk neonates are back transported to another hospital where ventilation or ototoxic therapy might be continued or initiated.

The second challenge is to consistently follow infants at risk for progressive hearing impairment. Risk factors for progressive hearing loss include family history of delayed onset hearing loss, meningitis, intrauterine infections, infants with chronic lung disease, pulmonary hypertension, degenerative disease, and ototoxicity. Thus, in our experience, hearing status is often not clear at hospital discharge. Even among infants failing a hearing screening in the hospital and requiring a single audiologic assessment, follow-up rates are typically less than 50%. The logistical problems associated with follow-up are more serious for infants at risk for progressive hearing loss who passed the hearing screening yet require repeated audiologic assessments during the first year of life. We found that only 13% of these infants returned regularly for their follow-up assessments. The lack of a documented link between some of these progressive risk factors and infant hearing impairment may contribute to the low return rate.

CONCLUSIONS

The 1990 Joint Committee recommendations have now been published widely. They should immediately replace the 1982 Joint

Committee recommendations. Adherence to 1990 Joint Committee recommendations substantially increases the amount of time needed for infant chart review and will increase the number of infants identified as at risk for hearing impairment. For most of these additional infants, the risk factor is exposure to ototoxic drugs. Perhaps the major clinical implication of 1990 versus 1982 Joint Committee recommendations is the challenge of long-term monitoring of infants at risk for progressive hearing impairment.

ACKNOWLEDGMENTS

This work was funded in part by a Vanderbilt University School of Medicine NIH Biomedical Research Support Grant (RR05424-29).

REFERENCES

Colding, H., Andersen, E.A., Prytz, S., Wulffsberg, H., and Andersen, G.E. 1989. Auditory function after continuous infusion of gentamicin to high-risk newborns. *Acta Paediatrica Scandinavica* 78:840-843.

Gerkin, K.P. 1984. The high risk register for deafness. *Asha* 26:17-23.

Griffin, J.P. 1988. Drug-induced ototoxicity. *British Journal of Audiology* 22: 195-210.

Hall, J.W. III. 1992. *Handbook of auditory evoked responses*. Needham, Mass.: Allyn and Bacon.

Hall, J.W. III, Brown, D.P., and Mackey-Hargadine, J. 1985. Pediatric applications of serial auditory brainstem response measurements. *International Journal of Pediatric Otorhinolaryngology* 9:201-218.

Hall, J.W. III, Winkler, J.B., Herndon, D.N., and Gary, L.B. 1986. Auditory brainstem response in young burn wound patients treated with ototoxic drugs. *International Journal of Pediatric Otorhinolaryngology* 12:187-203.

Hall, J.W. III, Winkler, J.B., Herndon, D.N., and Gary, L.B. 1987. Auditory brainstem response in auditory assessment of acute severely burned children. *Journal of Burn Care and Rehabilitation* 8:195-198.

Halpern, J., Hosford-Dunn, H., and Malachowski, N. 1987. Four factors that accurately predict hearing loss in "high risk" neonates. *Ear and Hearing* 8:21-25.

Joint Committee on Infant Hearing. 1982. Position statement. *Ear and Hearing* 4:3-4.

Joint Committee on Infant Hearing. 1991. 1990 Position statement. *Audiology Today* 3(4):14-17.

McCracken, G.G. 1986. Aminoglycoside toxicity in infants and children. *American Journal of Medicine* 80(Suppl. 68):172-178.

Temtamy, S.A., and Miller, J.D. 1974. Extending the scope of the VATER association: Definition of a VATER syndrome. *Journal of Pediatrics* 85:345.

Chapter 11

A Model for Neonatal Hearing Screening

M. Wende Yellin and Faith C. Wurm

INTRODUCTION

With the expanded 1990 Joint Committee risk criteria (Appendix 1), more infants are at risk for hearing loss. Consequently, neonatal hearing screening programs are faced with new challenges. Programs must screen more and more infants quickly and accurately before hospital discharge and also provide these screening services at minimum costs. This paper will describe a program that is successfully meeting these challenges.

PROGRAM SETTING

Parkland Memorial Hospital (PMH) is part of the Dallas County Hospital District. Hospital policy states that no person residing in Dallas County can be denied services at Parkland. Therefore, a large number of patients with limited financial resources and/or no insurance come to PMH for medical services.

The newborn nursery at PMH is one of the largest in the country. PMH records approximately 1,300 births per month, with the majority of these infants placed in the well-baby nursery for discharge soon after birth. However, approximately 100 babies per month develop problems that require placement in the special care nursery (SCN). The SCN is divided into three units. The neonatal intensive care unit (NICU) receives infants who require close medical attention and strict monitoring to ensure their survival. The acute care nursery (ACN) receives infants who must be monitored but whose health is not so fragile. The critical care nursery (CCN) receives graduates from the NICU and ACN, and infants who require observation following birth. Most of the infants in the CCN are in stable condition but need time to mature before hospital discharge. Infants admitted to the SCN may stay for a few days or for several months, depending on the severity of their problems. The goal is to discharge healthy, thriving infants as quickly as possible.

PROGRAM DEVELOPMENT

Developing a hearing screening program at PMH was a difficult undertaking to the audiologic staff. Approximately 95% of the SCN infants meet one or more of the Joint Committee risk criteria, but financial resources support only one part-time audiologist. The hospital provided the screening program with Crib-O-Grams, assuming that a large number of infants could be quickly screened by a limited staff. Infants who failed this behavioral test were to receive threshold ABR testing. However, in this population of sick and medicated infants, approximately 50% of the infants were referred for further testing based on Crib-O-Gram outcome. Time constraints prevented threshold testing on such a large group. A successful screening program needed to be structured to accurately screen a large number of infants at risk for hearing loss in a timely manner so that follow-up services could be provided.

Table 1
Prioritization of Infants for Screening

Priority I	Birth weight ≤ 1000 grams
	IVH Grade III/IV
	Congenital acquired infection
	Family history of hearing loss
	Anatomic malformation: major CNS or external ear abnormality
	Hyperbilirubinemia to exchange level
	Meningitis
	Asphyxia
Priority II	Birth weight 1001-1250 grams
Priority III	Birth weight 1251-1500 grams
Priority IV	Birth weight 1501-2000 grams

To ensure that infants most at risk for hearing loss were screened before hospital discharge, help was solicited from the pediatric nurse practitioners (PNPs). The PNPs are familiar with every infant admitted to the nursery. A system was established for prioritizing infants for screening based on Joint Committee risk criteria (table 1). Infants who have one or more of the risk factors receive Priority I status. Infants whose birth weight is between 1001 and 1250 grams are classified as Priority II; between 1251 and 1500 grams are Priority III; between 1501 and 2000 grams are Priority IV. Although the goal of the program is to screen every infant before discharge, this prioritization was necessary because of the large number of infants involved.

Table 2
ALGO-1 Plus Parameters

Bandpass filter	5-1500 Hz
Click duration	100 μsec
Intensity	35 dB nHL
Polarity	Alternating
Click rate	37.3/sec
Analysis time	25 msec
Samples/Sweep	100

To reduce the number of babies failing the hearing screening, a more accurate screening technique was sought. Through the University of Texas Southwestern Medical Center, the SCN acquired an ALGO-1 Plus Infant Hearing Screener.[1] This equipment records the ABR of neonates and infants using a 35 dB nHL click stimulus (table 2). When signal averaging is completed, a readout of "Pass" or "Refer" and a ratio of averaged responses are provided to the tester (see Appendix 3). Using this method, referrals for further testing decreased to approximately 10%. However, many infants were discharged before screening was performed, and follow-up services were limited because of time restrictions placed on the audiologist.

To increase the number of infants being tested, staff size had to increase, but budget limitations prevented the hiring of another audiologist. Therefore, volunteers were sought to perform the infant screening. Infant screening is amenable to the schedules of most people in today's busy world—infants are in the nursery 24 hours a day, 7 days

---

[1] ALGO-1 Plus™ Infant Hearing Screener Natus Medical Incorporated, Forest City, California.

a week. The ALGO-1 Plus lends itself well to volunteers, since responses are not interpreted by the tester, and with training, a nonprofessional can become competent in performing the test. Several volunteer organizations in the Dallas community were approached. After following the application process, the Infant Hearing Program was accepted as a service project of the National Council of Jewish Women-Dallas Section (NCJW).

PROGRAM IMPLEMENTATION

To organize the volunteers for the screening program, a volunteer coordinator was appointed by NCJW. This individual's responsibilities include soliciting volunteers and coordinating schedules. The volunteer coordinator also acts as liaison to the supervising audiologist, reporting problems that may arise and providing feedback to and from the other volunteers.

With the volunteer coordinator appointed, training began. Individuals interested in participating in the Infant Screening Program attend a three-hour training workshop and receive a training manual prepared by staff audiologists. Topics covered include basic concepts of hearing, diagnosis of hearing loss, operation of screening equipment, protocols of the screening program, and guidelines of the SCN. At the conclusion of the workshop, volunteers are asked to make a commitment for a minimum of three hours, one day a week to the program. Seven volunteers are currently participating in the program.

The workshop introduces the volunteers to the testing procedures, but the audiologist's involvement does not stop there. Before a volunteer is allowed to work independently, screening is performed in the SCN under the supervision of a staff audiologist. An audiologist is also always available through either the telephone or the hospital paging system. The audiologist who directs the program meets with the volunteer liaison at least once a month to discuss problems. A newsletter is published once a month that includes the number of babies tested and identified as hearing impaired, follow-up services that have been initiated or provided to those infants with hearing loss, and helpful tips that might resolve a screening problem. At the end of each year, the audiologists have a luncheon in appreciation of the volunteers' service.

PROGRAM PROTOCOL

A structured protocol was established to guarantee that screening and follow-up services were provided in a timely manner. Volunteers screen the infants based on priority stickers located on each infant's crib card. If an infant passes the screening in both ears, a "pass" result sticker is placed in the chart. "Pass" letters that have been written in both English and Spanish are placed on the crib to notify the parents of the results (Appendix A). An auditory development chart is also provided so that parents will be aware of hearing problems that may develop following discharge. If an infant is referred by the screening, a "refer" result sticker is placed in the chart, and the need for follow-up services is indicated in two ways. First, a referral note is placed on the outside of the chart, which alerts the PNP that threshold ABR testing is needed. Second, results are recorded in a master log, which is checked daily by the nursery audiologist. This method guarantees that either the PNP or the audiologist will be aware of the screening results and the need for threshold ABR testing.

Threshold ABR testing was initially scheduled on an outpatient basis to prevent delays in hospital discharge. However, six months after the program was established, a problem became evident. Although the volunteers had screened 266 babies and referred 58 for follow-up testing, only 10 babies arrived for follow-up appointments. Poor follow-up was negating the hard work of the volunteer screeners. The protocol was, therefore, revised. Currently, babies are scheduled for threshold ABR testing before hospital discharge. Since the initiation of this procedure, 79 babies have been screened, 17 referred, and 12 evaluated with threshold ABR. Five babies were discharged before threshold ABR testing could be completed, and they have been scheduled as outpatients. We hope that these infants will return for their follow-up appointments.

DISCUSSION

Now that the program in the SCN is established, plans have been initiated to expand services to the well-baby nursery. Infants placed in this nursery are healthy, and their risk for hearing loss may be overlooked. However, many have a family history of hearing loss, malformations or abnormalities of the external ear, or short-term regimen of potentially ototoxic drugs. PNPs who are responsible for infants in the well-baby nursery will identify the infants at risk and refer them to the audiologists for screening and follow-up.

Establishing a neonatal screening program at PMH has provided a challenge to the Audiology Service. Volunteers have offered an invaluable service to the program by increasing staff size. Nursery personnel have been crucial to ensure that each infant receives the appropriate attention. Other programs faced with minimum funds and financial resources should consider enlisting volunteers. However, the audiologists must be available to provide training and guidance to non-professional support.

SUMMARY

Establishing a neonatal screening program in a large nursery can present a special challenge. Infants must be tested as soon as possible after birth to prevent any delay in their discharge, so trained personnel and reliable equipment must be consistently available. A hospital providing indigent care may be faced with additional financial limitations. The need for early identification may be recognized, but funding may make it infeasible to acquire adequate staff and equipment to establish a large-scale program in difficult economic times.

The Audiology Service at Parkland Memorial Hospital has met these challenges by incorporating the services of volunteers into its screening program. Trained volunteers screen infants so that the audiologists' time can be concentrated on diagnostic testing for the infants referred. The audiologists also will be able to initiate and perform follow-up services in a more timely manner.

Establishing a volunteer neonatal hearing screening program requires strong commitment and dedication from all involved. Incorporating volunteers has allowed our service to meet its goal of screening infants quickly and accurately before hospital discharge within the financial limitations of a county hospital.

REFERENCE

Joint Committee on Infant Hearing. 1991. 1990 position statement. *Audiology Today* 3(4):14-17.

Appendix A
Sample Letter

Dear Parent:

Your child was given a hearing screening as part of the SCN care at Parkland Hospital. We are pleased to inform you that your child passed.

This test shows us that your child can hear moderately loud sounds. You should still be aware that this test does *not* rule out:

1. A progressive hearing loss (good hearing that gets worse over time);
2. A mild hearing loss (cannot hear soft sounds);
3. Ear infections;
4. Problems understanding speech.

If you have any questions about your child's hearing now or as he gets older, please ask your pediatrician or call the audiologist at Parkland at 590-5604.

Audiologist

Estimados Padres:

Al nino(a) suyo sele ha hecho un examen del oido como parte del cuidado de la Guarderia de Cuidado Especial del Hospital Parkland. Nos da placer informarles que su nino paso la prueba.

Este examen nos dice que su nino(a) es capaz de oir sonidos moderadamente altos. Todavia debe de tomar en cuenta que esto *no* quiere decir que no puede tener los problemas signientes:

1. Buen oido que a traves del tiempo se empeorece;
2. Incapacidad de oir sonidos suaves;
3. Infecciones del oido;
4. Problemas an entender palabras.

Si tiene preguntas encuanto al oido del nino(a) ahora o despues de que tenga mas edad favor de hablarle al pediatra o al audiologo en Parkland al 590-5604.

El Audiologo

Chapter 12

Infant Hearing Screening in Ohio

Gayle Riemer and Susan Farrer

INTRODUCTION

Devastating consequences can result from failure to identify and treat hearing impairment at a very early age. A child may never reach normative language proficiency even with intensive therapy if he does not develop these skills during the first few years of life. The importance of screening for hearing impairment cannot be overestimated.

The process of identifying children with hearing disorders in Ohio often began with the physician's examination, questioning the parents, or a variety of screening procedures. But in March 1988, an act was signed into law requiring hearing screening of infants born in the state of Ohio (revised Code Sections 3701.503 through 3701.507). Although the bill was enacted in 1988, the mandated screening process did not begin until February 1990. The Bureau for Children with Medical Handicaps' Medical Advisory Board appointed a subcommittee on Infant Hearing Screening and Assessment to assist the Ohio Department of Health (ODH) in implementing the program. This subcommittee used data collected from funded statewide programs to develop the procedures and criteria for the mandated state program.

In May 1988, the permanent subcommittee began its work. It was comprised of an otolaryngologist, a neonatologist, a pediatrician, a neurologist, a hospital administrator, four audiologists, a speech pathologist, a parent of a hearing-impaired child, and a teacher of hearing-impaired children (Ohio Department of Health 1989).

THE SCREENING

The law requires a two-tiered process: (1) a high-risk questionnaire, which is referred to as the "risk screening," and (2) the "assessment" (or screening test) process. Each infant in the hospital nursery must receive a risk screening unless his parents, guardian, or custodian objects for religious reasons. The hospital completing the risk screening must promptly notify the infant's primary care physician and the ODH of the infant's and parents' names and address. The parents must be informed of the factors or conditions for suspecting a possible hearing loss. A two-page state form must be used for these reporting activities.

The parents must also be informed of the effects of such a loss on a child's language development. The ODH distributes to the hospitals free of charge the developmental checklist handouts, parent letters, and forms. Hospitals may choose to provide hearing assessments of those infants identified as at risk or furnish the parents with a list of providers. The ODH must be notified of the assessment and will provide reimbursement for it under strict guidelines.

All hospitals with newborn nurseries must provide the risk screening. The last hospital from which the child is discharged into the care of the parents, or the hospital that the child has remained in until 6 months of age, is responsible for completing the risk screening. Each hospital must use the state's two-page form and complete it appropriately. Hospitals must also designate specific individuals to ensure the forms are distributed, completed, and reviewed. Individuals reviewing the questionnaires must successfully complete the special instructions course provided by ODH. A record of the completed questionnaire must be kept in the child's medical record.

Part I of the questionnaire is to be completed by the baby's parents (table 1). In addition to the identifying information of numbers 1, 2, and 3, two questions are asked. First: "While pregnant, did the baby's mother have any of the following conditions?" The parent checks "yes" or "no" and circles any of the appropriate conditions among the following: three-day measles/German measles/rubella, chickenpox, syphilis, active herpes infection, cytomegalovirus. And second: "Have any of the baby's blood relatives had a permanent hearing loss or nerve hearing loss before they were 7 years old?" In addition to checking "yes," "no," or "unknown," there is a table of relatives and hearing

Table 1
Infant Hearing Risk Questionnaire

Part I

1) Baby's name, birthdate, and sex as appears on birth certificate
2) Mother's and father's name
3) Address where baby will be living
4) Questions of prenatal conditions and family history of hearing loss
5) Consent for release of information

Part II

1) Birthweight, gestational age, Apgars
2) Resuscitation in delivery room
3) Prenatal illness of mother
4) Defects of head and neck
5) Meningitis
6) High bilirubin level, exchange transfusion
7) Conditions associated with hearing loss

---

history questions to complete. The parents are also asked for the name and address of the doctor or clinic where they will be taking the baby for checkups and medical care. The consent for release of information is so that the ODH can send information on the screening form to persons or agencies that participate in the assessment program.

Part II of the questionnaire is to be filled out by someone working at the hospital (table 1). There is considerable latitude as to who will have this responsibility, but hopefully, hospitals choose someone who is familiar with the baby and is able to interpret abbreviations and handwriting in the baby's records. This part of the form appears straightforward at first glance, but there is growing controversy over the intent of some categories. Resuscitation in the delivery room is particularly subject to interpretation. Number 7 in Part II is an open-ended category. It states that the "health care management team deems the infant to be at risk for hearing impairment because of the following condition(s) or suspected condition(s): treatment with aminoglycosides, neonatal sepsis, parental consanguinity, persistent pulmonary hypertension, bronchopulmonary dysplasia, result of high-risk pregnancy, syndrome associated with hearing impairment, and other."

Table 2
High-Risk Criteria

---

1) Asphyxia, 1 minute Apgar 0-3 or 5 minute Apgar 0-5 or resuscitation in delivery room
2) Meningitis
3) Congenital perinatal infection
4) Defect of the head and neck
5) Elevated bilirubin (exchange transfusion or indirect level exceeding 20 mg/dl)
6) Family history of childhood hearing loss
7) Birth weight less than 1500 grams
8) Conditions deemed by health care management team to place infant at risk

---

Interpretation of the data on the screening questionnaire is relative to the high-risk criteria listed in table 2. The definition of resuscitation has proven to be the biggest problem. For example, in a number of hospitals, resuscitation is done to some extent in all C-section births. The ODH is reviewing this factor and will be issuing more specific criteria. The ODH has listed syndromes that should be included as placing an infant at risk for hearing loss (table 3). Since many syndromes may not be identified prior to the completion of the screening questionnaire, pediatricians are urged to be suspicious of any possible syndrome as placing a child at risk for hearing loss and further investigate the implications of hearing involvement.

Table 3
Syndromes Associated with Hearing Loss

Achondroplasia	Long Arm 18 Delet. Syndrome
Apert's Syndrome	Madelung's Deformity
CHARGE Association	Marfan's Syndrome
Cleidocranial Dysostosis	Mohr Syndrome
Crouzon's Syndrome	Osteogenesis Imperfecta
Down's Syndrome	Pierre Robin Syndrome
Duane's Syndrome	Pyle's Disease
Hallgren's Syndrome	Treacher Collins Syndrome
Hand-Hearing Syndrome	Trisomy 13-15
Goldenhar's Syndrome	Trisomy 18
Klippel-Feil Syndrome	Waardenburg's Syndrome

(ODH 1989)

THE ASSESSMENT

The law states that assessments can be provided only by an Ohio licensed audiologist, board-certified otolaryngologist, or board-certified neurologist. Hospitals can decide whether or not to provide assessments but cannot discriminate on which infants they will do the assessment. Hospitals must assess either all infants or none. The screening test method used must identify failure to respond consistently to signals presented to each ear at 35 dB HL in the frequency range of 1000 to 4000 Hz.

The assessment portion of the state screening program also has a specific form that must be completed and distributed to the ODH, primary care physicians, parent, and medical record. In addition to the patient's identifying information, the reasons for the assessment are checked or written in. The test procedure used, either behavioral audiometry or auditory brainstem response (ABR), and the consistency of the response at 35 dB HL are noted. If the baby does not pass, recommendation for retesting, referral for further evaluation, or the "other" (with a description) must be made. The provider information at the bottom of the form is a cross-check with the state's list of providers and informs the parent and primary care physician of the provider in case there are any questions.

Two methods have been recognized for the assessment part of the program: behavioral observation audiometry and ABR. There are two obvious problems with the behavioral method. First, newborns do not normally respond to sounds at 35 dB HL. Also, it is difficult to keep earphones appropriately placed on an awake newborn. Each of the two programs using the behavioral technique in Ohio has two audiologists and conducts testing in sound-treated rooms. This is expensive and time consuming.

ABR screening is the method recommended by the 1990 Joint Committee on Infant Hearing (Appendix 1). Expense of equipment is one obvious drawback of ABR. The baby's neurologic status plays a significant part in the ABR screening process, but failure for this reason is acceptable since it can indicate a central nervous system auditory disorder. ABR screening has been effective only when the infant is asleep. The accuracy of this test method, however, outweighs its drawbacks (see Appendix 3).

The ALGO-1[1] Infant Hearing Screener was selected for the assessment tool. This unit uses a template matching detection algorithm to determine the presence of an ABR (Appendix 3). The design of the template is based on the morphology of a normal, near-threshold infant ABR. There are nine data points weighted according to their relative contribution to the identification of a response. Wave V and the trailing negative voltage trough are weighted relatively high. This template shifts in 0.25 msec steps across a 3 msec range, searching for the best fit. If the likelihood ratio reaches 160, there is a response at the 99.8% level of confidence. If the likelihood ratio does not reach 160 in 15,000 sweeps, data collected are not statistically different from a no-response condition at better than 99.8% level of confidence (Kileny 1988).

At Children's Hospital Medical Center, if the baby passes the paper screen, no follow-up testing is recommended. If the baby fails, the next step is the ABR screen. Again, if the baby passes, the assessment forms are mailed out, and no further testing is recommended. Failing the ABR screen, however, means the next step is a complete diagnostic ABR including threshold testing using broadband clicks, and 500 Hz and 4000 Hz tone pips. Babies who pass this portion of the assessment receive recommendations specific to the reason for referral. For example, babies with meningitis are retested six months later. Babies who fail the diagnostic ABR are channeled through our regular procedures for newly identified hearing-impaired children.

RESULTS

Children's Hospital Medical Center is a nonmaternity hospital. Babies in the newborn intensive care unit are the only ones to receive the paper screen. Other infants admitted to the Children's Hospital Medical Center had been previously discharged to home prior to their readmission to Children's. Over the calendar years 1989 and 1990, 1,270 babies had the paper screen. As a result of this paper screen, 591 babies were referred for the ABR screen (figure 1). Of those 591, 100 babies failed the ABR screen and were referred for a diagnostic ABR.

---

[1]ALGO-1™ Infant Hearing Screener Natus Medical Incorporated, Forest City, California.

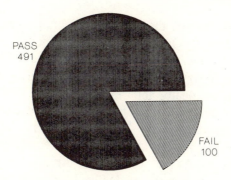

Figure 1. Distribution of results from the ABR screen. Results are based on a sample of 591 babies.

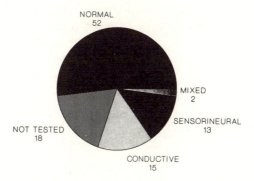

Figure 2. A full diagnostic ABR was recommended for 100 babies. The distribution of diagnostic test results is illustrated in this figure.

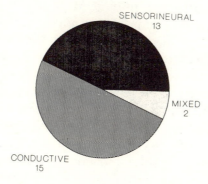

Figure 3. In this study, 30 babies were identified as having hearing loss by diagnostic ABR. The distribution of type of hearing loss is illustrated in this figure.

There were 100 babies, then, for whom a full diagnostic ABR was recommended (figure 2). Of that number, roughly half (52) had normal hearing. Many had waveforms that apparently were not accepted by the ALGO-1 template. In some cases, the reason for failing the ABR screen was clearly a neurologically abnormal ABR, with hearing sensitivity estimated as within normal limits. Thirty babies were identified as having hearing loss on the diagnostic ABR (figure 3). An equal number of babies had conductive hearing loss (15) as had combined sensorineural and mixed losses (15). At the beginning of this screening program, we suspected that large numbers of conductive hearing losses due to middle ear involvement would be identified. In fact, 15 babies in two years is surprisingly low. Eighteen of the 100 babies did not have the diagnostic ABR at Children's. Of those 18 who were not tested, 5 were completely lost to follow-up. The other 13 had multiple broken appointments, were tested at another facility, or had behavioral testing instead (at their physician's request).

In summary, 30% of the infants referred for diagnostic testing had hearing losses, and only 15 of them were sensorineural or mixed. The sensorineural losses were almost equally divided between bilateral (8) and unilateral (7) losses.

DISCUSSION

Our screening process began with 1,270 infants and ultimately identified 15 with significant hearing losses. Although the number may appear small, the 15 infants may have otherwise gone unidentified for a devastatingly significant length of time. Medical staff pediatricians are encouraged to review state forms and confirm that the information is correct. If additional risk factors are identified, further action should be taken to have the infant screened before 6 months of age. Risk screening still misses a large number of congenitally hearing-impaired children. The most common cause of congenital hearing impairment (40% of the hearing-impaired children followed at Children's Hospital Medical Center) is genetic deafness of autosomal recessive origin. If the parents are unaware of the genetic risk, children with such hearing impairments are cleared by a high-risk register. Monitoring of auditory behaviors and speech development in each child is recommended as part of the well-baby checkup.

SUMMARY

In order to comply with Ohio law (revised Code Sections 3701.503 through 3701.507), Children's Hospital began a new infant hearing screening and assessment program in 1989. A total of 1,270 infants were reviewed over a two-year period with 591 of them referred for auditory brainstem response screening. Of those 591, 100 failed the screening and were referred for diagnostic evoked potential testing. The end result of this two-year screening process was the identification of 30 hearing-impaired infants. Only 15 of them had significant sensorineural hearing losses.

Although this statewide assessment program is still in its formative years, it is already fulfilling its goal of early identification. Children's Hospital has fully implemented the screening and assessment protocols and identified 15 hearing-impaired newborns in a two-year period. These children have the unquestioned advantage of early amplification and a head start on speech and language acquisition.

REFERENCES

Kileny, P.R. 1988. New insights on infant ABR hearing screening. *Scandinavian Audiology* Suppl. 30:81-88.

Ohio Department of Health (ODH). 1989. *Infant hearing screening and assessment program manual.*

Ohio Revised Code Sections 3701.503 through 3701.507.

Chapter 13

Orienting as a Means of Assessing Hearing in Newly Born Infants

Richard S. Bernstein and Judith S. Gravel

INTRODUCTION

This chapter will describe our efforts toward the development of a behavioral examination of the hearing of newly born infants. Overt (i.e., behavioral) responses to sound may be affected by the integrity of both peripheral and central functions. Thus, an examination based on behavior is, in principle, capable of identifying infants with either peripheral or central auditory dysfunctions. By their nature, behavioral techniques complement peripheral assessments based on recordings of evoked brainstem responses and otoacoustic emissions.

CHOICE OF BEHAVIOR

Three interrelated factors must be considered in the design of a behavioral assessment technique. The behavior, the method to monitor the behavior, and the eliciting stimulus must be chosen so as to yield a valid and sensitive indicator of clinically significant dysfunction. Because newborns spend the majority of their time sleeping, there have been several attempts at assessing hearing by examining the ability of sounds to arouse or startle an infant. Procedures have been developed using both human (e.g., Downs and Hemenway 1969; Mencher 1976) and automated (Simmons 1977; Bennett 1979) observers. These procedures have been criticized because of an insensitivity to less than severe deficits and because of high rates of identifying normal hearing infants as being impaired (Durieux-Smith et al. 1987).

We have chosen a different approach. Newborns are capable of being awake, quiet, and alert. Although in this state for only short periods of time, newborns exhibit a remarkable range of organized behaviors and are responsive to both visual and auditory stimulation. If an object is moved from one side to the other, an alert infant will often follow the object with his or her eyes. Similarly, if a sound is played from one side, an alert infant will often attempt to turn (orient) toward the sound (Muir and Field 1979). Because of the high degree of organization inherent in visual and auditory orienting, these behaviors are included in several neurobehavioral examinations of newborns (Brazelton 1973; McCarton-Daum et al. 1977).

An infant that orients to sound demonstrates, at a minimum, the capability to detect the presence of the sound and determine its location as well as sufficient sensory/motor integration to permit an attempt at seeing the sound source. Dysfunction in any process underlying these capabilities should disrupt orienting. There is some evidence that poor orienting ability is related to newborns having neurobehavioral deficits (Kurtzburg et al. 1979) and later impaired cognitive and linguistic function (Wallace et al. 1982). Properly exploited, orienting seems to be a behavior well suited for an examination of auditory system integrity.

MONITORING OF BEHAVIOR

An observer faced with the task of determining if a newborn infant can hear must somehow decide if the baby is responding or not. Newborn infants tend to perform certain behaviors as a consequence of sound being presented (e.g., eye and head movements) and have a lesser tendency to perform the same behaviors in the absence of an eliciting sound. Presentation of the same sound repeatedly may elicit a variety of responses. Signal Detection Theory (Green and Swets 1974) provides a framework for test-structure and data analysis of binary decisions based on variable information. Accordingly, two types of trials are used; the eliciting sound is presented on test-trials and is omitted on catch-trials. Observers are required to decide, on each trial, whether or not the eliciting sound was presented. Decisions are to be based solely on the observation of infants' behaviors. If decisions about responses are congruent with the sequence of trials, the infant is regarded as having responded to sound. The amount of congruence between the examiner's judgments and trial type is indicative of the robustness of responses.

THE ELICITING STIMULUS

The final factor that must be considered is the choice of stimulus used to elicit responding. Although orienting responsivity is known to vary with stimulus parameters (Clarkson et al. 1991), characteristics that yield best-responding have yet to be determined. Thus, we regard the choice of stimulus as an empirical issue. Neurobehavioral evaluations of orienting have used eliciting sounds (e.g., speech, rattle, bell) with energy at both low and high frequencies. Since hearing loss most often includes the high frequencies, these are not optimal for audiometric purposes. Eisenberg (1976) has noted that awake and alert newborns are most responsive to natural speech and to patterned (i.e., time-varying) acoustic stimulation. Several studies have shown that infants are best aroused by complex sounds (e.g., Bench and Mentz 1975; Gerber and Mencher 1979; Gerber and Dobkin 1984). Based on these considerations, we are evaluating two types of time-varying (patterned) sounds restricted to the high frequencies and broadband natural speech as elicitors.

METHOD

SUBJECTS

Healthy newborn infants between 1 and 3 days old were recruited from the well-baby nursery of an affiliated hospital. Selection criteria included uncomplicated antenatal course, full-term gestation, uneventful labor, vaginal delivery, Apgar score of 8 or above at 1 and 5 minutes, and the absence of neonatal complications.

APPARATUS

The goal is the development of a practical means to identify newborns with auditory disorders in the nursery. The technique must therefore be compatible with the activity of an inner-city hospital. Nurseries are hostile places for hearing evaluations. It became apparent during pilot work that testing must be performed in a well-controlled environment. The test apparatus had to be transportable since permanent test space was not available. We developed an enclosure that has been dubbed the NEST—an acronym for Neonatal Environment for Sensitivity Testing.

The NEST was designed to provide a controlled auditory and visual environment. Since echo-suppression mechanisms are not operative in newborns (Clifton et al. 1984), the NEST is lined with 3" acoustic foam (Sonex) to minimize echoes. Loudspeakers are mounted on two walls of the NEST at the level of the head of the baby. Provisions have been made to support the infant on a (slightly) inclined mattress and to image the infant's head with a closed circuit television (CCTV). The NEST and necessary electronics are mounted on a laboratory cart for portability.

PROCEDURE

Awake and alert infants were placed semisupine on a mattress in the NEST facing a back-illuminated bull's-eye (see figure 1). The observer

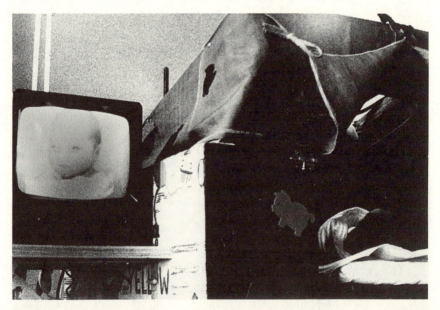

Figure 1. An awake and alert infant placed semisupine in the NEST. A trial is initiated by the examiner when the infant is gazing upward at a back-illuminating bull's-eye target. A quasi-random sequence is used to determine type of trial (test or catch) and side of presentation (left or right). The "deafened" examiner monitors the infant's head with a closed circuit TV. On each trial the examiner (based on only the infant's behavior) judges whether or not the eliciting sound was presented. Testing continues until the infant's awake and alert state cannot be maintained.

initiated a trial when the infant was in the proper state and gazing at the bull's-eye. When a trial was initiated, one of three events occurred: (1) the elicitor was presented from the left; (2) the elicitor was presented from the right; or (3) the elicitor was omitted. On 60% of the trials (test-trials), the eliciting sound was presented for 12 seconds (Clarkson et al. 1985) at the appropriate level. On the other 40% of the trials (catch-trials), the eliciting stimulus was omitted. Trial type was chosen at random with the constraint that no more than two catch-trials occurred in succession.

Based on the behavior of the baby, the examiner decided whether the eliciting sound was presented and was given immediate feedback. On both test- and catch-trials, the examiner heard the elicitor binaurally (through headphones) to ensure that decisions were based only on the behavior of the baby. Having the examiner initiate the trial, marking every observation interval with the test sound, and providing immediate performance feedback were intended to maximize the ability of the observer to detect responses by reducing observer uncertainty. When necessary, an assistant adjusted the infant's position and manipulated the infant in order to maintain the appropriate state. Testing continued until the awake and alert state could no longer be obtained. Typically, 15 to 20 trials were obtained in a 15-minute session.

RESULTS AND DISCUSSION

Following the nomenclature of Signal Detection Theory, the cluster of behaviors emitted in response to sound is referred to as the signal (sn-). Neonatal responses to sound always occur in the presence of ongoing activity, which is uncorrelated with the presentation of sound and may include some or all components of the signal. Again following Detection Theory nomenclature, this background activity is referred to as noise (n-). Each opportunity to classify an observation is defined as a trial. Trials were classified as either response present (sn-trial) or response absent (n-trial). Judgments were made for trials in which the sound was presented (test-trials) and also for trials with the elicitor omitted (catch-trials).

To evaluate performance we compute (1) the probability of classifying a trial as an sn-trial given the sound was presented and (2) the probability of classifying a trial as an sn-trial given the sound was omitted. The two conditional probabilities, p(sn-trial | test-trial) and p(sn-trial│catch-trial), are known as the hit and the false alarm rate, respectively. For each eliciting sound, the hit rate is plotted against the false alarm rate to form a Receiver Operation Characteristic (ROC). Each point represents the data from an individual infant.

According to Signal Detection Theory, points falling along the negative diagonal represent chance performance. The hit rate equals the false alarm rate. Points above the chance line represent detectable responses. Figure 2 (left panel) displays the results obtained from healthy newborn infants presented with the "spectrally patterned" elicitor. The eliciting sound was presented at 70 dB SPL and consisted of a tone whose frequency was modulated sinusoidally between 1500 and 4000 Hz. The rate of modulation was 10 Hz. All infants yielded points above the chance diagonal. Figure 3 (left panel) displays results obtained with the same stimulus presented at 80 dB SPL. Inspection reveals that all 7 infants yielded points above the chance line.

A single parameter detectability score (d') may be obtained by transforming the hit and false alarm rates to standard scores (z-scores) and computing the difference (i.e., $d' = z[p(hit)] - z[p(false\ alarm)]$). A d' value of 0 indicates that the observer could not discriminate test-trials from catch-trials. Detectable responses to sound will yield values of $d' > 0$. The right panels of figures 2 and 3 present histograms of d' values

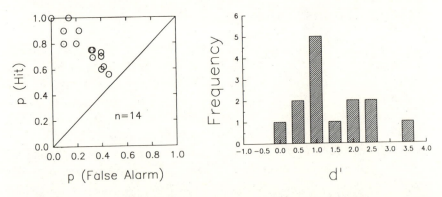

Figure 2. Data from 14 infants obtained using spectrally patterned elicitor presented at 70 dB SPL. On the left are plotted the hit and false alarm rates yielded by each infant to form a Receiver Operation Characteristic (ROC) curve. Points falling along the negative diagonal represent chance performance. Detectable responses yield points above the chance line. Greater detectabilities yield points closer to the left-hand corner of the ROC. Hit and false alarm rates from each infant were used to calculate response detectability. A histogram of d's is presented on the right.

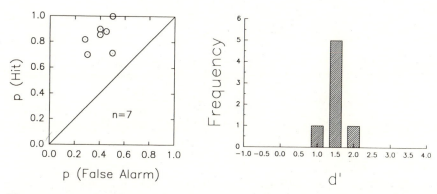

Figure 3. Data from 7 infants using the spectrally patterned sound presented at 80 dB SPL. (See figure 2 for detail).

yielded by each presentation level. Because data were collected while our method was evolving and because only small numbers of infants were tested, we must be cautious in comparing these data sets. Nevertheless, inspection of the ROCs and histograms above suggests that orienting detectability depends on the presentation level of the elicitor. Infants respond more robustly to the louder stimulus.

Figure 4 presents data from the 26 infants tested with a "temporally patterned" stimulus presented at 80 dB SPL. The stimulus was generated by amplitude modulating a bandlimited noise. The lower and upper bandlimits were 1500 and 4000 Hz, respectively. All but one infant yielded points above the chance line.

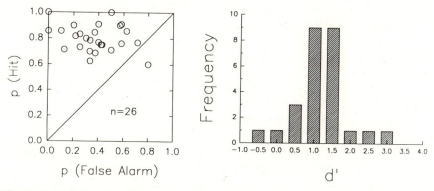

Figure 4. Data from 26 infants using a temporally patterned sound presented at 80 dB SPL. (See figure 2 for detail).

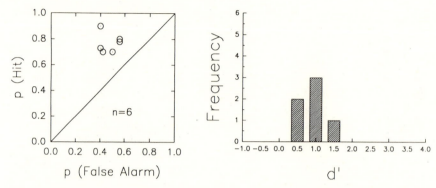

Figure 5. Data from 6 infants using a sample of recorded speech presented at 75 dB SPL. (See figure 2 for detail).

Figure 5 presents data obtained with a sample of natural speech serving as the elicitor. A short phrase was recorded and was presented at 75 dB SPL. All infants yielded points above the chance diagonal. The type of stimulus (spectrally, temporally patterned, or speech) does not seem to exert a strong influence.

The vast majority of healthy infants tested to date have yielded points above the chance line. This encourages us to continue developing this method. However, much work needs to be done. We are expanding testing to include at-risk infants and are arranging for longitudinal assessments of hearing, cognition, and language development so that we may examine the extent that early orienting responsivity is associated with later clinically significant dysfunction. It is our hope that measures of early orienting ability may provide useful information about the integrity of the auditory system and aid in the detection of infants at risk for communication disorders.

Summary

This chapter has described our efforts toward the development of a behavioral assessment technique suitable for administration prior to discharge from the nursery. According to our analysis, the design of a behavior-based evaluation requires decisions involving three major factors, namely: (1) the behavior to be monitored; (2) the method to monitor the behavior; and (3) the stimulus to elicit the behavior.

We have chosen to evaluate the robustness of auditory orienting. Orienting is a highly organized behavior, which should be disrupted by peripheral and also by central dysfunctions. Thus, orienting seems to be a behavior well suited for evaluating auditory system integrity. Since a newborn's responses to sound are variable, we scale responsivity with measures derived from Signal Detection Theory. Currently, we are investigating the use of several different classes of stimuli as elicitors. To date, we have observed responding to a sample of natural speech and to "patterned" stimuli bandlimited to the high frequencies. Although much work needs to be done, the findings thus far suggest that evaluations of orienting may be useful for the early detection of auditory dysfunction.

ACKNOWLEDGMENTS

We would like to express gratitude to Dr. Robin Cooper for generously sharing her expertise in testing newborn infants, and for the many hours spent observing orienting responses during a feasibility study. This work has been supported by a grant from the Deafness Research Foundation.

REFERENCES

Bench, J., and Mentz, L. 1975. Stimulus complexity, state and infants' auditory behavioral responses. *British Journal of Disorders of Communication* 10:52-60.

Bennett, M.J. 1979. Trials with the auditory response cradle; 1. Neonatal responses to auditory stimuli. *British Journal of Audiology* 13:125.

Brazelton, T.B. 1973. *Neonatal behavioral assessment scale. Clinics in developmental medicine, no. 50.* London: S.I.M.P. with Heinemann Medical; Philadelphia: J.B. Lippincott.

Clarkson, M.G., Clifton, R.K., and Morrongiello, B.A. 1985. The effects of sound duration on newborns' head orientation. *Journal of Experimental Child Psychology* 39:20-39.

Clarkson, M.G., Swain, I.U., Clifton, R.K., and Cohen, K. 1991. Newborns' head orientation towards trains of brief sounds. *Journal of the Acoustical Society of America* 89(5):2411-2420.

Clifton, R., Morrongiello, B., and Dowd, J. 1984. A developmental look at an auditory illusion: The precedence effect. *Developmental Psychobiology* 17:519-536.

Downs, M., and Hemenway, W.G. 1969. Report on the hearing screening of 17,000 neonates. *International Audiology* 8:72-76.

Durieux-Smith, A., Picton, T.W., Edwards, C.G., MacMurray, B., and Goodman, J.T. 1987. Brainstem electric-response audiometry in infants of a neonatal intensive care unit. *Audiology* 26:284-297.

Eisenberg, R.B. 1976. *Auditory competence in early life*. Baltimore: University Park Press.

Gerber, S.E., and Mencher, G.T. 1979. *Arousal responses of neonates to wide band and narrow band noise*. Paper presented at the convention of the American Speech-Language-Hearing Association, Atlanta, Ga.

Gerber, S.E., and Dobkin, M.S. 1984. The effect of noise bandwidth on the auditory arousal response of neonates. *Ear and Hearing* 5:195-198.

Green, D.M., and Swets, J.A. 1974. *Signal detection theory and psychophysics*. New York: Kreiger Press.

Kurtzberg, D., Vaughan, H.G., Jr., McCarton-Daum, C.M., Grellong, B.A., Albin, S., and Rotkin, L. 1979. Neurobehavioral performance of low birth weight infants at 40 weeks conceptional age: Comparison with normal full term infants. *Developmental Medicine and Child Neurology* 21:590-607.

McCarton-Daum, C.M., Grellong, B., Kurtzberg, D., et al. 1977. *Einstein neonatal neurobehavioral assessment scale*. Unpublished manuscript.

Mencher, G.T. 1976. On beyond the cochlea: Auditory perceptual disorder. In G.T. Mencher (ed.), *Early identification of hearing loss* (pp.1-13). Basel, Switzerland: Karger AG.

Muir, D., and Field, J. 1979. Newborn infants orient to sounds. *Child Development* 50:431-436.

Simmons, F.B. 1977. Automated screening test for newborns: The Crib-O-Gram. In B.J. Jaffe, (ed.), *Hearing loss in children* (pp. 87-98). Baltimore: University Park Press.

Wallace, I.F., Escalona, S.K., McCarton-Daum, C.M., and Vaughan, H.G. 1982. Neonatal precursors of cognitive development in low birth weight children. *Seminars in Perinatalogy* 6:327-333.

Chapter 14

Otoacoustic Hearing Screening in Newborns: Optimization

G. Salomon, B. Anthonisen, J. Groth, and P.P. Thomsen

INTRODUCTION

Increased awareness of the impact of even moderate hearing impairment on a child's development of speech and language, cognitive and social skills has motivated investigators to devise better methods of identifying hearing impairment at as early an age as possible. It is commonly believed that the earlier a hearing impairment is identified and habilitation begun, the better are the chances for normal development of the aforementioned skills.

In Denmark, 96% of births occur in hospitals, where the ensuing length of stay ranges from one to six days. Furthermore, the population is quite stable, which affords a unique opportunity for establishing a newborn hearing screening and follow-up program. The basic aim of the investigation presently under way is to develop an automated hearing screening procedure based on evoked otoacoustic emissions (EOAE) (Johnsen et al. 1983; Elberling et al. 1985; Kemp et al. 1986; Bray and Kemp 1987; Bonfils et al. 1988; Stevens et al. 1991) and to evaluate the possibility of the screening being performed by a nonprofessional but trained individual (Vohr et al. 1990).

One consideration of such a screening procedure is how long postnatally the screening should take place. Results from other investigations (Vohr et al. 1990; Hogan and Callaghan 1990; Kok et al. 1990) indicate that the specificity of EOAE as a screening instrument may be lacking when the procedure is performed during the first postnatal day. It has been speculated that this may be due to a lack of ventilation of the middle ear during the first day of life (Kok et al. 1990; Kemp et al. 1990).

This chapter deals with the biologic findings of a pilot study focusing on the optimal time and stimulus parameters for the screening. Specifically, the relationship between middle ear conditions and presence of EOAE are examined.

METHOD

SUBJECTS

Subjects were 209 infants ranging from 8 hours to 8 days in age.[1] The subjects were neither selected for nor excluded from participation on the basis of any established criteria. Rather, all consecutively born babies at the hospital where the study was conducted were included when it was possible to secure parental consent. It should be noted, however, that because this hospital has only a well-baby nursery, no neonatal intensive care unit (NICU) babies were included in the present investigation.

INSTRUMENTATION AND STIMULI

The probe used in this study was constructed with a miniature microphone (Knowles EA 1843) and an earphone (Knowles BK 1615) as described by Johnsen and Elberling (1982). The acoustic stimulus was a click of 250 μs (10^{-6}sec) in duration. Synchronization of stimulus generation and data recording were accomplished by an IBM compatible PC. The signals from the microphone were sampled at 20 kHz in a time window beginning simultaneously with the stimulus presentation and lasting 26 msec. In the time frame from 0 to 3.5 msec poststimulus, the signal was kept at a constant level to avoid overloading of the filtering and amplification system.

Two times 1000 sweeps were averaged in the computer following appropriate amplification and bandpass filtering (500 Hz/6 dB per octave, 5 KHz/24 dB per octave). Fixed artifact rejection was implemented in the computer along with a rejection based on the magnitude of the control tone, which should have indicated whether the volume of the cavity sealed by the probe was probable for neonate ears.

---

[1] One subject included in the present study was 7½ weeks of age at the time of testing.

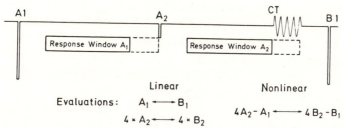

Figure 1. Illustrates a stimulus cycle, subtraction procedure for determining the nonlinear component of the response and comparisons made in evaluating responses. A and B refer to the averaged signal of the two groups of 1000 stimulus cycles presented. 1 and 2 refer to the click stimuli where 1 (69 dB pe SPL) is four times more intense than 2. CT refers to the control tone. In evaluating whether or not a response was present, a reproducible waveform meeting the established criteria for visual scoring must have been identifiable in at least one of the comparisons.

The click-evoked otoacoustic emissions were elicited using a stimulus pattern as shown in figure 1. One stimulus cycle had a duration of approximately 120 ms. A click of approximately 69 dB pe SPL (measured in a Zwislocki coupler) was delivered, and after a 26 msec pause, a four times less intense stimulus with the same polarity was presented. The less intense stimulus was followed by presentation of a control tone of approximately the same intensity as a large magnitude otoacoustic emission (i.e., 35 dB SPL RMS) to check for correct placement of the probe. After 7 msec, this sequence of stimuli was repeated. One thousand stimulus cycles were presented twice, resulting in two averaged responses, which we have called the A-buffer and B-buffer. In each buffer, three waveforms were displayed: two representing responses to the two different intensity stimuli, and a third representing the nonlinear components of the signal. This final average was arrived at using a subtraction procedure similar to that described by Kemp and his colleagues (Kemp et al. 1986).

PROCEDURE

Testing was performed in a quiet but not sound-treated room with the infants lying in open cradles. The intention was to screen for presence of EOAE and to perform tympanometry on each infant three times. The first screening was to take place during the first postnatal day, the second between 24 and 48 hours of age, and the final screening after the infant was older than 48 hours. Independent visual judgments of the data were performed by two of the authors (BA and JG) according to the following procedure. Each of the averaged response signals representing both the linear and the nonlinear elements of the response in the A-buffer was compared to the corresponding signals in the B-buffer (see figure 1). The presence of one "match" between A1 versus B1, A2 versus B2, or A3 versus B3 was deemed sufficient to determine that an EOAE was present. A "match" was judged when at least one of the following criteria was met:

1. Presence of a sinus-shaped configuration consisting of three sequential peaks and three troughs appearing either after the exponential ringing of the stimulus had ceased or clearly distinguishable from the ringing (figure 2).

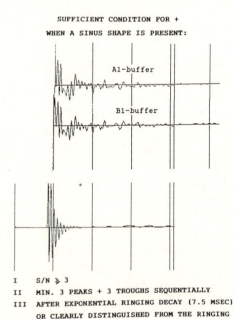

I   S/N ≥ 3
II   MIN. 3 PEAKS + 3 TROUGHS SEQUENTIALLY
III   AFTER EXPONENTIAL RINGING DECAY (7.5 MSEC)
     OR CLEARLY DISTINGUISHED FROM THE RINGING

Figure 2. Example of a signal meeting the sinus-shaped configuration criteria (see text). The bottom curve is an example of ringing of the stimulus and would not be interpreted as a response.

SUFFICIENT CONDITION FOR + WHEN A PATTERN (A MIX OF
FREQUENCIES MOSTLY LOW) IS PRESENT

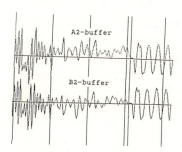

I THE PATTERN MUST BE CLEARLY PRESENT THROUGHOUT
10 MSEC.

II OBVIOUS ARTIFACTS MUST BE REJECTED
(EXAMPLE: A_1 ⟷ B_1 OK
A_1 ⟷ A_2: NO RESEMBLANCE)

Figure 3. Example of a signal fulfilling the criteria (see text) for judging that a response is present based on identification of a reproducible waveform.

NONLINEAR RESPONSES

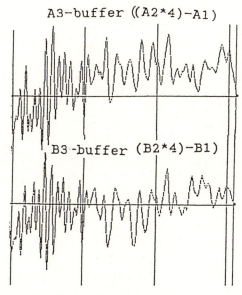

Figure 4. Example of a signal where both a sinus-shaped configuration and an identifiable pattern in the waveform are present.

2. Presence of a pattern with a duration of at least 10 msec consisting of a mixture of high and low frequencies clearly not attributable to artifact (figure 3). For example, artifact appeared to be responsible in the case where a match was judged to be present between A1 and B1, but no resemblance could be observed between A1 and A2.

A further criterion for all responses was that the signal-to-noise ratio was at least 3:1. Frequently, as illustrated in figure 4, both a sinus-shaped configuration and a pattern of at least 10 msec in duration could be identified.

Fourteen trials in which no stimulus had been present were randomly distributed among the tests to be judged. Furthermore, no information pertaining to subject age at time of testing or stimulus conditions was available to the examiners during the judgment task.

RESULTS

SUBJECT ATTRITION

Due to practical problems including a limited time period in which to perform the examinations each day and scheduling conflicts, not to mention fussy babies, it was seldom possible to complete the screening

Table 1

Examples of the Evoked Otoacoustic Emissions (EOAE) and Tympanometry Results Obtained for the Individual Infants

Patient Number	Age (hours)											
	8-24				24-48				>48			
	OAE		TYMP (MM)		OAE		TYMP (MM)		OAE		TYMP (MM)	
	R	L	R	L	R	L	R	L	R	L	R	L
83	−	−	0	+75		+		0	+	+	+25	0
79	−	−	0	+25	+	−	0	0				
67									+	+		−200
77	−	−	50	0	−				+			
34					+	+		−100				

OAE: Otoacoustic emission, + indicates OAE, − indicates no OAE, No entry: not tested, R: right ear, L: left ear, TYMP: middle ear pressure.

of all subjects on three consecutive days. Screening for EOAE and tympanometry was performed on the three consecutive days for only seven infants. Table 1 shows examples of the results obtained for the individual infants. For instance, the full test protocol was completed on all three days with subject 83, whereas the next subject had results from only the first two days, and the next from only the third day of life. Subsequently, the data have been pooled, and group trends have been examined in the present study.

RELIABILITY OF VISUAL INSPECTION

It was possible to evaluate 403 measurements from 346 different ears. Data were discarded as "unjudgeable" when a high artifact rejection rate resulted in less than 1000 stimulus cycle sweeps in each buffer and a clear response was not readily identifiable. Data were also discarded when poor probe fit was suspected based on a control tone that was extremely large and only a long-lasting ringing of the stimulus could be identified in the averaged signal. Such a control tone was interpreted as an indication that the probe was obstructed or that it was directed toward the wall of the ear canal—in other words, that it was not coupled ideally with the tympanic membrane. Another indication of poor probe fit that resulted in the data being discarded was an extremely small control tone, that was seen when there was a lack of a good seal or when the probe had fallen out of the ear canal.

In addition to the criteria for visual scoring described previously, a global evaluation based on identification of a reproducible response pattern was included in assessing the data. This allowed us to include several measurements in which, although the response appeared clear-cut, the signal-to-noise ratio and/or duration requirements were not fulfilled.

The 403 measurements (which include the no stimulus trials) were independently scored with identical results by the two investigators in 90% of the total cases. Interexaminer agreement was 100% in judging "no response" when no stimulus had been presented. Subsequent to a joint review of the measurements that had been scored differently by the two examiners, concurrence on the presence or absence of a response was attained in all but 1% of the total cases. In these ambiguous cases, another of the investigators (GS) made the final decision regarding presence or absence of a response. All of these cases were judged as not showing a response.

SCREENING RESULTS

Presence of EOAE

Table 2 shows the results obtained from 346 ears: 28 ears were tested within the first 24 hours of life, 96 ears between 24 and 48 hours, and 265 ears after 48 hours. No EOAE was identifiable in 43% (n=12) of ears tested during the first 24 hours postnatally. It was not possible to elicit EOAE from 15% (n=14) of ears tested during the second day of life and from 14% (n=38) of ears tested after 48 hours postnatally. Overall, EOAE was never observed in any of the measurements in 14% (n=50) of all ears tested.

Three ears were tested only during the first 24 hours postnatally. Our results strongly suggest that, had these ears been retested later, a response would likely have been present. If these 3 ears are excluded, the total percentage of ears tested in which a response was never obtained drops to 13.7% (47 of 343 different ears).

The criterion for passing the screening was established to be the presence of EOAE in at least one ear. Table 3 shows the positive screening results in infants in the present study. No response bilaterally constituted a positive screening. Of the infants tested during the first postnatal day, 27.8% (n=5) were positive, while 6.3% (n=4) of the

Table 2

Evoked Otoacoustic Emissions (EOAE) Screening Results Obtained from 346 Neonate Ears in Terms of Age in Hours

	Age (hours)			No. of tested ears	
	8-24	24-48	>48		
No. of tests	28	96	265	346	
No OAE	12	14	38	60*	50**
% Pos. screening	43	15	14	17*	14**

OAE: Otoacoustic emission; Pos. screening: positive screening, no OAE in test ear.
*: No OAE at one test.
**: No OAE at any test.

second day and 7.5% (n=12) of the third day screenings were positive. In all, screening was positive in 15 (7.2%) of 209 infants. Two babies who failed the screening were tested only during the first 24 hours of life. As mentioned previously, it appears likely that these children would have passed the screening if retested at a later date. Thus, if the data from these children are not considered, a positive screening was the result in only 6.3% of the subjects.

It should be noted that, at present, 3 of the 15 subjects for whom EOAE screenings were positive have been further tested using ABR and determined to have normal hearing. Due to our relatively small sample size and the small probability of hearing loss among these infants, we have operated under the assumption that the other 12 also are normal hearing, and we attribute screening failure to methodological problems.

Tympanometry and presence of EOAE

A total of 389 measurements of EOAE data and 371 tympanograms was obtained from 346 different ears. These data are shown in table 4. In all but 5 ears (6 measurements) in which tympanometry was performed, middle ear pressure was found to be normal. One baby (3 measurements) had flat tympanograms, and negative middle ear pressure was only recorded in three babies, all of whom were older than 24 hours.

A total of 59 measurements demonstrated no EOAE despite normal middle ear pressure. In contrast, EOAE was identified in all of three ears

Table 3
Evoked Otoacoustic Emissions (EOAE) Screening Results Obtained with Neonates in Terms of Age in Hours

	Age (hours)				
	8-24	24-48	>48	Total	>24
N	18	64	160	209*	207**
No OAE	5	4	12	15	13
% Pos. screening	27.8	6.3	7.5	7	6

OAE: Otoacoustic emission; Pos. screening: positive screening, no OAE in either ear.
* 234 children participated; 25 were excluded due to insufficient data.
** 2 children, only tested <24 hours showed no emissions.

Table 4*

The Results of Tympanometry and Evoked Otoacoustic Emissions (EOAE) Screening Obtained
from Neonate Ears in Terms of Age in Hours
("+" or "−" indicates presence or absence of EOAE)

| | Age (hours) | | | |
	0-24	24-48	> 48	No. (%)
No. of ears / Tympanometry	28	96	265	346 different ears / 389 measurements
p> −50 mm	−11(39%) / +14(50%)	−13(14%) / +78(81%)	−35(13%) / +225(85%)	−59/389 (15%) / +317/389 (82%)
−50 >p> −100 / −100 >p> −200	0 / 0	+1 / 0	+1 / +1	+2 / +1
Flat Tympanogram	0	−1	−2	−3 (0.8%)
p unknown	−1 / +2	−0 / +3	−1 / +11	−2 / +18

* The three flat tympanograms were obtained from one infant on two separate days.

with negative middle ear pressure. No EOAE response was obtained in the ears exhibiting flat tympanograms. In two cases where EOAEs were not present, tympanometry was not performed. There were an additional 16 cases where EOAE was identified in which tympanograms were not obtained. Overall, negative middle ear pressure and flat tympanograms were each demonstrated in only 0.8% of the total number of measurements.

DISCUSSION

A failure rate of 43% of ears (28% of babies) tested during the first 24 hours of life is in agreement with results reported by other investigators (Vohr et al. 1990; Hogan and Callaghan 1990; Kok et al. 1990; see chapter 15). The positive screening results of 6.3% in babies older than 24 hours found in the present study are also comparable to the results of the mentioned groups, with the exception of Kok and his colleagues, who reported that "prevalence of an EOAE was close to 100%." However, our circumstances call for a false positive screening rate not greater than 2% due to escalating costs involved in follow-up examinations.

At least two explanations are offered for the discrepancy between our results and our ideal of ≤2% false positives for a screening instrument. First, the present investigation employed a stimulus intensity of only 69 dB pe SPL in an attempt to avoid awakening and arousing the infants. This is approximately 10 dB less intense than the stimulus reportedly used in Kemp's and others' studies. It is conceivable that the stimulus intensity used in this study in some cases was too low to elicit the nonlinear components of the EOAE, and that the linear components of the response could not be clearly distinguished from stimulus ringing. It is therefore our intent to experiment with raising the stimulus intensity a bit to maximize the possibility of eliciting an identifiable response.

Second, the methods of noise reduction employed in the present study have proven insufficient. In many cases, our measurements were contaminated by environmental noise, which not only complicated evaluation of the response but frequently made evaluation impossible. We have since begun performing screening with the infants in a closed cradle in an attempt to reduce environmental noise, and the results appear promising. We further intend to introduce a weighted average in the signal processing, which should also help in improving the signal-to-noise ratio.

As previously stated, it has been suggested that the high rate of screening failures observed in babies younger than 24 hours could be due to a negative middle ear pressure or middle ear effusion. Our results do not lend support to this notion, in that we found no clear relationship between conditions in the middle ear and presence of EOAE. The vast majority of ears that failed EOAE screening had normal middle ear pressure, and in the few ears demonstrating negative pressure, it was nevertheless possible to elicit EOAE. Furthermore, there was no tendency for ears younger than 24 hours to have a higher prevalence of abnormal tympanograms. On the contrary, negative middle ear pressure was only found in babies older than 24 hours. It was only in the case of flat tympanograms that failed EOAE screening appeared to be positively correlated with abnormal middle ear conditions. Tos and his colleagues (Tos et al. 1979; Poulsen and Tos 1978) reported that middle ear effusion in neonates was rare, which further supports our assertion that the high rate of EOAE screening failures in very young infants is generally not attributable to this condition.

One might also hypothesize that structural developmental changes in the middle ear are responsible for the high proportion of false positive EOAE screening in infants tested during the first 24 hours of life. However, this appears unlikely as well, based on our results. Several investigators (Keith 1973; 1975; Bennett 1975) have reported that a substantial proportion of newborns have notched tympanograms, and this has also been our observation. Since the bony floor of the ear canal has not yet formed in the newborn, the ear canal wall is quite compliant. Thus, tympanograms obtained from newborns likely reflect complex interactions of external and middle ear properties and are not easily interpreted (Margolis and Shanks 1985). However, our observation was that, for any given ear, there was no change in tympanogram shape from day to day in spite of the fact that the ear could fail EOAE screening one day and pass the next. This indicates that, whatever the structural conditions in the external and middle ear, they do not apparently change significantly from one day to the next, and therefore, such changes cannot explain the differences in EOAE screening results from day to day.

Moreover, it does not appear that structural developmental changes in the cochlea can explain such differences in EOAE screening results. Evidence contradicting this concept can be found in the work of Lary and his colleagues (Lary' et al. 1985) who reported that structural maturization accounts for only a 2 dB improvement per week in the hearing threshold (determined using ABR) of preterm babies after birth from the 28th gestational week. This indicates that maturization of cochlear structures occurs too slowly to account for the differences in EOAE screening that have been observed from day to day.

We propose that the high prevalence of failed EOAE screenings in infants younger than 24 hours could be related to the oxygen tension in the neonatal ear. According to Metcalfe et al. (1967), the umbilical vein delivers oxygenated blood to the fetal ear with an oxygen pressure of less than 20 mm Hg, which corresponds to an oxygen saturation of about 30%. In cats, an oxygen saturation of only 30% has been demonstrated to produce a reversible (Evans 1974), specific auditory hearing loss of 10 to 50 dB, without any concurrent changes in somatosensory, visual, or vestibular responsiveness (Sohmer et al. 1986). The extreme sensitivity of the mammalian cochlea is a result of the endocochlear potentials (Sellick and Bock 1974) and the active function of the outer hair cells. Sohmer et al. (1986) found that, in animals, a 30% reduction in oxygen saturation depresses the cochlear microphonic potentials. Likewise, Sellick et al. (1982) demonstrated reduced motion of the basilar membrane in the guinea pig consequent to a reduction in oxygen saturation. Sohmer and Freeman (1991) therefore postulate that the child in utero has a hearing loss of at least 20 dB due to the reduced level of oxygen saturation in its blood supply.

Oxygen tension in neonatal blood rises to approximately 100 mm Hg immediately after onset of normal breathing. However, our suggestion is that the cochlear potential and active function of the outer hair cells require a critical period of time with normal oxygen tension before the electrogenic pump begins to operate efficiently, enabling elicitation of full-scale EOAE. This notion finds further support in the fact that, for ears demonstrating no response during the first day of life but with a response on subsequent days, small deflections could occasionally be identified in the first day's averaged signal, which corresponded temporally to the response identified in later measurements.

In conclusion, it would appear that it is possible to elicit EOAE from virtually all normally hearing newborns over 24 hours of age, given that methodological problems such as environmental noise, stimulus level, and probe fit do not interfere. Furthermore, it does not seem that the high rate of EOAE screening failures in infants tested during the first 24 hours of life is generally due to negative middle ear pressure, middle ear effusion, or structural developmental changes in the neonatal auditory system. Whatever the reason for this finding, it is clear that hearing screening of newborns based on EOAE should be performed on infants older than 24 hours to reduce the number of false positives and thus maximize efficiency of the screening.

Summary

Preceding a systematic hearing screening of newborns based on evoked otoacoustic emissions (EOAE), a pilot study including 209 newborn babies showed that using a proper stimulation pattern, a reliable visual, double-blind scoring of presence/nonpresence of EOAE was possible in 99% of 403 tests. Twenty-eight percent of the babies showed no EOAE in either ear the first 24 hours of life versus 6% from the second day on.

A systematic tympanometry excluded correlation between middle ear condition and missing OAE the first day. Based on the low oxygen pressure reported in fetal life, and the hypofunction of the cochlear mechanisms in utero, it is suggested that the bioelectric and biomechanical active cells need a critical period of time with normal oxygen tension before full-scale emissions can be observed, and this latency varies from few to 24 hours.

ACKNOWLEDGMENTS

The authors would like to thank Professor H. Sohmer, Department of Physiology, Hadassa Medical School, Jerusalem, for helpful comments and fruitful discussions.

The authors are further indebted to the staff of the Obstetric Department, Gentofte University Hospital. This study would not have been possible without their committed assistance.

REFERENCES

Bennett, M.J. 1975. Acoustic impedance bridge measurements with the neonate. *British Journal of Audiology* 9:117-124.

Bonfils, P., Uziel, A., and Pujol, R. 1988. Screening for auditory dysfunction in infants by evoked otoacoustic emissions. *Archives of Otolaryngology Head and Neck Surgery* 114:887-890.

Bray, P., and Kemp, D. 1987. An advanced cochlear echo technique suitable for infant screening. *British Journal of Audiology* 21:191-204.

Elberling, C., Parbo, J., Johnsen, N.J., and Bagi, P. 1985. Evoked acoustic emission: Clinical application. *Acta Otolaryngology* Suppl. 421:77-85.

Evans, E.F. 1974. Functions of the cochlear nerve. In R.J. Bench, A. Pye, and J.D. Pye (ed.), *Sound reception in mammals*. London: Academic Press.

Hogan, S.C.M., and Callaghan, D.E. 1990. A detailed analysis of the neonatal histories of infants screened using an otoacoustic emission measurement system and the effect on outcomes. Paper read at XXth International Congress of Audiology, October 1990, Puerto de la Cruz, Spain.

Johnsen, N.J., and Elberling, C. 1982. Evoked acoustic emissions from the human ear. I. Equipment and response parameters. *Scandinavian Audiology* 11:69-77.

Johnsen, N.J., Bagi, P., and Elberling, C. 1983. Evoked acoustic emissions from the human ear. III. Findings in neonates. *Scandinavian Audiology* 12:17-24.

Keith, R.W. 1973. Impedance audiometry with neonates. *Archives of Otolaryngology* 97:465-467.

Keith, R.W. 1975. Middle ear function in neonates. *Archives of Otolaryngology* 101:376-379.

Kemp, D., Bray, P., Alexander, L., and Brown, A.M. 1986. Acoustic emission cochleography-practical aspects. *Scandinavian Audiology* Suppl. 25:71-95.

Kemp, D., Siobhan, R., and Bray, P. 1990. A guide to the effective use of otoacoustic emissions. *Ear and Hearing* 11:93-105.

Kok, M.R., Brocaar, M.P., and van Zanten, G.A. 1990. Evoked otoacoustic emissions in healthy newborns. Paper read at XXth International Congress of Audiology, October 1990, Puerto de la Cruz, Spain.

Lary, S., Briassoulis, G., de Vries, L., and Dubowitz, V. 1985. Hearing threshold in preterm and term infants by ABR. *Journal of Pediatrics* 107:593-599.

Margolis, R., and Shanks, J. 1985. Tympanometry. In J. Katz (ed.), *Handbook of clinical audiology*. 3d ed. Baltimore: Williams and Wilkins.

Metcalfe, J., and Bartels, H., and Moll, N. 1967. Gas exchange in the pregnant uterus. *Physiology Review* 47:147-152.

Poulsen, G., and Tos, M. 1978. Screening tympanometry in newborn infants and during the first six months of life. *Scandinavian Audiology* 7(3):159-166.

Sellick, P.M., and Bock, G.R. 1974. Evidence for an electrogenic potassium as an origin of the positive component of the endocochlear potential. *Flüggers Archives* 352:351-361.

Sellick, P.M., Patuzzi, R., and Johanstone, B.M. 1982. Measurements of basilar motion in the guinea pig using Mössbauer technique. *Journal of the Acoustical Society of America* 72:131-141.

Sohmer, H., Freeman, S., and Malachi, S. 1986. Multimodality evoked potentials in hypoxemia. *Electroencepholography and Clinical Neurophysiology* 64:328-333.

Sohmer, H., and Freeman, S. 1991. Hypoxia induced hearing loss in animal models of the fetus in-utero. *Hearing Research* 55:92-97.

Stevens, J.C., Webb, H.D., Hutchinson, J., Connell, J., Smith, M.F., and Buffin, J.T. 1991. Evaluation of click-evoked oto-acoustic emissions in the newborn. *British Journal of Audiology* 25(1):11-14.

Tos, M., Poulsen, G., and Hancke, A.B. 1979. Screening tympanometry during the first year of life. *Acta Otolaryngology* 88:388-394.

Vohr, B., Kemp, D., White, K., Blackwell, P., Johnsen, M.J., Maxon, A., Cronan, R., and Clarkson, R. 1990. Auditory screen trials for neonates.

Paper read at XXth International Congress of Audiology, October 1990, Puerto de la Cruz, Spain.

Chapter 15

Neonatal Hearing Screening Using Evoked Otoacoustic Emissions: The Rhode Island Hearing Assessment Project

Karl R. White, Antonia B. Maxon, Thomas R. Behrens, Peter M. Blackwell, and Betty R. Vohr

INTRODUCTION

Although everyone agrees that early identification of hearing loss is important, currently available procedures in the United States have not been successful in identifying the majority of hearing-impaired children during the first year of life. This chapter describes the procedures and preliminary results of the Rhode Island Hearing Assessment Project (RIHAP), which was designed to evaluate the use of evoked otoacoustic emissions (EOAE) to screen all live births for hearing loss.

The average delay between birth and the confirmation of significant sensorineural hearing loss in the United States is 2½ years or more (Academy of Otolaryngology-Head and Neck Surgery 1990; Commission on Education of the Deaf 1988; Pappas and Mundy 1981). For children born with significant sensorineural hearing loss, this delay may unfortunately extend well into the critical early years of language and speech development. The developmental and psychosocial impact of delayed identification of hearing loss is often devastating because the ability to hear during the first 3 years of life is critical for the acquisition of spoken language.

Failure to identify hearing loss and provide intervention (amplification, parent management, speech and language management, and/or sign language instruction) within the first year of life has needless negative effects on other areas besides language because adequate communication skills are basic to future psychosocial, educational, and vocational development (Bebout 1989; Downs 1986; Madell 1988; Sacks 1989; Schum 1987; Ross 1990). Fortunately, if hearing loss is identified early, many of the negative effects of hearing impairment can be ameliorated or eliminated. For example, Clark (1979) demonstrated that hearing-impaired children who receive intervention before 2½ years of age have significantly better communicative skills than children who receive similar intervention at later ages.

The importance of identifying hearing-impaired children at an earlier age is also underscored by the government's recently issued plan to improve significantly the nation's health over the coming decade (*Healthy People 2000: National Health Promotion and Disease Prevention Objectives*, U.S. Department of Health and Human Services 1990). One goal of that plan is to "reduce the average age at which children with significant hearing impairment are identified to no more than 12 months." The document goes on to state:

> The future of a child born with a significant hearing impairment depends to a very large degree on early identification (i.e., audiological diagnosis before 12 months of age) followed by immediate and appropriate intervention. If hearing-impaired children are not identified early, it is difficult, if not impossible, for many of them to acquire the fundamental language, social, and cognitive skills that provide the foundation for later schooling and success in society. When early identification and intervention occurs, hearing-impaired children make dramatic progress, are more successful in school, and become more productive members of society. The earlier intervention and habilitation begins, the more dramatic the benefits. (P. 460)

How likely are we to accomplish the goal of earlier identification if present policies and procedures are continued? At first glance, it appears that substantial progress is being made. A recent article by Blake and Hall (1990) noted that 14 states now have a legislative mandate to do neonatal hearing screening and 12 additional states have a policy or program in place, even though no legislative mandate exists. Unfortunately, the current status is not as positive as these numbers suggest. Six of the 14 states have not actually implemented screening programs because no funds have been appropriated. Of the 12 states that have a policy or a program but no legislative mandate, most have only a policy that acknowledges the importance of early identification. Of the programs in existence, all limit screening to a small number of high-risk babies. Unfortunately, recent research (Elssmann, Matkin, and Sabo 1987; Mauk, White, Mortensen, and Behrens 1991) has demonstrated that at least half of all children with sensorineural hearing loss never exhibit any of these high-risk characteristics.

ALTERNATIVE METHODS FOR EARLY HEARING SCREENING

Although there is a great deal of interest in identifying children earlier, most currently used screening procedures are either too expensive to implement or miss such large numbers of children that it is unlikely that such techniques would lead to reduction of the average age of identification to 12 months of age, even if they were used by every state. The most frequently used methods available for early identification of hearing loss include the following.

BEHAVIORAL TESTING BY HOME VISITORS

Where it is feasible to make home visits to most children in the population, e.g., a country such as England with socialized medicine, this technique is very effective (Barr 1980; Bentzen and Jensen 1981; McCormick 1983). A trained home visitor uses simple behavioral testing techniques to observe whether the child responds to various noises such as rattles or bells, which are presented so that the child's hearing instead of visual responsiveness is tested. In countries where universal home visits are done, behavioral testing for hearing is very economical. In countries without universal home visiting, such as the United States, the costs would be prohibitive.

HIGH-RISK REGISTRIES

In 1982, the Joint Committee on Infant Hearing identified seven risk factors associated with hearing impairment in young children (family history of deafness, congenital infections, anatomic malformations of the head or neck, birth weight less than 1500 g, hyperbilirubinemia, bacterial meningitis, and severe asphyxia). More recently, the 1982 criteria have been updated and expanded (Joint Committee on Infant Hearing 1991). By focusing screening only on children who exhibit one or more of these risk factors, the costs of screening are minimized. Such screening programs have been implemented where information about the risk factors is collected from the legally required birth certificate (Mahoney and Eichwald 1986; 1987) or as a questionnaire, which is completed by the mother or the hospital staff (Epstein and Reilly 1989; Schuyler and Rushmer 1987). Although children who exhibit one of these risk factors are more likely to be hearing impaired, most hearing-impaired children never exhibit any of these risk factors (Elssmann et al. 1987; Mauk et al. 1991). More widespread implementation of screening programs for children with such risk factors would certainly reduce the average age of identification. However, it is unrealistic to expect that the goal of reducing the average age of identification to 12 months of age can be accomplished by such programs since so many hearing-impaired children do not exhibit any of these risk factors.

CRIB-O-GRAM

A hospital-based alternative (Miller and Simmons 1984) uses a cradlelike device that is sensitive to movements of the baby and that can emit sound at predetermined levels and times. By monitoring whether movements of the baby correspond to the times that sound was emitted, it was hoped that early detection of hearing impairment could be possible. Unfortunately, data on the validity of such techniques have been disappointing (Shimizu et al. 1985).

AUDITORY BRAINSTEM RESPONSE (ABR)

Numerous researchers (e.g., Galambos and Despland 1980; Kileny 1988; Levi, Tell, Feinmesser, Gafni, and Sohmer 1983; Murray, Javel, and Watson 1985) have demonstrated that ABR testing is useful in identifying hearing impairment in very young children. Generally, an initial test is done a few days before the child is released from the hospital, and those who fail are rescreened several weeks later to correct for the high false positive rate of the initial screen. A very high percentage of those who fail both tests will have significant hearing impairment. The technique is accurate, but the expense and the substantial training and experience necessary for operators mean that traditional ABR testing is not feasible as a mass hearing screen (American Speech-Language-Hearing Association 1989). Recently introduced portable ABR equipment and equipment that includes automated scoring routines may bring the costs down, but further research is necessary (Jacobson, Jacobson, and Spahr 1990; Kileny 1988). Some hospitals have also used ABR screening only for children who exhibit high-risk characteristics, but even that is more expensive than desired and has the added disadvantage of missing those hearing-impaired babies who do not exhibit any of the risk variables.

PURPOSE

The problems noted above with each of the most widely used screening techniques for early identification of hearing loss have probably contributed to the lack of success in substantially reducing the average age at which hearing-impaired children are identified. The purpose of the Rhode Island Hearing Assessment Project (RIHAP) was to determine whether evoked otoacoustic emissions (EOAEs) could be used with every live birth to reduce the average age of identification for significant hearing impairment. In other words, is a neonatal hearing screening program using EOAE feasible, valid, and cost-efficient?

FEASIBILITY

The evaluation of feasibility was based on whether it was possible to organize the logistical and procedural details of conducting a large-scale screening program in a busy hospital, and whether appropriate staff could be hired, trained, and appropriately supervised to test that many babies. Data regarding feasibility were collected by screening over 3,000 babies in regular and special care nurseries.

VALIDITY

It is also important to know whether EOAE-based screening correctly identifies children who have hearing losses, and correctly passes most children who do not have hearing losses. To determine the validity of the EOAE procedure: (*a*) data were collected for a subsample of infants with both EOAE and ABR; (*b*) the number of children with hearing losses identified with EOAE is being documented; (*c*) information is being collected about how many of those children would not have been identified using other techniques; and (*d*) information about hearing status at 5 years of age for all children screened will be collected and referenced to the initial screening results. The follow-up data are possible because of the unusual degree of cooperation between the Departments of Education and Health in Rhode Island, and because the Rhode Island School for the Deaf is already conducting a very comprehensive screening program for all kindergarten-age children in the state. Thus, it will be possible to cross-reference all of the children who were originally screened with EOAE to their results 5 years later in kindergarten.

COST-EFFICIENCY

A screening program may be feasible and produce valid results but may be too expensive. The cost-efficiency of an EOAE screening program can be determined by analyzing whether the costs of implementing the program are reasonable, given available resources and in light of the benefits associated with early identification. The cost of screening each baby will be calculated using an ingredients approach (Levin 1983), and the cost of identifying each hearing-impaired child will be calculated by dividing the total cost of the program by the number of children identified.

PROCEDURE

Before describing the procedures used in screening infants, it is important to provide a brief explanation of what evoked otoacoustic emissions are and how they are measured. This will be followed by a summary of how the project was designed and the procedures used to collect data.

EVOKED OTOACOUSTIC EMISSIONS

Evoked otoacoustic emissions (EOAEs) are acoustic responses associated with the normal hearing process. EOAEs are produced in the inner ear by physiologic activity of the cochlea (outer hair cells) and can be measured with a low-noise microphone placed in the ear canal (Kemp 1978). EOAEs can be evoked by various stimuli in virtually all normally hearing individuals. Substantial evidence now shows that EOAEs are a property of the healthy, normal-functioning cochlea, generated by active, frequency-selective, nonlinear elements within the cochlear partition. These elements enhance the cochlear response to sound by a positive feedback mechanism, thus improving sensitivity and frequency selectivity. Substantial recent research has shown that EOAEs are not present in adults or children with hearing loss greater than 30 dB HL (Bray and Kemp 1987; Kemp, Bray, Alexander, and Brown 1986; Probst, Lonsbury-Martin, Martin, and Coats 1987; Rutten 1980).

The physical mechanisms of the middle ear and cochlea serve to collect and concentrate sound energy onto the sensory hair cells. Vibrations generated inside the cochlea are magnified by the middle ear and transmitted into the air as sound. By placing a receiver-microphone probe into the ear canal, sounds made by the cochlea can be evoked by external sound and recorded from virtually any ear with normal mid-frequency hearing (Kemp 1989). Consequently, several researchers have suggested that EOAEs may be a valuable noninvasive, objective tool for evaluating cochlear status in infants and young children (Bonfils, Uziel, and Pujol 1988; Elberling, Parbo, Johnsen, and Bagi 1985; Johnsen, Bagi, and Elberling 1983; Kemp 1988; Lutman, Mason, Sheppard, and Gibbin 1989; Stevens et al. 1991).

The ease with which EOAEs can be measured led to the development of a commercially available device that is appropriate for screening infants (Kemp 1988). The Otodynamic Analyzer (ILO88) works by placing a probe in the ear of the child to be evaluated (see figure 1). A series of clicks is then sent into the ear canal, delayed EOAEs are recorded in the ear canal following the click stimuli, and responses are analyzed by the ILO88.

The ILO88 produces information like that in figure 2, which shows the results for a normal hearing neonate. The information in the upper

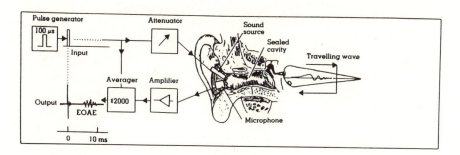

Figure 1. Basic method of recording evoked otoacoustic emissions (EOAEs) stimulated by transient sound. Reproduced from Kemp, D.T. 1989, with permission.

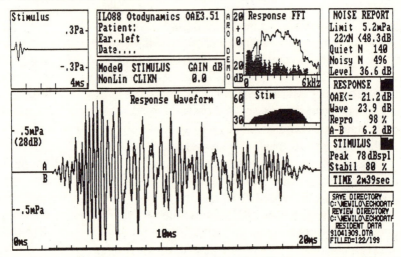

Figure 2. Example of evoked otoacoustic emissions (EOAE) from a neonate with normal hearing.

right-hand corner that shows the clear wave above the dark wave indicates that the child has hearing across the frequency range from 1 to 5 kHz. In contrast, figure 3 shows the response of a neonate who failed the screening test as indicated by the information in the upper right-hand corner where there is no waveform evident above the dark wave.

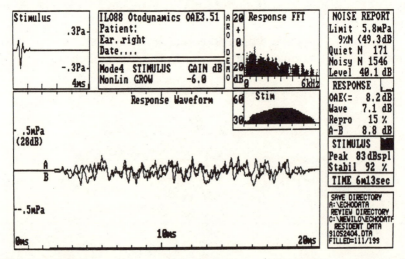

Figure 3. Example of evoked otoacoustic emissions (EOAE) from a neonate with impaired hearing.

Based on previous research with small samples, the use of EOAE in a neonatal hearing screening program has the following apparent advantages:

1. Simple. No advanced technical training is required for administration.
2. Fast. Detection of EOAEs can be achieved in less than 15 minutes for both ears.
3. Noninvasive. The acoustic probe is placed into the external ear canal using an impedance probe protector without support.
4. Objective. A visual record of cochlear response is provided for future reference.
5. Sensitive. The method is sensitive to small hearing losses (25 dB HL) over a 2 to 3 octave range.

However, EOAEs have not been used in the United States in a large-scale screening program to determine whether such an application is feasible, produces valid results, and is cost-efficient. The Rhode Island Hearing Assessment Project provides the basis for such an evaluation.

DESIGN

The RIHAP design and timelines for assessments are shown in figure 4. As can be seen, children included in the screening can be divided into two groups. Some children receive both EOAE and ABR regardless of their results on either test. If they fail either or both, they are referred for rescreening at 4 to 6 weeks. In the second group, children are first screened initially with the EOAE. If they fail the EOAE, they are tested with ABR. Whether or not they pass the ABR, they are referred for rescreening at 4 to 6 weeks.

All children who are rescreened at 4 to 6 weeks receive both EOAE and ABR. Although a number of variables influence the decision of whether to refer for further testing from this point forward, the general guidelines are as follows. If they fail either test, they are referred for further evaluation. Children who fail the ABR at 60 dB or greater are referred for sedated ABR at 12 to 16 weeks of age. If they fail the sedated ABR at 60 dB or greater, they are referred immediately for behavioral audiometry, diagnosis, and habilitation. If they fail the sedated ABR at less than 60 dB, they are referred for further behavioral audiometry at 6 months of age.

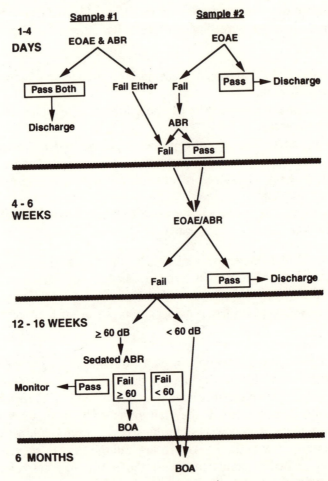

Figure 4. Design for the Rhode Island Hearing Assessment Project (RIHAP) hearing loss screening using evoked otoacoustic emissions (EOAE). ABR=auditory brainstem response; BOA=behavioral observation audiometry.

All children included in the sample were born at Women and Infants Hospital of Rhode Island (WIHRI). Approximately 70% of all births in the state of Rhode Island are at WIHRI. Because of the small geographical size of the state, virtually all children in the sample lived within a one-hour drive. At the present time, approximately 3,000 children have been screened. Because it took several months for screeners to become proficient with the techniques, the data reported in this chapter are based on approximately 2,000 infants who were screened after the third month of the project and who are now old enough to have completed the sedated ABR testing if that was indicated. It should also be emphasized that the confirmation of hearing loss using behavioral audiometry will not occur for several months for most of these children. Thus, the results concerning hearing loss reported in this chapter are based primarily on the results of sedated ABR testing. Further information about confirmation testing will be contained in future reports.

DATA COLLECTION PROCEDURES

For EOAE screening, the ILO88 Otodynamic Analyzer (Kemp 1988) produced by Otodynamics, Ltd. was used. ABR screening was done using the GSI-55. Further information concerning the protocols for each test is available elsewhere (Maxon, White, Norton, and Behrens 1991).

Testing was scheduled by examining the log of births and expected release dates each day, identifying babies who were appropriate for testing, obtaining informed consent from their mothers, and coordinating the schedule of screeners with scheduled hospital procedures. Babies were brought by schedulers into a relatively quiet room to which acoustic tiles and room dividers had been added. The baby was placed in an isolette that could be closed, and testing was done by screeners who had been trained for that purpose.

Screeners with different types of training and experience were intentionally used (i.e., registered nurses, audiologists, and paraprofessionals). Extensive training was provided, and each potential screener had to complete a certification process before beginning screening. Regular monitoring of performance and, where necessary, corrective feedback were given by a certified audiologist.

Babies who failed the initial screen were invited back to the hospital at 4 to 6 weeks of age for further testing as depicted in figure 4. In those cases where transportation would be a financial hardship, the parents were reimbursed for travel costs. Letters were sent to the primary care physician for all children who failed the initial screen, and the help of the pediatrician was enlisted in those cases where it was difficult to get the parent to bring the child back. Approximately 70% of the children who failed the initial screen were successfully rescreened.

RESULTS

The results reported here are preliminary. Not only is further confirmatory testing being done with those children tentatively identified as having hearing losses, but additional children are being screened. This section summarizes the lessons learned thus far from the project concerning the conduct of a neonatal hearing screening program based on EOAE and provides preliminary information regarding the feasibility, validity, and cost-efficiency of doing mass neonatal hearing screening using EOAE.

PROCEDURAL LESSONS LEARNED

Because EOAEs have not previously been used in a large-scale neonatal hearing screening program, there are a number of valuable lessons that have been learned about conducting an EOAE screening program. Several of the most important lessons are summarized below.

Training and monitoring of screeners. Although the use of the EOAE screening equipment is simple and straightforward, it is absolutely essential that procedures be established for structured training of screeners (including didactic presentation of information, observation, and experiential learning), and that regular monitoring procedures be implemented thereafter. Unless such training and monitoring occur, there will be an unnecessarily high rate of invalid results. It is very unlikely that a child with a hearing loss will pass the screen if the testers are not using appropriate techniques, but there will be an unnecessarily high rate of false positives (children who fail the test even though their hearing is normal).

Qualifications and experience of screeners. Screeners with varying types of experience and qualifications were intentionally used to determine if some were more successful than others. A certified audiologist who had extensive experience testing babies observed each screener on a regular basis for adherence to the protocol and mastery of testing procedures, and data were collected for each screener about the percentage of children who failed or had uninterpretable results. Based on those data, no particular prior training or expertise is required to be a successful EOAE screener. Surprisingly, the category of screeners that turned over most frequently and encountered the most difficulty with the screening protocol was the certified audiologists—probably because the screening protocol limited their ability to function as an audiologist (i.e., they wanted to proceed beyond screening to diagnosis, habilitation, and work with the child and parent). In all cases, it was clear that expertise of the screeners improved dramatically with experience. Screeners who worked 20 hours or more per week were much more successful than those who worked fewer than 10 hours a week.

Time of testing. Children in the regular care nursery were tested at whatever time was convenient prior to being discharged. After an examination of the failure and pass rates for children according to their age in days when testing occurred, it was discovered that the failure rate was strongly correlated with the age at which testing occurred. Children tested within 24 hours of birth had a failure rate of 30%, while the failure rate for children tested three to four days following birth was only 18%. Thus, it is clear that the false positive rate (and thus the cost of the screening program) can be substantially reduced by scheduling screening sometime following the first 24 hours of birth but prior to the time that the child is released from the hospital.

Environmental noise. Although a soundproof room is not required for EOAE testing, environmental noise can interfere with testing if precautions are not taken. One of the most important sources of environmental noise comes from the baby. If testing can be conducted when the baby is in a quiet state, such as shortly after feeding, the time required to do testing is substantially reduced, and the pass rate is substantially increased. Testing was also more successful if it was done in an isolette that could be covered to block out other environmental noise in the room. The ILO88 equipment has built-in noise artifact rejection, but arranging to do the testing in a place that is reasonably quiet is well worth the effort.

Debris in the ear. Because they are tested so soon after birth, many babies had obstructions in the ear canal (e.g., vernix, wax, birthing debris), or their ear canals were partially collapsed. Based on a carefully controlled subsample, it was discovered that the failure rate could be reduced by as much as 60% by removing the debris from the canal or using the probe to "open" the canal. Because of time limitations and other logistical considerations, these procedures were not used for the majority of the babies in this data set, but they are procedures that should be considered as a part of the protocol in designing EOAE screening programs.

Scheduling and transportation. In budgeting for the EOAE screening program, it is critical to remember that babies will have to be transported from the nursery to the testing location, and someone will have to be responsible for coordinating all of the scheduling. In this project, scheduling and transportation required as much time and resources as actually doing the testing.

Increased community awareness—A fringe benefit. At the beginning of the project, letters were sent to all pediatricians in the community to explain the purpose and activities of RIHAP. Meetings were also held with the hospital staff (nurses, residents, administrators). After screening was initiated, letters were sent to the primary care physician whenever a baby failed the initial screen or any subsequent screen. In addition, when RIHAP staff experienced difficulty in scheduling a child for follow-up testing, the primary care physician was contacted to request assistance in having the parent bring the baby back for testing. Information about the project also appeared in the newspaper and on the local television news. The awareness created by these activities has had a substantial impact on early identification of hearing loss beyond the children actually identified through screening. Over the year and a half since RIHAP began, the enrollment in the infant program (birth to 2 years of age) at the Rhode Island School for the Deaf has more than quadrupled over the average enrollment for the past seven years. Officials at the school attribute this enrollment increase to the awareness in the community about hearing loss that has happened as a result of RIHAP.

FEASIBILITY OF USING EOAE IN NEONATAL HEARING SCREENING

Thus far, the project has screened over 3,000 babies, including children in regular and special care nurseries. The average time required to do screening has been 12 minutes per child in the regular care nursery and 14 minutes per child in the special care nursery. Approximately 18% of the children in the regular care nursery fail the initial screen and are referred for further testing, while 25% of the children in the special care nursery require further testing.

The project has clearly demonstrated that it is possible to screen large numbers of infants (as many as 25 per day). It is feasible to manage the logistical and procedural details of scheduling infants for testing, transporting them to the testing location, coordinating screening with necessary medical procedures, and accomplishing the testing prior to discharge. With the trend toward shorter stays in the hospital, a few babies will be missed. But the results of this project demonstrate that EOAE techniques can be used to screen over 95% of all babies in regular and special care nurseries.

VALIDITY OF USING EOAE IN NEONATAL HEARING SCREENING

Although the data reported here are preliminary and information about hearing loss is, in many cases, based only on the results of the sedated ABR, EOAE appears to be a very promising technique for use in screening programs to identify hearing loss. Considering those data collected after the time that the operational procedures for the project were refined, just under 2,000 babies have been screened and are now old enough to have received a sedated ABR if one was indicated. Based on that sample, 9 children with suspected sensorineural hearing loss and 12 children with fluctuating conductive hearing losses have been identified. Thus, the EOAE screening program is identifying almost 5 children per 1,000 with a sensorineural hearing loss. This prevalence of sensorineural hearing loss is two to three times what is typically expected in the general population (Bergstrom 1982; Parving 1985). This is strong evidence that EOAE can be successfully used to identify children who have a hearing loss.

If only the sample of children who received both an EOAE and an ABR at the initial screen is considered, the agreement between initial EOAE and initial ABR is quite good as shown in figure 5. The agreement between initial EOAE and rescreen ABR and rescreen EOAE and rescreen ABR is even better.

About half of the children with suspected sensorineural hearing loss would not have been identified using other typically used approaches to early identification. Four of the nine children with suspected sensorineural hearing losses exhibited none of the high-risk factors recommended by the Joint Committee on Infant Hearing (1983), and six of the nine children did not spend any time in the special care nursery. Thus, a screening program that focused only on children who exhibited one or more of the risk factors or children in a special care nursery would have missed a substantial number of these children. One of the nine children identified through EOAE would not have been identified based on the results of the initial ABR.

Initial ABR

		Fail	Pass	
Initial EOAE	Fail	50	162	Sensitivity=60%
	Pass	34	826	Specificity=84%

(only includes infants who received both tests regardless of results)

Rescreen ABR

		Fail	Pass	
Initial EOAE	Fail	31	210	Sensitivity=91%
	Pass	3	79	Specificity=27%

Rescreen ABR

		Fail	Pass	
Rescreen EOAE	Fail	30	40	Sensitivity=94%
	Pass	2	215	Specificity=84%

Figure 5. Agreement between evoked otoacoustic emissions (EOAE) and auditory brainstem response (ABR) (data based on ears for period from June 1, 1990, to April 30, 1991).

All of these children were identified as having a suspected sensorineural hearing loss before 4 months of age. Although final confirmation of hearing loss must be based on the results of behavioral testing, it is expected that such confirmation will happen well before the goal of 12 months established by the U.S. Department of Health and Human Services (1990) in the *Healthy People 2000* goals.

COST-EFFICIENCY OF USING EOAE IN NEONATAL SCREENING

The cost of screening every live birth using EOAE will vary to some degree depending on the specific protocol used, who does the testing, and the prevailing pay-scale in a particular location. For example, if screening is done by audiologists or registered nurses, it will be much more expensive than if paraprofessionals are used. Furthermore, if ABR testing is routinely incorporated as a part of a 4- to 6-week rescreen, the cost of screening will be more expensive than if only EOAE is used at both the initial screen and the subsequent rescreen.

Using an ingredients approach to cost-analysis (Levin 1983), we estimated the costs of a screening program similar to RIHAP using paraprofessionals to do all testing and using only the EOAE at both the initial and the rescreen tests. Including the costs of screening, scheduling and transportation, coordination, and training and monitoring of the project by an audiologist, the cost of such screening would be approximately $20 per child. Thus, the cost of identifying each child with sensorineural hearing loss is approximately $4,500.

Precise information is not available about the benefits of identifying children with sensorineural hearing loss at 6 months of age instead of 24 to 30 months of age (as is currently the case). However, given the devastating consequences on all aspects of life of not acquiring appropriate language skills, it seems that this initial cost of identification would be easily recovered in terms of reduced costs for special education, increased productivity, and more complete participation in society. Further analyses of the cost-benefit ratios are clearly needed, but the costs of identifying sensorineural hearing loss in children in this project certainly seem reasonable. If one considers the benefits of also identifying children with conductive losses earlier, the cost-benefit ratios are even more favorable.

SUMMARY

There is universal agreement that significant hearing loss should be identified as early as possible, preferably before 12 months of age (American Speech-Language-Hearing Association 1989; U.S. Department of Health and Human Services 1990). Unfortunately, existing techniques, such as the use of high-risk registers, ABR testing, or behavioral screening, have not been successful in identifying the majority of children in the United States with significant hearing loss at such a young age. The Rhode Island Hearing Assessment Project (RIHAP) was designed to evaluate the use of evoked otoacoustic emissions (EOAE) in a mass neonatal hearing screening program. Based on the data collected thus far, the preliminary results are encouraging.

Using the EOAE techniques, approximately two to three times as many children with a suspected sensorineural hearing loss have been identified as would typically be expected. The results of the EOAE agree substantially with the results of ABR screening for those children for whom both tests were done. Furthermore, about half of the children identified using EOAE did not exhibit any of the 1982 high-risk criteria and would not have been identified using ABR screening methods with high-risk children or children in a special care nursery. The fact that the results of this project demonstrate that EOAE is feasible to use in a screening program for every live birth clearly demonstrates that this technique deserves further investigation and evaluation.

Much additional research is necessary before concluding that EOAE is the screening technique of choice. The data reported in this article are preliminary, yet promising. The project continues to screen children so that the sample sizes will be larger, many of the results reported here concerning hearing loss are based only on sedated ABRs and must be confirmed through behavioral testing, and further analyses will be done after the sample sizes are complete. Nonetheless, this project demonstrates the feasibility of implementing such a program and suggests that a substantial number of hearing-impaired children, who otherwise would have been missed, are being identified using EOAE-based screening. The cost of such a program is reasonable compared to other screening programs.

Since this is the first effort in the United States to implement EOAE screening on a large scale, many questions still remain. Not only should the additional data collection and analysis referred to above be conducted, but it is important that other sites replicate the techniques used in RIHAP. Additional questions remain concerning the exact nature of the protocol to be used; techniques for reducing the relatively high rate of false positives; who should do testing; and how results should be scored and interpreted. In spite of the need for further research and refinement, the results of this project suggest that EOAE is a viable and promising technique for use in neonatal hearing screening programs.

ACKNOWLEDGMENTS

Supported in part by project #MCJ-495037 from the Maternal and Child Health program (Title V, Social Security Act), Health Resources and Services Administration, Department of Health and Human Services.

REFERENCES

American Academy of Otolaryngology—Head and Neck Surgery. 1990. Infant hearing screening program launched. *Bulletin of the American Academy of Otolaryngology Head and Neck Surgery* 9:46-47.

American Speech-Language-Hearing Association. 1989. Guidelines for audiologic screening of newborn infants who are at risk for hearing impairment. *Asha* 31(3):89-92.

Barr, B. 1980. Early identification of hearing impairment. In I.G. Taylor and A. Markides (eds.), *Disorders of auditory function*, vol. 3 (pp. 33-42). New York: Academic Press.

Bebout, J.M. 1989. Pediatric hearing aid fitting: A practical overview. *The Hearing Journal* 49:13-14.

Bentzen, O., and Jensen, J.H. 1981. Early detection and treatment of deaf children: A European concept. In S.E. Gerber and G.T. Mencher (eds.), *Early management of hearing loss* (pp. 85-103). San Francisco: Grune and Stratton.

Bergstrom, L. 1982. Otolaryngology. In G.M. English (ed.), *Congenital deafness* (pp. 1-20). Philadelphia: Harper and Row.

Blake, P.E., and Hall, J.W. 1990. The status of state-wide policies for neonatal hearing screening. *Journal of the American Academy of Audiology* 1(2):67-74.

Bonfils, P., Uziel, A., and Pujol, R. 1988. Screening for auditory dysfunction in infants by evoked oto-acoustic emissions. *Archives of Otolaryngology and Head and Neck Surgery* 114:887-890.

Bray, P., and Kemp, D.T. 1987. An advanced cochlear echo technique suitable for infant screening. *British Journal of Audiology* 21(2):191-204.

Clark, T.C. 1979. *Language development through home intervention for infant hearing—impaired children*. Chapel Hill, N.C.: University of North Carolina. University Microfilms International no. 80-13, 924.

Commission on Education of the Deaf. 1988. *Toward equality: Education of the deaf*. Washington, D.C.: U.S. Government Printing Office.

Downs, M.P. 1986. The rationale for neonatal hearing screening. In E.T. Swigart (ed.), *Neonatal hearing screening* (pp. 3-16). San Diego: College Hill Press.

Elberling, C., Parbo, J., Johnsen, N.J., and Bagi, P. 1985. Evoked acoustic emissions: Clinical application. *Acta Otolaryngologica* 421:77-85.

Elssmann, S.F., Matkin, N.D., and Sabo, M.P. 1987. Early identification of congenital sensorineural hearing impairment. *The Hearing Journal* 40:13-17.

Epstein, S., and Reilly, J.S. 1989. Sensorineural hearing loss. *Pediatric Clinics of North America* 36:1501-1520.

Galambos, R., and Despland, P.A. 1980. The auditory brainstem response (ABR) evaluates risk factors for hearing loss in the newborn. *Pediatric Research* 14:159-163.

Jacobson, J.T., Jacobson, C.A., and Spahr, R.C. 1990. Automated and conventional ABR screening techniques in high-risk infants. *Journal of the American Academy of Audiology* 1:187-195.

Johnsen, N.J., Bagi, P., and Elberling, C. 1983. Evoked acoustic emissions from the human ear: III. Findings in neonates. *Scandinavian Audiology* 12:17-24.

Joint Committee on Infant Hearing. 1983. Position statement—1982. *Ear and Hearing* 4:3-4.

Joint Committee on Infant Hearing. 1991. 1990 position statement. *Asha* 33(Suppl. 5):3-6.

Kemp, D.T. 1978. Stimulated acoustic emissions from the human auditory system. *Journal of Acoustical Society of America* 64:1386-1391.

Kemp, D.T. 1988. Developments in cochlear mechanics and techniques for non-invasive evaluation. *Advances in Audiology* 5:27-45.

Kemp, D.T. 1989. Otoacoustic emissions: Basic facts and applications. *Audiology in Practice* 6(3):1-4.

Kemp, D.T., Bray, P., Alexander, L., and Brown, A.M. 1986. Acoustic emission cochleography—Practical aspects. In G. Cianfrone and F. Grandorl (eds.), *Cochlear mechanics and otoacoustic emissions* (pp. 71-94). Stockholm: Almquist and Wiksell Periodical Company.

Kileny, P.R. 1988. New insights on infant ABR hearing screening. *Scandinavian Audiology* Suppl. 30:81-88.

Levi, H., Tell, L., Feinmesser, M., Gafni, M., and Sohmer, H. 1983. Early detection of hearing loss in infants by auditory nerve and brainstem responses. *Audiology* 22:181-188.

Levin, H.M. 1983. *Cost-effectiveness: A primer.* Beverly Hills, Calif.: Sage.

Lutman, M.E., Mason, S.M., Sheppard, S., and Gibbin, K.P. 1989. Differential diagnostic potential of otoacoustic emissions: A case study. *Audiology* 28:205-210.

McCormick, B. 1983. Hearing screening by health visitors: A critical appraisal of the distraction test. *Health Visitor* 56:449-451.

Madell, J.R. 1988. Identification and treatment of very young children with hearing loss. *Infants and Young Children* 1:20-30.

Mahoney, T.M., and Eichwald, J.G. 1986. Model Program V: A high-risk register by computerized search of birth certificates. In E.T. Swigart (ed.), *Neonatal hearing screening* (pp. 223-241). San Diego: College Hill Press.

Mahoney, T.M., and Eichwald, J.G. 1987. The ups and "downs" of high-risk hearing screening: The Utah statewide program. *Seminars in Hearing* 8:155-163.

Mauk, G.W., White, K.R., Mortensen, L.B., and Behrens, T.R. 1991. The effectiveness of screening programs based on high-risk characteristics in early identification of hearing impairment. *Ear and Hearing* 12:312-319.

Maxon, A.B., White, K.R., Norton, S.J., and Behrens, T.R. 1991. *Evoked otoacoustic emissions in neonatal screening and follow-up: Clinical trials.* Seminar (½ day) presented at the annual meeting of the American Speech-Language-Hearing Association, Atlanta, Ga.

Miller, K., and Simmons, F.B. 1984. A retrospective and an update in the Crib-O-Gram neonatal hearing screening audiometer. *Seminars in Hearing* 5:49-56.

Murray, A.D., Javel, E., and Watson, C.S. 1985. Prognostic validity of auditory brainstem evoked response screening in newborn infants. *American Journal of Otolaryngology* 6:120-131.

Pappas, D.G., and Mundy, M.R. 1981. Sensorineural hearing loss in young children: A systematic approach to evaluation. *Southern Medical Journal* 74:965-967.

Parving, A. 1985. Hearing disorders in childhood, some procedures for detection, identification and diagnostic evaluation. *International Journal of Pediatric Otorhinolaryngology* 9:31-57.

Probst, R., Lonsbury-Martin, B.L., Martin, G.K., and Coats, A.C. 1987. Otoacoustic emissions in ears with hearing loss. *American Journal of Otolaryngology* 8:73-81.

Ross, M. 1990. Implications of delay in detection and management of deafness. *Volta Review* 92:69-79.

Rutten, W.L.C. 1980. Evoked otoacoustic emissions from within normal and abnormal ears: Comparison with audiometric and electrocochleographic findings. *Hearing Research* 2:263-271.

Sacks, O. 1989. *Seeing voices.* Berkeley, Calif.: University of California Press.

Schum, R.L. 1987. Communication and social growth: A developmental model of deaf social behavior. In M.S. Robinette and C.D. Bauch (eds.), *Proceedings of a symposium in audiology* (pp. 1-25). Rochester, Minn.: Mayo Clinic-Mayo Foundation.

Schuyler, V., and Rushmer, N. 1987. *Parent-infant habilitation: A comprehensive approach to working with hearing-impaired infants and toddlers and their families.* Portland, Oreg.: Infant Hearing Resource Publications.

Shimizu, H., Walters, R.J., Kennedy, D.W., Allen, M.C., Markowitz, R.K., and Luebkert, F.R. 1985. Crib-O-Gram vs. auditory brainstem response for infant hearing screening. *Laryngoscope* 95:806-810.

Stevens, J.C., Webb, H.D., Hutchinson, J., Connell, J., Smith, M.F., and Buffin, J.T. 1991. Evaluation of click evoked otoacoustic emissions in the newborn. *British Journal of Audiology* 25:11-14.

U.S. Department of Health and Human Services, Public Health Service. 1990. *Healthy people 2000: National health promotion and disease prevention objectives*. Washington, D.C.: U.S. Government Printing Office.

Chapter 16

Sensorineural Hearing Loss
in High-Risk Infants

Diane L. Sabo, David R. Brown, and Jon F. Watchko

INTRODUCTION

Sensorineural hearing loss continues to be a serious long-term neurodevelopmental sequela of neonatal intensive care. The prevalence of hearing loss is estimated to be between 2.5% and 10% among infants who manifest any of the risk factors recommended by the 1982 Joint Committee on Infant Hearing (Anagnostakis et al. 1982; Astbury et al. 1983; Bergman et al. 1985; Duara et al. 1986; Pettigrew, Edwards, and Henderson-Smart 1988; Salamy, Eldredge, and Tooley 1989; Stein et al. 1983). Hyperbilirubinemia (Bergman et al. 1985; de Vries, Lary, and Dubowitz 1985; Perlman et al. 1983; Vohr, Lester, and Rapisardi 1989; Wennberg et al. 1982), perinatal asphyxia (Duara et al. 1986; Barden and Peltzman 1980), and the general medical condition of the infant (Bergman et al. 1985; Duara et al. 1986; Pettigrew et al. 1988) have been implicated as the causes of sensorineural hearing loss without consensus being reached. Therefore, we studied 35 children with sensorineural hearing loss and 70 matched controls to determine the independent effects of conventional risk factors for hearing impairment.

METHODS

Auditory brainstem responses (ABRs) have been used at Magee-Womens Hospital since 1980 as a screening method for hearing loss. Infants were selected for screening based on 1982 Joint Committee's risk

229

Table 1

Criteria for ABR Screening

Asphyxia
Bacterial meningitis
Congenital perinatal infections
Defects of the head and neck
Elevated bilirubin
Family history of hearing loss
Gram birth weight less than 1500
Respiratory distress
Aminoglycosides > 72 hours
Seizures or neurologic insult
Persistent pulmonary hypertension of the newborn

---

criteria and, in addition, history of seizures or neurologic insults, prolonged respiratory distress, and aminoglycoside therapy (table 1). Most neonates who were screened were admitted to Magee-Womens Hospital neonatal intensive care unit (NICU). During the calendar years 1981 through 1984, 1,160 neonates were screened, representing 3.1% of live births, 31.5% of NICU admissions, and 35.2% of NICU survivors.

Testing was done with a Madsen 74 during 1981 and a Cadwell 5200 during 1982 through 1984. The ABRs were recorded bedside during natural sleep, following a feeding, and when the patient was considered ready for discharge. Single channel ABRs were recorded with electrodes on the forehead (midline at the hairline, noninverting electrode) and mastoid of the ear being stimulated (inverting electrode). The common (ground) electrode was on the contralateral mastoid. Responses were bandpass filtered from 130 to 3200 Hz with the Madsen 74 evoked response system (in 1981) and 100 to 2000 Hz for the Cadwell 5200 system (in 1982 to 1984). Click stimuli, generated by delivering rectangular pulses of 100 μsec duration and alternating in polarity, were delivered via TDH 49 earphones at 60 and 30 dB nHL (1981) or at 70 and 35 dB nHL (1982 to 1984). Each response was averaged for 2000 stimulus presentations. Each response was replicated once to assess reproducibility.

Failure of the ABR screening was defined as no reproducible response at the higher intensity level for at least one ear. Included in the study were 35 infants who failed the screening. Infants who failed and

Table 2*
Clinical Variables

Deafness (Y/N)	Polycythemia (Hct < 65) (Y/N)
Race (white, black, other)	Virus Infection (specify)
Maternal Age (yrs)	Sepsis (Y/N)
Maternal Gravidity	Apnea and/or Bradycardia (Y/N)
Maternal Parity	Hypocalcemia (Ca <7.0) (Y/N)
Maternal Abortions	Hypokalemia (K <3.0) (Y/N)
Labor Inhibition (Y/N)	Hyperkalemia (K >7.0) (Y/N)
Beta-Methasone (Y/N)	Hypoglycemia (glucose <40) (Y/N)
Gestational Age by Dates (wks)	Hyperglycemia (glucose > 200) (Y/N)
Gestational Age by Exam (wks)	Hyponatremia (Na <126) (Y/N)
Birth Date	Hypernatremia (Na >149) (Y/N)
Place of Birth	Exchange Transfusion (number)
Birth Order	Total Phototherapy (hrs)
Sex	Peak Total Bilirubin (mg/dl)
Birth Weight (g)	Peak Direct Bilirubin (mg/dl)
Rupture of Membranes (hrs)	Umbilical Arterial Blood Gases before
Apgar Score, 1-minute	6-10-82 (number)
Apgar Score, 5-minute	Non-umbilical Arterial Blood Gases
Mode of Delivery	before 6-10-82 (number)
Length of Hospital Stay (days)	Admission Rectal Temp (°C)
Aspiration Pneumonia (Y/N)	Days in O^2
Infectious Pneumonia (Y/N)	Days on Respirator
Pulmonary Hemorrhage (Y/N)	Days in Incubator
Air Leak Syndrome (Y/N)	Aminophylline (# of doses and total
Rh Disease (Y/N)	dose)
ABO Disease (Y/N)	Ampicillin (# of doses and total dose)
Retinopathy of Prematurity (stage)	Calcium Gluconate (# of doses and total
Rickets (Y/N)	dose)
Seizures (Y/N)	Curare (# of doses and total dose)
Intraventricular Hemorrhage (grade)	Chlorothiazide (# of doses and total
Necrotizing Enterocolitis (Y/N)	dose)
Other GI Disease (Y/N)	Diazepam (# of doses and total dose)
Patent Ductus Arteriosus (Y/N)	Digoxin (# of doses and total dose)
Congenital Heart Disease (Y/N)	Dopamine (# of doses and total dose)
Infant of a Diabetic Mother (class)	Furosemide (# of doses and total dose)
Congenital Anomaly (specify)	Gentamicin (# of doses and total dose)
Early Anemia (Hct <40, Age <24	Indomethacin (# of doses and total dose)
hr) (Y/N)	Kanamycin (# of doses and total dose)
Late Anemia (Hct <30, Age > 14	Methicillin (# of doses and total dose)
days) (Y/N)	Nafcillin (# of doses and total dose)

Table 2
Clinical Variables (Continued)

Phenobarbital (# of doses and total dose)	Spironolactone (# of doses and total dose)
Phenytoin (# of doses and total dose)	Tolazoline (# of doses and total dose)
Primidone (# of doses and total dose)	Theophylline (# of doses and total dose)
Bilirubin Value (date of each test; value [mg/dl])	Vitamin E (# of doses and total dose)
	Blood or Colloid Transfusion (ml)
	Discharge Weight (g)

* Reproduced from Brown et al. 1991, with permission.

had a positive family history of hearing loss or anomalies of the ear, nose, or throat were excluded. Two control patients were selected for each patient with sensorineural hearing loss and were matched for time of birth and birth weight. Initial follow-up evaluation, conducted at Children's Hospital of Pittsburgh, included both age-appropriate behavioral audiologic testing and a complete ABR using click stimuli and 500 Hz tone bursts to further define the nature, degree, and configuration of impairment.

Once the study population was defined, the medical records of the 105 patients were abstracted for the variables listed in table 2. Data were analyzed initially using Student's-t, Fisher's exact or chi-square tests and, subsequently, using the method of Mantel and Haenszel.

RESULTS

The 35 infants who failed ABR screening had at least one follow-up evaluation at our facility that confirmed the presence of a permanent auditory impairment. Long-term (greater than five years) follow-up data are available for 28. Of the 7 children without long-term follow-up information, 3 died between 1 and 2 years of age. Two had severe sensorineural hearing losses bilaterally and were fit with hearing aids before they were lost to follow-up at this facility. Two had mild impairments by ABR assessment at the three-month follow-up visit but did not return for further testing to allow us to more completely evaluate the hearing loss.

Of the remaining 28 children, 6 had asymmetrical hearing losses, and 22 had symmetrical hearing losses. Reliable, ear-specific information was obtained from all of these children. Two of the 6 with asymmetrical hearing loss had hearing levels that were normal in one ear through 2000 Hz, with severe sensorineural hearing losses at 4000 Hz and above. These infants had sloping mild-moderate-to-severe sensorineural hearing losses in the other ear and are wearing amplification in regular classroom settings and receive itinerant services for hearing, speech, and language. The remaining 4 children have varying degrees of hearing losses in both ears, are wearing at least one hearing aid, and are receiving services for the hearing impaired, either in a classroom for the hearing impaired provided by their school district or in a school for the hearing impaired.

Of the 22 children with symmetrical hearing losses, 8 have severe-to-profound bilateral hearing losses, and 7 have hearing losses with a sloping configuration characterized by mild-to-moderate low frequency hearing losses sloping to severe-to-profound high frequency hearing losses. Two have moderate and 5 have moderate-to-severe sensorineural losses of flat configuration. All of these children are wearing amplification and attend a school for the hearing impaired, are in a classroom for the hearing impaired, are mainstreamed with an interpreter in the classroom, or are in placements that address other needs (e.g., blindness and physical or mental handicaps) but also receive itinerant services for speech, language, and hearing.

Table 3*
Prevalence of Hearing Loss

Year	Number of Live Births		Number with Hearing Loss		Rate $/\times 10^{-3}$ Live Births	
	BW $\leq 2kg$	BW $> 2kg$	BW $\leq 2kg$	BW $> 2kg$	BW $\leq 2kg$	BW $> 2kg$
1981	375	8894	17	4	45.33	0.45
1982	365	8710	5	2	13.70	0.23
1983	421	9161	0	2	0	0.22
1984	448	9424	3	2	6.70	0.21
Total	1,609	36,189	25	10	15.54	0.28

BW = birth weight.
* Reproduced from Brown et al. 1991, with permission.

Table 4*
Independent Variables Related to Deafness, Univariate Analyses

Variable	DEAF		CONTROL		Fisher p
	No.+	No.−	No.+	No.−	
Blood Transfusion	32	3	42	28	0.0010
Seizure	18	17	11	59	0.0004
IVH (any grade)	12	23	7	63	0.0066
Early Anemia	11	24	6	64	0.0080
Hypocalcemia	30	5	31	39	<0.0001
Hyponatremia	15	20	5	65	<0.0001
Ampicillin ℞	34	1	49	21	0.0012
Calcium Gluconate ℞	29	6	31	39	0.0002
Dilantin ℞	11	24	2	68	0.0002
Kanamycin ℞	33	2	49	21	0.0060
Diazepam ℞	7	28	1	69	0.0036
Furosemide ℞	17	18	6	64	<0.0001
Phenobarbital ℞	18	17	12	58	0.0008
Primidone ℞	6	29	0	70	0.0020

* Reproduced from Brown et al. 1991, with permission.

There were 37,798 live births at Magee-Womens Hospital during the four-year study period (1981-1984), of which 1,609 (4.2%) weighed ≤ 2000 g at birth. During this four-year period, the overall prevalence of neonatal sensorineural hearing loss, excluding familial hearing loss and hearing loss related to physical anomalies of the ear, nose, or throat, was 0.93 per 1,000 births. The birth weight-adjusted estimated prevalence per 1,000 births was 15.54 for birth weight ≤ 2000 g and 0.28 for larger babies. The rate for smaller babies decreased from 45.33 to 6.70 from 1981 to 1984 while the estimated rate for the larger babies decreased from 0.45 to 0.21 per 1,000 births (table 3). There was a statistically significant temporal trend that can be accounted for by the high rate in 1981.

Univariate analyses were initially done on all the potential independent variables in this case-control study. Those variables for which there was a statistically significant difference ($p < 0.01$) are listed in table 4. From this subset of variables, furosemide was selected because it was one of the three variables most strongly associated with sensorineural hearing loss. Mantel-Haenszel analyses were performed on each of the remaining variables controlling for the effects of furosemide in each analysis. Early anemia, hypocalcemia, calcium gluconate, hyponatremia, blood transfusion, and ampicillin treatment continued to show a significant association with sensorineural hearing loss ($p < 0.05$) when furosemide use was controlled. When each of the seven variables was then analyzed for association with sensorineural hearing loss while controlling for the effects of the other six, only furosemide treatment continued to show a statistically significant effect.

DISCUSSION

Long-term follow-up of the infants who failed their ABR screening indicates that the majority have significant sensorineural hearing losses, require the use of amplification, and are in schools for the hearing impaired as their primary placement or are receiving hearing therapy services at a school that addresses other sensory, physical, or mental disability. The prevalence of hearing loss in our NICU population is of interest because, with the exception of the 4.5% rate in 1981 for patients weighing ≤ 2000 g at birth, the rates were never $> 2\%$ in this low-birth weight group. These figures do not include infants with familial history of sensorineural hearing loss or those with anomalies of the ear, nose, or throat. This is a much lower prevalence than has been reported by others (Anagnostakis et al. 1982; Astbury et al. 1983; Bergman et al. 1985; Duara et al. 1986; Pettigrew et al. 1988; Salamy et al. 1989). The decreasing prevalence of sensorineural hearing loss over time suggested to us the possibility that some change in nursery procedure might be responsible. The most noteworthy change between 1981 and 1984 was the elimination of benzyl alcohol from saline solutions used for mixing medications and for clearing umbilical arterial lines. Benzyl alcohol has been reported to be associated with intraventricular hemorrhage (Jardine and Rogers 1989) and neurologic handicap (Benda et al. 1986), and it seemed logical to incriminate it in the development of another central nervous system injury. We had no measurements of serum benzyl alcohol concentration for our patients, but we did calculate an index of benzyl alcohol exposure based on the number of umbilical arterial blood samples and the number of medication doses in which benzyl alcohol was a diluent. Although the temporal relationship was compelling, when we controlled for confounding factors, we were unable to show a relationship between benzyl alcohol exposure and sensorineural hearing loss.

The theoretical importance of bilirubin as a risk factor for sensorineural hearing loss has been extensively debated (Anagnostakis et al. 1982; Bergman et al. 1985; de Vries et al. 1985; Lenhardt et al. 1984; Nwaesei et al. 1984; Perlman et al. 1983; Salamy et al. 1989; Vohr et al. 1989; Wennberg et al. 1982). Serum bilirubin concentration has been inconsistently implicated as a risk factor for sensorineural hearing loss. Our data fail to support any relationship, although the mean peak serum concentration for all our neonates (13 mg/dl) was consistently nontoxic, even if bilirubin concentration is an important risk factor.

The potential importance of drug exposure in the pathogenesis of hearing loss has been widely discussed (Abramovich et al. 1979; Brummett et al. 1975; Brummett 1981; Brummett and Fox 1982; Finitzo-Hieber et al. 1985; Gottl et al. 1985; Marshall et al. 1980; McDonald 1964; Rybak 1985; Winkel et al. 1978). The role of drugs in producing hearing impairment among high-risk neonates, however, remains controversial and was not part of the neonatal risk factors for hearing loss until recently. The 1990 Joint Committee on Infant Hearing Position Statement includes ototoxic medications. Studies that have addressed the potential ototoxic effects of aminoglycosides in human newborns are inconclusive (Abramovich et al. 1979; Anagnostakis et al. 1982; Adelman, Linder, and Levi 1989; Finitzo-Hieber et al. 1985; Marshall et al. 1980; McDonald 1964; Meyerhoff et al. 1989; Winkel et al. 1978). However, findings from recent investigations suggest that combined use of aminoglycosides and furosemide (Salamy et al. 1989) or extensive use of aminoglycosides (Pettigrew et al. 1988) is associated with the development of sensorineural hearing loss in low-birth-weight infants. Ototoxic effects have resulted from use of diuretics such as furosemide in adult animals (Gottl, Roesch, and Klinke 1985; Rybak 1985). A synergistic interaction producing irreversible ototoxicity has been found between these diuretics and aminoglycoside therapy (Brummett et al. 1975; Brummett 1981; Brummett and Fox 1982; Rybak 1985).

Our study documents that furosemide, a drug commonly used in the care of neonates with chronic lung disease (Engelhardt et al. 1986), is independently associated with the development of sensorineural hearing loss and confirms a recent report on the importance of exposure to furosemide as a risk factor for sensorineural hearing loss (Salamy et al. 1989). That furosemide is an independent risk factor is a new finding in neonates but is consistent with previous findings in animals and adult humans (Rybak 1985). However, we were unable to confirm that the combination of furosemide and aminoglycoside antibiotics was a risk factor for sensorineural hearing loss in very-low-birth-weight neonates, as reported by Salamy et al. (1989).

The association of furosemide with sensorineural hearing loss will demand that we look more critically at the use of this drug in the NICU. Although furosemide has short-lived positive effects on pulmonary function in neonates with chronic lung disease (Kao et al. 1983), there are no reports of improvement in mortality or long-term morbidity. A large study is now warranted to confirm our findings. Ideally, this would be a cohort study, thus avoiding the biases inherent in selecting control patients.

REFERENCES

Abramovich, S.J., Gregory S., Slemick, M., and Stewart, A. 1979. Hearing loss in very low birth weight infants treated with neonatal intensive care. *Archives of Disease in Childhood* 54:421-426.

Adelman, C., Linder, N., and Levi, H. 1989. Auditory nerve and brain stem evoked response thresholds in infants treated with gentamicin as neonates. *Annals of Otology, Rhinology and Laryngology* 98:283-286.

Anagnostakis, D., Petmezakis, J., Papazissus, G., Messaritakis, J., and Matsaniotis, N. 1982. Hearing loss in low-birth-weight infants. *American Journal of Diseases of Children* 136:602-604.

Astbury, J., Orgill, A.A., Bajuk, B., and Yu, V.Y. 1983. Determinants of developmental performance of very low-birth-weight survivors at one and two years of age. *Developmental Medicine and Child Neurology* 25:709-719.

Barden, T.P., and Peltzman, P. 1980. Newborn brainstem auditory evoked responses and perinatal clinical events. *American Journal of Obstetrics and Gynecology* 136:912-919.

Benda, G.I., Hiller, J.L., and Reynolds, J.W. 1986. Benzyl alcohol toxicity: impact on neurologic handicaps among surviving very low birth weight infants. *Pediatrics* 77:507-512.

Bergman, I., Hirsch, R.P., Fria, T.J., Shapiro, S.M., Holzman, I., and Painter, M.J. 1985. Cause of hearing loss in the high-risk-premature infant. *Journal of Pediatrics* 106:95-101.

Brown, D.R., Watchko, J.F., and Sabo, D. 1991. Neonatal sensorineural hearing loss associated with furosemide: A case-control study. *Developmental Medicine and Child Neurology* 33:816-823.

Brummett, R.E. 1981. Effects of antibiotic-diuretic interactions in the guinea pig model of ototoxicity. *Review of Infectious Diseases* Suppl. 3:S216-S223.

Brummett, R.E., Traynor, J., Brown, R., and Himes, D. 1975. Cochlear damage resulting from kanamycin and furosemide. *Acta Otolaryngologica* 80:86-92.

Brummett, R.E., and Fox, K.E. 1982. Studies of aminoglycoside ototoxicity in animal models. In A. Welton and H.C. Neu (eds.), *The aminoglycosides: Microbiology, clinical use and toxicology.* New York: Marcel Dekker.

deVries, L.S., Lary, S., and Dubowitz, L.M.S. 1985. Relationship of serum bilirubin level to ototoxicity and deafness in high-risk low-birth-weight infants. *Pediatrics* 76:351-354.

Duara, S., Suter, C.M., Bessard, K.K., and Gutberlet, R.L. 1986. Neonatal screening with auditory brainstem responses: Results of follow-up audiometry and risk factor evaluation. *Journal of Pediatrics* 108:276-281.

Engelhardt, B., Elliot, S., and Hazinski, T.A. 1986. Short- and long-term effects of furosemide on lung function in infants with bronchopulmonary dysplasia. *Journal of Pediatrics* 109:1034-1039.

Finitzo-Hieber, T., McCracken, G.H. Jr., and Brown, K.C. 1985. Prospective controlled evaluation of auditory function in neonates given netilmicin or amikacin. *Journal of Pediatrics* 106:129-136.

Gottl, K.H., Roesch, A., and Klinke, R. 1985. Quantitative evaluation of ototoxic side effects of furosemide, piretanide, bumetanide, azosemide and ozolinone in the cat—a new approach to the problem of ototoxicity. *Archives of Pharmacology* 331:275-282.

Jardine, D.S., and Rogers, J. 1989. Relationship of benzyl alcohol to kernicterus, intraventricular hemorrhage and mortality in preterm infants. *Pediatrics* 83:153-160.

Joint Committee on Infant Hearing. 1982. Position statement. *Asha* 24(12):1017-1018.

Joint Committee on Infant Hearing. 1991. 1990 Position statement. *Asha* 33(Suppl. 5):3-6.

Kao, L.C., Warburton, D., Sargent, C.W., Platzker, A.C.G., and Keens, T. G. 1983. Furosemide acutely decreases airway resistance in chronic bronchopulmonary dysplasia. *Journal of Pediatrics* 103:624-629.

Lenhardt, M.L., McArtor, R., and Bryant, B. 1984. Effects of neonatal hyperbilirubinemia on the brainstem electric response. *Journal of Pediatrics* 104:281-284.

McDonald, A.D. 1964. Deafness in children of very low birth weight. *Archives of Disease in Childhood* 39:272-277.

Marshall, R.E., Reichert, T.J., Kerley, S.M., and Davis, J. 1980. Auditory function in newborn intensive care unit patients revealed by auditory brainstem potential. *Journal of Pediatrics* 96:731-735.

Meyerhoff, W.L., Maale, G.E., Yellin, W., and Roland, P.S. 1989. Audiologic threshold monitoring of patients receiving ototoxic drugs. Preliminary report. *Annals of Otology, Rhinology and Laryngology* 98:950-954.

Nwaesei, C.G., Van Aerde, J., Boyden, M., and Perlman, C. 1984. Changes in auditory brainstem responses in hyperbilirubinemic infants before and after exchange transfusion. *Pediatrics* 74:800-803.

Perlman, M., Fainmesser, P., Sohmer, H., Tamari, H., Wax, Y., and Pevsmer, B. 1983. Auditory nerve-brainstem evoked response in hyperbilirubinemic neonates. *Pediatrics* 72:658-686.

Pettigrew, A.G., Edwards, D.A., and Henderson-Smart, D.J. 1988. Perinatal risk factors in preterm infants with moderate-to-profound hearing deficits. *Medical Journal of Australia* 148:174-177.

Rybak, L.P. 1985. Furosemide ototoxicity: Clinical and experimental aspects. *Laryngoscope* 9(Suppl):1-14.

Salamy, A., Eldredge, L., and Tooley, W.J. 1989. Neonatal status and hearing loss in high-risk infants. *Journal of Pediatrics* 114:847-852.

Stein, L., Ozdamar, O., Kraus, N., and Paton, J. 1983. Follow-up of infants screened by auditory brainstem response in the neonatal intensive care unit. *Journal of Pediatrics* 103:447-453.

Vohr, B.R., Lester, B., and Rapisardi, G. 1989. Abnormal brain-stem function (brain-stem auditory evoked response) correlates with acoustic cry features in term infants with hyperbilirubinemia. *Journal of Pediatrics* 115:303-308.

Wennberg, R.P., Ahlfors, C.E., Bickers, R., McMurtry, C.A., and Shetter, J.L. 1982. Abnormal auditory brainstem response in a newborn infant with hyperbilirubinemia: Improvement with exchange transfusion. *Journal of Pediatrics* 100:624-626.

Winkel, S., Bonding, P., Larsen, P.K., and Roosen, J. 1978. Possible effects of kanamycin and incubation in newborn children with low birthweight. *Acta Paediatrica Scandinavica* 67:709-715.

PART III.

Screening Infants and Young Children for Auditory Function

Chapter 17

Screening for Hearing Loss:
Behavioral Options

Allan O. Diefendorf

INTRODUCTION

Screening for hearing loss in young children is the first step of early identification planning. Previous evaluations of the screening process (Paradise and Smith 1978; Jerger et al. 1983) have devoted considerable attention to the disease characteristics required for mass screening. In general, screening for sensorineural hearing impairment meets the specified prerequisites. Regardless of specific screening procedures, the principal objective of any hearing screening program is to correctly identify hearing loss in those infants who are truly hearing impaired while passing those with normal hearing. The focus of screening is not to specify the infant's hearing sensitivity but to determine whether or not a hearing loss exists.

The foundation underlying any screening program is largely determined by the goals and rationale for the screening program and the age at which children are to be screened. A program aimed at identifying severe sensorineural hearing loss would be approached differently from a program geared toward detecting milder hearing losses. Age is of crucial importance in determining program goals (Folsom 1990). For example, expectations regarding screening efficiency are different in a program designed to identify hearing loss in a neonatal population from those in a program designed to identify hearing loss in the school-age population. Some general guiding principles hold, however, and are virtually universal across identification programs: (1) identification of hearing loss at the earliest possible time, (2) rescreening or ongoing assessment of failures, (3) dissemination of information about hearing for parents of all infants screened, and (4) intervention protocols in place to serve those children who fail as well as their families.

PROGRAMMATIC AND PROCEDURAL CONSIDERATIONS

In general, early identification programs can be broken down into two categories: (1) neonatal screening, and (2) infant screening. Frequently, these categories evolve from hospitals' program priorities, health care financing, patient demographics, and personnel and equipment logistics.

Neonatal screening encompasses programs such as mass screening of all newborns, graduates of neonatal intensive care units (NICU), and infants from full-term nurseries (FTN) who have been selected on the basis of high-risk factors (see Appendix 1). For newborns and developmentally delayed infants, the screening test procedure of choice is the auditory brainstem response (ABR). Regardless of how the population is selected (mass newborn screening, NICU patients, or low-risk infants from the FTN selected by high-risk factors), the ABR offers the most efficient tool for screening this age group. Reliable estimates of peripheral hearing in newborns can be derived from these responses.

Infant screening programs are often associated with high-risk infant follow-up clinics. These clinics are designed to assess developmental landmarks in infants at risk for developmental delay (motor and/or cognitive). Infants who are graduates of a NICU, and other newborns selected by high-risk factors (see Appendix 1), are referred into these programs early in life and return for follow-up assessment at regular intervals.

With the realization that the ABR is an effective method of screening hearing in infants, interest in pursuing behavioral screening techniques has diminished. However, many of the problems of ABR screening (activity state, length of test, expense) are compounded for older infants. Scheduling, sedation, and cost may become prohibitive. Under these circumstances, ABR is no longer a reasonable screening procedure. By converging the requirements of screening (valid, reliable, efficient, inexpensive) with interests and abilities of young children, *behavioral* screening emerges as the choice with this age group.

BEHAVIORAL SCREENING TECHNIQUES

Three techniques should be viewed in the context of behavioral screening: behavioral observation audiometry (BOA), an observer-based psychoacoustic procedure (OPP), and visual reinforcement audiometry (VRA). Each technique has application in some aspect of pediatric assessment. However, the advantages and limitations of each technique with regard to hearing screening are notable.

BEHAVIORAL OBSERVATION AUDIOMETRY

BOA is an approach to hearing screening where a high-intensity (e.g., 90 dBA) narrow band noise is presented by a hand-held instrument positioned near the infant. The expected response includes localization, eye widening and other changes in facial expression, cessation of activity, crying, and gross startle responses. The determination of whether a response has occurred is highly subjective and can often be difficult even for experienced observers. As a result, there are serious concerns about the effectiveness of BOA for screening. For example, using BOA, Plotnick and Leppler (1986) identified only 2 severely hearing-impaired infants among 356 newborns screened in the NICU. Assuming a very conservative 2% prevalence of significant sensorineural hearing loss in the NICU, at least three times as many hearing-impaired infants should have been identified in the group tested. Because of the high stimulus intensity used, BOA is likely to miss an infant with a mild-moderate bilateral hearing loss as well as those with unilateral impairment. False negative rates of 40% to 86% have been reported for BOA (Alberti et al. 1983; Durieux-Smith et al. 1985; Jacobson and Morehouse 1984), meaning that a large number of infants with significant hearing loss pass behavioral screening and are thus lost to immediate intervention. The restrictions on validity and reliability imposed by stimulus and response factors when using BOA with newborns are not acceptable. Thus, BOA cannot be recommended for neonatal hearing screening. Although BOA is no longer viewed as an effective screening procedure, there are still some proponents of the technique as evidenced by a small hand-held screener currently being marketed as a convenient and inexpensive alternative to more elaborate and costly instrumentation.

OBSERVER-BASED PSYCHOACOUSTIC PROCEDURE

OPP (Olsho et al. 1987) combines features of the forced-choice preferential looking (FPL) technique and of VRA to determine infant hearing sensitivity. The FPL technique (Teller 1979) is based on an infant's tendency to attend preferentially to certain visual stimuli (presented left or right), as evidenced by looking toward and continuing to look at the preferred stimulus. An observer must judge the location of the stimulus based on the infant's gaze direction, and make a two-alternative (right vs. left) forced choice. Whereas FPL is a two-interval forced-choice procedure, OPP is based on an infant's tendency to respond to the presence of a single auditory stimulus. Thus, OPP is a single-interval, yes/no procedure. Additionally, reinforcement is not utilized in FPL, but it is a critical aspect of OPP.

For the infant, OPP is almost identical to visual reinforcement audiometry. The infant sits on the parent's lap while listening to sounds presented monaurally over lightweight earphones. The infant's attention is maintained at midline by an assistant manipulating noiseless toys. At certain times an auditory signal is presented. If the infant responds in such a way (i.e., responses similar to BOA) that the observer correctly decides that a signal has occurred, a mechanical toy is activated to reinforce whatever response was made by the infant. Clearly, OPP differs from BOA by developing specific rules and protocols for observers in order to control response bias, and by developing the assertion that auditory behaviors from very young infants can be influenced by reinforcement. In turn, reinforcement motivates responsiveness, minimizes habituation, and increases the likelihood and magnitude of subsequent responses.

OPP has been shown to be a valid technique for defining pure-tone sensitivity in normally hearing infants as young as 3 months of age (Olsho et al. 1987; Olsho et al. 1988). The current utilization of OPP is geared toward laboratory research into developmental questions of infant audition; therefore, clinical data are absent regarding the success of OPP with hearing-impaired infants. Yet, the average number of trials to obtain a single frequency threshold for normally hearing infants suggests that the OPP technique would be inefficient for hearing screening.

VISUAL REINFORCEMENT AUDIOMETRY

VRA has emerged as a valid and reliable behavioral procedure for infants and young children, 5½ months through 2 years of age. VRA is based on the premise that the discrimination of a change in the child's environment (detection of the presence of sound from no sound) results in reinforcement. The VRA procedure capitalizes on the child's natural inclination to turn toward a sound source. Through operant conditioning, the child learns that a head turn following the detection of a sound results in reinforcement.

The success of VRA is related to the fact that the response (head turn) and reinforcer (animated toy) are well suited to the developmental level of children within this age range. Once the child is under stimulus control, he will continue to respond at low sensation levels long enough to provide an estimate of threshold (minimum response level). In contrast to BOA, infants tested by VRA respond equally as well to pure tones as to signals with varying bandwidth, demonstrating that response behavior is shaped by reinforcement and not characteristics of the auditory signal (Wilson and Moore 1978; Thompson and Folsom 1985). Inter- and intra-infant data obtained with VRA are impressive. Not only are threshold estimates consistent from the same infant and similar to those obtained from other infants, but threshold data are similar to older children and adults. Moreover, due to low response variability using the VRA procedure, threshold elevations secondary to even mild peripheral hearing impairments are reliably detected. It is generally agreed that as long as the child is under stimulus control, thresholds are obtained quickly and provide, with a high degree of confidence, valid information for making diagnostic and management decisions.

VRA has one primary limitation as a screening technique. The procedure can be personnel intensive and expensive. Accurate VRA assessment depends in large part on the ability of one examiner to keep an infant appropriately attentive while another assumes the responsibility of audiometry and operant conditioning. The use of two examiners, however, reduces the efficiency of VRA. The procedure can be completed by a single examiner. A remote audiometer switching program or the use of a personal computer puts the control of the equipment into the hands of one audiologist who can be in direct contact with the child.

This approach enhances the examiner's direct interaction with the infant and minimizes random head turning and false responding.[1]

For each of these procedures, as with all psychophysical methods, several measures are useful for making comparisons and determining procedural choices: (1) validity, or the accuracy of the threshold estimate (minimum response level); (2) efficiency, defined as the greatest accuracy for effort expended (trials needed to estimate threshold); and (3) reliability of patient responses. Reliability can be further divided into intersubject reliability, intrasubject reliability across test sessions, and test-retest reliability within the same session. Single session results are of particular importance in the context of hearing screening where infants are presumably "tested" once and do not return multiple times.

Table 1 highlights the differences between the three techniques relative to validity, efficiency, and reliability. When screening young infants for hearing loss, VRA emerges as the most appropriate choice.

Table 1
Summary of Screening Test Requirements for the Different Behavioral Options

	VALIDITY	EFFICIENCY	RELIABILITY
BOA	-	+	-
OPP	+	-	+
VRA	+	+	+

FACTORS IN VISUAL REINFORCEMENT AUDIOMETRY

Infant hearing screening using VRA does not follow a standard protocol across clinical settings. Varying strategies are employed by clinicians and researchers. Conditioning criteria, the type of test stimuli, and the starting intensity used in screening or evaluation vary from setting to setting. Stopping rules (terminating threshold exploration for

---

[1] A single examiner can use a "centering toy" for maintaining a child's attention at midline. However, this approach removes the examiner from the test room, creates noisy competition with the "test" signal, and results in increased false responses.

a given stimulus) and the application of reinforcement also vary. A variety of schemes are used for implementing control trials. These factors and their interactions must be considered when developing behavioral protocols for infant hearing screening using VRA.

CONDITIONING CRITERIA

The first phase of VRA is the conditioning process. Response shaping is critical to the success of the operant procedure. This phase of the testing is completely under the examiner's control. Thus, the examiner must be skilled in response training and sensitive to the various stages of response acquisition. Two different approaches that can be attempted in the first phase of VRA are (1) pairing the stimulus with the reinforcer and (2) observing a spontaneous response from the infant followed by reinforcement. Following several "training trials," a criterion of several consecutive head-turn responses must be met prior to moving to the second phase of actual test trials. Successful completion of training occurs when the infant is making contingent responses and random head turning is at a minimum. If criterion is not reached, phase one retraining must occur until criterion is met. The number of training trials needed before phase two trials begin differs among infants. However, the training phase is usually brief.

A spontaneous head turn is not going to be elicited from children who, because of hearing loss or central auditory problems, have not developed auditory localization skills. When training children suspected of hearing loss or other developmental problems in phase one, it is preferable to administer several paired conditioning trials at suprathreshold levels. This strategy will probably be required to teach the head-turn response prior to stage two threshold exploration. Failure to condition rapidly should alert the examiner to a potential auditory problem or other factors (physical, cognitive, social) that affect the child's behavior.

Primus and Thompson (1985) investigated three stimulus conditions (complex noise presented at 50 dB nHL, complex noise presented at 25 dB nHL, and a 1500 Hz warble tone presented at 50 dB nHL) on the conditioning rate in VRA with 1-year-old children. These authors concluded that variation in stimulus properties (stimulus type and starting intensity) had no effect on the rate of conditioning in their sample of children. Thirty-two of 36 infants satisfied the conditioning criteria (three consecutive correct responses) immediately following two training trials. The remaining four subjects required four training trials (paired presentations of stimulus and reinforcement) prior to reaching the conditioning criteria. These findings provide evidence that examiners need not compromise signal parameters in the assessment of infants so long as the children condition well to the VRA task.

Thompson and Folsom (1984) compared the effects of two conditioning procedures in VRA with 1- and 2-year-old children. One conditioning procedure used an initial stimulus presentation of 30 dB HL and only two conditioning trials prior to threshold exploration. The second procedure used a 60 dB HL initial presentation level and five conditioning trials prior to threshold exploration. The stimulus was complex noise, filtered to pass frequencies primarily in the 500 to 2000 Hz range. This study revealed no differences between the two conditioning procedures with regard to minimum response levels or the number of stimulus presentations required to establish minimum response levels (discounting conditioning trials). Results from the Primus and Thompson study and the Thompson and Folsom study lead to the inference that signal type or starting intensity has minimal effect on conditioning success or response consistency.

Eilers et al. (1991a) used computer simulation to evaluate several parameters of an automated hearing test algorithm with an infant response model. Starting intensity was one of the parameters of interest. Results of simulations with normal hearing and hearing-impaired pseudosubjects showed that, in general, starting intensities close to true threshold yield more accurate estimates of threshold than distant starting intensities. That is, there was a small advantage in accuracy with a 30 dB HL starting intensity for normal subjects and a larger disadvantage for these same subjects with a 50 dB HL starting intensity. These data suggest that the farther the test starting intensity is from the subject's true threshold, the more opportunity the subject has to make a response error (fail to respond to a detectable signal). Greater numbers of response errors lead to less accurate thresholds. In a companion article, Eilers et al. (1991b) compared the computer simulation data to response patterns for infants. In an actual test situation, starting intensity had little practical significance. Minimum response levels differed across starting levels by approximately 3 dB, a value less than one measurement step.

Individual circumstances in hearing screening may dictate the use of various starting intensities. However, given that the majority of infants can be expected to have normal hearing, the most efficient test is one that uses a low screening level. Another test situation that warrants a low screening level (i.e., 30 to 40 dB) is when children cannot be conditioned to respond satisfactorily to the VRA procedure and demonstrate only a few spontaneous responses prior to habituation. In this situation, it is clinically more productive to obtain responses at lower intensity levels as opposed to higher intensity levels.

STOPPING RULES

Following a training procedure, the test phase of VRA begins. Depending on response outcome during the test phase, signal intensity is either attenuated after every "yes" response or increased after every "no" response. An adaptive threshold search is initiated until a stopping criterion is met. For example, stimulus intensity is attenuated in 10 dB steps until the infant makes the first "miss" (no response to a signal trial). A miss is followed by an increase in signal intensity. Two correct responses are followed by a decrease in signal level. After a specific number of reversals, the threshold search is terminated. Threshold (minimum response level) is then defined as the mean of the reversal points (figure 1).

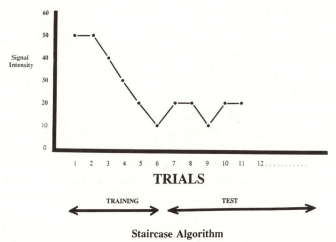

Staircase Algorithm

Figure 1. Adaptive test procedure with 10 dB step size; threshold (minimum response level) based on the mean of four reversals. In this case the MRL was approximately 15 dB HL.

How many reversals should be required before stopping a threshold search? Too few may sacrifice response accuracy. However, too many may reduce efficiency as well as the number of trials that can be spent obtaining thresholds to other stimuli before an infant tires of testing. Eilers et al. (1991a, b), using computer simulation and infant counterparts, suggest that a range of three to six reversals has little impact on test accuracy; that is, less than a 3 dB difference in minimum response levels across the range of stopping rule conditions (3, 4, 5, 6 for computer simulation and 3 and 6 for infants). Thus, beyond three to four reversals, little accuracy is gained. However, these authors demonstrate that stopping rules do have a significant effect on test length. Tests with a three-reversal stopping rule were significantly shorter than those with six reversals. As stopping rules are increased from three to six, there is about a 50% increase in the number of test trials without any practical change in response accuracy. These results suggest that by using relatively few reversals to estimate minimum response levels a staircase algorithm may be shortened without sacrificing accuracy.

REINFORCEMENT SCHEDULES AND NOVELTY

A critical feature of the VRA procedure is that the reward for correct responding is highly appealing. Maintaining response behavior over repeated trials depends on the use of appropriate reinforcement. Moore, Thompson, and Thompson (1975) demonstrated the strength of visual reinforcement (a lighted three-dimensional animated toy) over a flashing light and over social reinforcement in maintaining response motivation of infants 12 to 18 months of age. The strength of the "complex" visual reinforcer was subsequently demonstrated with normally developing 5-month-old infants.

In general, a 100% reinforcement schedule (reinforcement for every correct response) results in more rapid conditioning, yet more rapid habituation. Conversely, an intermittent reinforcement schedule produces slower conditioning but also a slower rate of habituation. Consequently, most clinicians recommended a protocol that begins with a 100% reinforcement schedule and then gradually shifts to an intermittent reinforcement schedule.

In an effort to investigate the influence of reinforcement schedules on the VRA procedure, Primus and Thompson (1985) compared a 100% reinforcement schedule to an intermittent reinforcement schedule with 2-

year-old children. The two reinforcement schedules revealed no differences in the infant's rate of habituation or on the number of infant responses during stimulus trials. These findings provide an excellent guideline for reinforcing questionable infant responses. That is, reinforcement should be withheld when clinicians are uncertain about reinforcing delayed or ambiguous head-turn responses. The risk of reinforcing a false response is that it may lead to confusion for a child under stimulus control. Thus, this error in reinforcement must be avoided. Failure to reinforce a correct response, however, does not degrade performance. In this particular situation, withholding reinforcement is actually viewed as intermittent reinforcement, which will not interfere with subsequent infant responses.

The use of novelty in a reinforcement protocol is an effective technique for improving responses. In addition to slowing the decline in response rate, novelty can renew a subject's interest in the experimental task and revive response behavior (Bond 1972; Lipsitt and Werner 1981; Primus and Thompson 1985). Evidence shows that infants and young children attend more to novel versus familiar stimuli, and are more willing to respond appropriately to elicit novel stimuli (Caron and Caron 1968; 1969; Lewis and Goldberg 1969; Lipsitt and Werner 1981).

The availability of multiple visual reinforcers (stacked and housed in separate compartments) in VRA enhances novelty and, therefore, the impact of reinforcement. Switching between the toy reinforcers enhances reinforcement by increasing novelty and uncertainty. The primary benefit of novel reinforcement in VRA is an increased amount of information about hearing in a single test session. This is an especially valuable advantage when one screens children who may be unable to return for multiple visits.

CONTROL TRIALS

False positive responses must be monitored by means of control trials when assessing infant hearing. This is true for both screening and diagnostic applications of VRA. Both test trials (signal presented) and control trials (no signal presented) occur during threshold exploration. Either trial initiates an observation interval during which responses are judged. If a response occurs during a signal trial, it is considered a correct detection. A response occurring during a control trial, however, is considered a false response. Control trials are interspersed among actual stimulus trials on a random schedule. The assumption is that infants produce a comparable number of incorrect head turns during both control and test trials. Therefore, it is possible to estimate chance responding to test trials by monitoring responses during control trials. The purpose of the control trial is to assess the reliability of responses. Test results on any infant who reaches an unacceptable false response rate are excluded. In clinical and research protocols, test results are frequently discounted if a criterion of greater than 25% incorrect controls is exceeded (Nozza and Wilson 1984; Primus and Thompson 1985).

MODIFICATIONS IN VRA FOR SCREENING

Clinical investigators have reported modifications of traditional VRA procedures to allow a single examiner to conduct a screening test. Popejoy et al. (1988) developed a remote audiometer switching program (RASP). With this approach, a microcomputer interfaced with a clinical audiometer can be remotely accessed from the test room where the examiner is seated with the child. This arrangement eliminates the need for a second "examiner," thereby improving the efficiency of VRA in a standard clinical setting.

Hardware modifications, including the use of personal computers to automate the VRA procedure, increase the possibility of large-scale screening applications. Weber (1987a; 1987b) described his efforts with the public health service in Colorado. A portable screening VRA unit was designed for use primarily in public health nursing offices. Switches are mounted on a hand-held control paddle for activating test stimuli and reinforcement. A distracting toy is fastened to the opposite side of the paddle. Calibrated test signals are presented via audiocassette tape. Of 25,000 youngsters screened, almost 4,000 (16%) were referred for medical consultation, and 30 children were found with significant sensorineural hearing loss. These data reinforce the need for outreach screening efforts in rural areas where an efficient and cost-effective procedure is required. They also illustrate that a portable VRA screening system can be successful as a valid, reliable, and efficient screening procedure with infants and toddlers.

Widen (1990) reported on the effectiveness of VRA screening with a large population of at-risk infants in Miami using a computer-based system. Software programs were written for four components of the screening process: calibration, storage of patient information, testing, and reporting. An Apple II was programmed to choose stimulus type and level, activate reinforcement, keep track of responses, calculate threshold, and print a report.

To pass the screening, an infant was required to respond three out of four times to each of two stimuli (speech noise and a 4000 Hz narrow band noise). These stimuli were chosen as the best two choices to rule out either low- or high-frequency loss of hearing sensitivity. As soon as screening was completed, threshold estimation was attempted. Screening and threshold testing for the two stimuli were accomplished in 7 to 11 minutes. VRA task success was defined when the infant was conditioned and yielded a threshold for at least one stimulus, or passed the screening for the two stimuli, in one session. Of the infants who were screened, a high percentage failed the screening levels for one or both stimuli. One-third of the 6-month-old infants and nearly a one-fourth of the 12-month-old infants failed the screening. Widen (1990) suspected that a high prevalence of otitis media in this population was responsible for the screening failures.

To determine the accuracy of the VRA screening outcome, results were compared to tympanometric screening data. For those children who passed the behavioral screening, 72% had normal tympanograms, 23% showed negative pressure (> -150 daPa), and 5% revealed flat tympanograms. For the children who failed the behavioral screen, only one child had a normal tympanogram while 80% had flat tympanograms. These results reflect the sensitivity of Widen's procedure, particularly for screening those children who may have hearing loss due to otitis media with effusion. Moreover, the screening test was cost-effective and completed in a short time.

The most recent improvement in infant hearing assessment is the development of a screening algorithm called "classification of audiograms by sequential testing," or CAST (Eilers et al. 1989a; Eilers et al. 1989b; Ozdamar et al. 1990). This approach utilizes the VRA procedure, but does not result in a pass-fail determination or a threshold determination. Rather, CAST attempts to find an audiogram pattern (figure 2) that most closely conforms to a patient's response pattern. Four frequency audiogram prediction is based on probability of occurrence that is designed to maximize the information obtained from each preceding trial.

In testing children, most clinicians use their knowledge of the auditory system, patient history, possible configurations of hearing loss

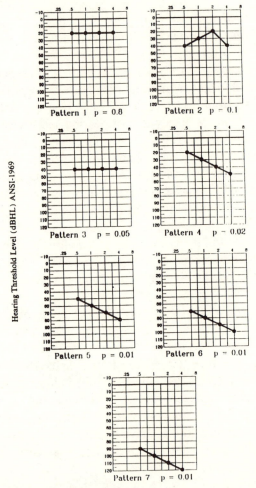

Figure 2. Patterns of Audiometric Prediction from "classification of audiograms by sequential testing" or CAST. Reproduced from Ozdamar, Eilers, Miskiel, and Widen 1990, with permission.

associated with specific etiologies, and the child's response behavior to determine the best choice of signal parameters for assessment. As testing progresses, likely future responses are determined from preceding responses. Taken together, clinicians are able to make predictions about audiogram outcomes. The CAST algorithm formalizes some of the intuitive capacities of experienced clinicians and thereby reduces the total number of trials necessary to estimate an infant audiogram. For example, if an infant responds correctly at 20 dB HL to a 1000 Hz signal, the likelihood of that infant's having a pattern consistent with normal hearing is quite high.

With CAST, the frequency and intensity of a test signal are chosen to maximize information obtained from the subject. Signal trials are presented and head-turn responses are elicited. The weights of the audiometric patterns are updated using subject response outcome. If one of the weights exceeds the criterion value, then a pattern is chosen from among the other patterns as the infant's most likely audiogram. If no pattern weight exceeds the criterion value, the procedure is continued. The average number of total trials for audiogram prediction ranges from 13 to 20.

In order to evaluate the capability of CAST to predict infant audiogram patterns correctly, computer simulations (see Eilers et al. 1991a; 1991b) were performed. Each pseudotest continued until the procedure's stopping criterion was met, and then an audiogram pattern was predicted. Computer simulations revealed that CAST was 100% sensitive. Not one of the hearing-impaired pseudosubjects was passed as normal. CAST did, however, yield some false positives and some misclassifications under conditions of high pseudosubject variability. While CAST shows promise as a screening test for predicting four frequency audiograms in infants and toddlers, clinical trials must be documented to determine its actual capabilities.

A long recognized need for early identification of and intervention for children with hearing impairment may soon be realized through the impetus of Public Law 99-457. The earlier in life that intervention can be initiated, the greater the opportunity to mitigate the impact of the impairment on speech, language, and learning. With an anticipated increase in the number of infants with hearing loss, coupled with changes in health care reimbursement, efficient and cost-effective programs are essential. Therefore, infant hearing screening must be approached with an appropriate balance between electrophysiologic and behavioral procedures.

SUMMARY

This chapter has focused on behavioral options for hearing screening. Moreover, for infants 6 months of age (corrected) and older, the conditioned head-turn response is the most appropriate procedural screening tool. However, knowledge of operant conditioning, the effects of reinforcement, and infant's response behavior must be applied by clinicians in order to maximize this test strategy. Finally, any program of early identification must have a systematic follow-up and intervention program in place for children with hearing impairment identified by the screening process.

REFERENCES

Alberti, P.W., Hyde, M.L., Riko, K., Corgin, H., and Ambramovich, S. 1983. An equivalent of BERA for hearing screening in high-risk neonates. *Laryngoscope* 93:1115-1121.

Bond, E.K. 1972. Perception of form by the human infant. *Psychological Bulletin* 77:225-245.

Caron, R.F., and Caron, A.J. 1968. The effects of repeated exposure and stimulus complexity on visual fixation in infants. *Psychonomic Science* 10:207-208.

Caron, R.F., and Caron, A.J. 1969. Degree of stimulus complexity on visual fixation in infants. *Psychonomic Science* 14:78-79.

Durieux-Smith, A., Picton, T., Edwards, C., Goodman, J.T., and MacMurray, B. 1985. The Crib-O-Gram in the NICU: An evaluation based on brain stem electric response audiometry. *Ear and Hearing* 6:20-24.

Eilers, R.E., Ozdamar, O., Miskiel, E., and Widen, J.E. 1989a. Innovations in infant audiometry: Classification of audiograms by sequential testing (CAST). Paper presented at the American Speech-Language-Hearing Association Convention, St. Louis.

Eilers, R.E., Miskiel, E., Widen, J.E., and Lopez, C. 1989b. Optimization of automated hearing test algorithms: Simulations using an infant response model. Paper presented at the American Speech-Language-Hearing Association Convention, St. Louis.

Eilers, R.E., Widen, J.E., Urbano, R., Hudson, T.M., and Gonzales, L. 1991a. Optimization of automated hearing test algorithms: A comparison of data from simulations and young children. *Ear and Hearing* 12(3):199-214.

Eilers, R.E., Miskiel, E., Ozdamar, O., Urbano, R., and Widen, J.E. 1991b. Optimization of automated hearing test algorithms: Simulations using an infant response model. *Ear and Hearing* 12(3):191-198.

Folsom, R.C. 1990. Identification of hearing loss in infants using auditory brainstem response: Strategies and program choices. *Seminars in Hearing* 11:333-341.

Jacobson, J.T., and Morehouse, C.R. 1984. A comparison of auditory brainstem response and behavioral screening in high risk and normal newborn infants. *Ear and Hearing* 5:247-253.

Jerger, J., Howie, V., Bess, F., et al. 1983. Panel VI: Diagnosis and screening. Proceedings of the Third International Research Conference on Recent Advances in Otitis Media with Effusion, Fort Lauderdale, Fla.

Joint Committee on Infant Hearing. 1991. 1990 position statement. *Asha* 33(Suppl. 5):3-6.

Lewis, M., and Goldberg, S. 1969. The acquisition and violation of expectancy: An experimental paradigm. *Journal of Experimental Psychology* 1:75-86.

Lipsitt, L.P., and Werner, J.S. 1981. The infancy of human learning processes. In E.S. Gollin (ed.), *Developmental plasticity: Behavioral and biological aspects of variations in development* (pp. 101-133). New York: Academic Press.

Moore, J.M., Thompson, G., and Thompson, M. 1975. Auditory localization of infants as a function of reinforcement conditions. *Journal of Speech and Hearing Disorders* 40:29-34.

Nozza, R.J., and Wilson, W.R. 1984. Masked and unmasked pure-tone thresholds of infants and adults: Development of auditory frequency selectivity and sensitivity. *Journal of Speech and Hearing Research* 27:613-622.

Olsho, L.W., Koch, E.G., Halpin, C.F., and Carter, E.A. 1987. An observer-based psychoacoustic procedure for use with young infants. *Developmental Psychology* 23(5):627-640.

Olsho, L.W., Koch, E.G., Carter, E.A., Halpin, C.F., and Spetner, N.B. 1988. Pure tone sensitivity of human infants. *Journal of the Acoustical Society of America* 84:1316-1324.

Ozdamar, O., Eilers, R.E., Miskiel, E., and Widen, J. 1990. Classification of audiograms by sequential testing using a dynamic Bayesian procedure. *Journal of the Acoustical Society of America* 88(95):2171-2179.

Paradise, J., and Smith, C.G. 1978. Impedance screening for preschool children—state of the art. In E. Harford et al. (eds.), *Impedance screening for middle ear disease in children* (pp. 113-124). New York: Grune and Stratton.

Plotnick, C.H., and Leppler, J.G. 1986. Infant hearing assessment: A program for identification and habilitation within four months of age. *The Hearing Journal* 39:23-25.

Popejoy, E., DeRuyter, F., and Gordon, C. 1988. Computer assisted pediatric audiologic evaluations through remote switching. Paper presented at American Speech and Hearing Foundation Technology Conference, Mesa Ariz.

Primus, M.A., and Thompson, G. 1985. Response strength of young children in operant audiometry. *Journal of Speech and Hearing Research* 28:539-547.

Teller, D.Y. 1979. The forced-choice preferential looking procedure: A psychophysical technique for use with human infants. *Infant Behavior and Development* 2:135-153.

Thompson, G., and Folsom, R.C. 1984. A comparison of two conditioning procedures in the use of visual reinforcement audiometry (VRA). *Journal of Speech and Hearing Disorders* 49:241-245.

Thompson, G., and Folsom, R.C. 1985. Reinforced and nonreinforced head-turn responses of infants as a function of stimulus bandwidth. *Ear and Hearing* 6:125-129.

Weber, H. 1987a. Ten years of searching for the hearing-impaired infant in rural Colorado. *Seminars in Hearing* 8:149-154.

Weber, H. 1987b. Colorado's statewide hearing screening program utilizing visual reinforcement audiometry. *Hearing Instruments* 38(9):22-23.

Widen, J.E. 1990. Behavioral screening of high-risk infants using visual reinforcement audiometry. *Seminars in Hearing* 11(4):342-356.

Wilson, W.R., and Moore, J.M. 1978. Pure-tone earphone thresholds of infants utilizing visual reinforcement audiometry (VRA). Paper presented at the American Speech and Hearing Association Convention, San Francisco.

Chapter 18

The Infant Hearing Program (IHP) of Arkansas: Its Past, Present, and Future

Terrey Oliver Penn

INTRODUCTION

The Infant Hearing Program (IHP) of Arkansas has been identifying infants at risk for hearing loss since 1979. The program currently is supported by the Arkansas Department of Health and is administered by its Office of Hearing, Speech & Vision Services. The program's history, its current status, and its future direction will be discussed in this report. But before I begin to describe the IHP specifically, I would like to illustrate why we believe it is extremely critical for Arkansas to have an early identification program for hearing loss.

The interrelationships of low economic status, limited prenatal health care, teenage pregnancy, and incidence of at-risk newborns are documented (Reed and Stanley 1977; Raju 1986). Unfortunately, Arkansas has its share of health concerns and economic difficulties. For instance, Arkansas ranks 48th in the nation in per capita income (U.S. Bureau of the Census 1990). It ranks 46th for the number of mothers receiving prenatal care (National Center for Health Statistics 1990a). Another dismaying statistic for Arkansas is its position as 2d in the nation in the number of births to teenage mothers (National Center for Health Statistics 1990a). In fact, 20% of all births in the state are to mothers who are 19 years of age and younger. These three factors contribute to Arkansas' overall ranking of 5th in the nation for percentage of low-birth-weight (LBW) infants (National Center for Health Statistics 1990b). LBW infants account for 8.3% of all births in the state. Sadly, some eastern counties of Arkansas, located near the Mississippi River, have LBW rates as high as 11%. The end result is that there are a number of "unhealthy" infants born in Arkansas—many of whom will be at risk for hearing loss.

A BRIEF HISTORY

The Children's Hearing and Speech Clinic,[1] located within the Arkansas Department of Health (ADH), was one of the pioneers in providing hearing services for the children of Arkansas. Before 1978, very few facilities were available within Arkansas to provide pediatric audiology services, and even fewer facilities were available to objectively assess the hearing of infants (i.e., ABR testing).

In 1979, in commemoration of the 20th Anniversary of the Declaration of the Rights of Children, the United Nation's General Assembly declared that year the International Year of the Child. Arkansas Governor Bill Clinton appointed his wife, Hillary Rodham Clinton, as spokesperson for Arkansas' efforts in this regard. She worked cooperatively with Maternal and Child Health specialists from the ADH to determine the need and feasibility of numerous preventive health proposals for children. Several projects were discussed, but through the efforts of the mother of a hearing-impaired child, Mrs. Clinton chose to emphasize an early identification program for hearing loss. A committee was formed, the Governor's Council on Hearing Loss, composed of professionals and others interested in hearing, hearing loss, and children. Through the efforts of Mrs. Clinton and this council, the development of a program to identify infants at risk for hearing loss flourished. This was the beginning of the Infant Hearing Assessment Program.[2]

PROGRAM DEVELOPMENT

The initial project was divided into four phases:

Phase 1: Informational brochures regarding auditory development were distributed at local fairs and the state fair.

---

[1] Currently identified as the Arkansas Department of Health, Hearing & Speech Clinic.

[2] Currently identified as the Infant Hearing Program (IHP) of Arkansas.

Phase 2: Informational brochures were distributed in educational packets given to new mothers.

Phase 3: Public awareness concerning the need for early detection of hearing loss was spotlighted. Public service announcements emphasizing this need and describing the milestones in auditory development were created and broadcast across the state.

Phase 4: Using risk factors compiled by the Joint Committee on Infant Hearing (ASHA 1974), a high-risk registry system was developed.

After these four phases were completed, implementation of the early identification program began. However, although this project received enormous statewide enthusiasm, no budget was allocated. Therefore, implementation and coordination of the program depended upon volunteers. Three lead volunteers coordinated the program with a pool of additional volunteers managing the registry. All volunteers received intensive training in pertinent aspects of hearing and hearing loss.

Initially, the program originated in one hospital in the Little Rock area, but within one year several Arkansas hospitals, including one outside the Little Rock area, were participating in the Infant Hearing Assessment Program. Hospital staff completed a high-risk form for every live birth at their facility. The trained volunteers sorted through the forms and identified those infants at risk.

Once an infant was found to be at risk, the parents and the infant's physician were notified. Through the use of telephone questionnaires, parents were questioned regarding their infant's auditory behavior at 3, 6, 12, and 24 months of age. If the parents' responses suggested a hearing problem, then the volunteers would refer the child for an audiologic evaluation. Table 1 lists the questions that were asked at the appropriate age of the infant.

Approximately two years into the program, two significant problems became obvious. First, families were often difficult to locate by telephone. Many families either moved during the questionnaire's timetable (3 through 24 months of age) or did not own a phone. Second, in many cases the parents did not exhibit concern about their child's hearing. Parents almost invariably stated that their child's hearing was *normal*. These two problems led to two further complications: (1) the diagnostic portion of the program was essentially nonexistent, and (2) the volunteer turnover was great. Volunteers had joined the IHP to help identify hearing-impaired infants and help their families receive services.

Table 1
Questions Included in the 3, 6, 12, and 24 Month Telephone Questionnaires

Age of Infant	Question
3 Months	When your baby is asleep in a quiet room, does he/she move or begin to wake up when there is a sudden loud noise?
	Does your baby startle when there is a sudden loud sound?
	Have you had any worry about your child's hearing?
6 Months	When your baby is asleep in a quiet room, does he/she move or begin to wake up when there is a sudden loud noise?
	Does your baby startle when there is a sudden loud sound?
	Does your baby turn his/her head when his/her name is called or there is an interesting sound?
	Have you had any worry about your child's hearing?
12 Months	Does your baby imitate simple words or sounds?
	Can your baby point to or look at familiar objects or people when asked to do so?
	Does your baby turn his/her head in various directions to find a noise or someone calling his/her name?
	Does your baby understand common words, such as "no" or "bye bye" (without gestures)?
	Have you had any worry about your child's hearing?
24 Months	Does your child repeat words or phrases?
	Does your child follow simple commands, such as "Close the door"?
	Will your child point to body parts when asked (without gestures)?
	Have you had any worry about your child's hearing?

When they saw that they were unable to do so, they became quickly disenchanted with the program and withdrew from participation. In addition, in those infrequent cases in which an infant was identified as needing audiologic services, often there was not a service provider available within reasonably close proximity.

In order to address these concerns, some changes were made within the IHP and the ADH. The difficulty of follow-up by telephone and the lack of parental concern were combated by obtaining ABR equipment to assess infants at the earliest possible age. Equipment was made available through the Infant Hearing Assessment Foundation (Concord, Calif.) and was placed in the ADH Hearing & Speech Clinic in Little Rock. In this way, infants could be tested within the first 3 months of life, and the subsequent telephone follow-ups at 6, 12, and 24 months would no longer be necessary. Further, to encourage volunteer stability, volunteers were recruited to conduct the hearing screenings. The volunteers were trained to prepare the infants for screening and to use the ABR equipment. These trained volunteers, under the supervision of an audiologist, began screening infants at risk for hearing loss at the Little Rock Hearing & Speech Clinic in 1982. This development was a turning point for early identification of hearing loss in Arkansas. Soon thereafter, in order to address the availability problem of service providers, the ADH opened two Hearing & Speech Clinics in areas of the state particularly void of such services.

As screenings were being conducted at the ADH Clinic, plans were under way to begin hearing screenings in hospital intensive care nurseries (ICNs). From 1984 through 1986, the program rapidly expanded into these settings. By late 1986, hearing screenings were being conducted in five hospital ICNs. In 1987, one hospital (Arkansas Children's Hospital) withdrew from the program and began providing its own screening services. Today, the IHP tests infants in six hospital nurseries—four located in Little Rock and two in northwest Arkansas.

CURRENT STATUS OF THE IHP

The IHP has grown significantly since 1979. Today, 16 hospitals participate in this extremely important program. These hospitals and their general locations are illustrated in figure 1. A large majority of the state is covered by the program; however, we are concerned about two areas: the north central and southern portions of the state. Although these two

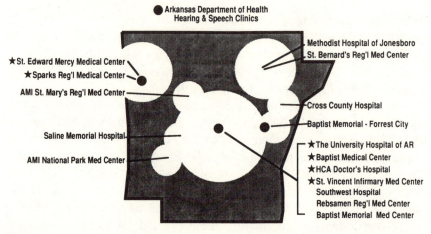

Figure 1. A map of the state of Arkansas identifying locations of the 16 hospitals affiliated with the Infant Hearing Program and the three ADH Hearing & Speech Clinics (●). Stars (★) identify the hospitals where on-site ABR screening occurs.

regions are relatively sparsely populated, they must be addressed in the near future.

Figure 2 describes the mechanics of the IHP of Arkansas. As with most infant screening programs, infants are identified while in the hospital. Once identified, they are screened, either while hospitalized or later at one of the ADH Hearing & Speech Clinics. ABR testing is conducted on all infants under 3 months of age (without sedation). After this age it is very difficult to encourage sleep, so we attempt to evaluate the infant's hearing behaviorally at approximately 6 months of age. Depending on the initial screening results, an infant is rescreened or receives a follow-up evaluation. Currently, parents of all infants who pass the initial screening are asked to return for follow-up assessment (behavioral and immittance testing) when the child is 8 to 12 months of age. Plans are under way to use a questionnaire system for follow-up of the infants who passed the initial screening and are not at risk for progressive or late onset hearing loss.

Since 1982, nearly 4,000 infants have received ABR screening by the IHP. Figure 3 shows the number of infants tested and their test outcomes from 1987 through 1990. As the figure illustrates, approximately 500 to 600 infants are tested each year. The hatched portion of the bars indicates the number of infants who pass the screening each year. The

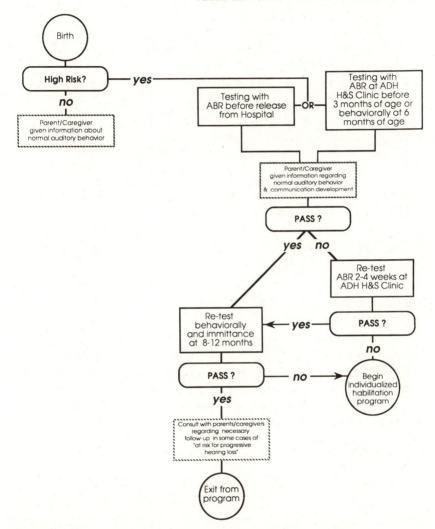

Figure 2. Flowchart of the Infant Hearing Program (IHP) of Arkansas.

black portion indicates the number who fail. Two screens are always conducted before an infant is considered as having a "fail" outcome. For each of the past four years, approximately 2% to 4% of all infants tested have failed. The white portion of the bars indicates the number of questionable outcomes. To receive a questionable outcome, an infant must have failed the initial screening but was not rescreened for one

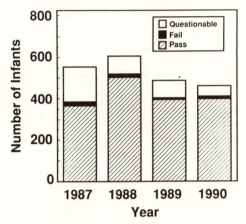

Figure 3. Total number of infants tested by the Infant Hearing Program (IHP) of Arkansas from 1987 through 1990. The number of passing, failing, or questionable screening outcomes is designated.

reason or another. Since 1988, we have focused our efforts on reducing the number of questionable outcomes, but to do so, because of the limited resources available, we have also had to reduce the number of overall screenings. The narrowing of the white bar with time indicates that we have improved our ability to reconcile these questionable outcomes. Therefore, we will now rededicate ourselves to increasing the number of infants tested each year while still attempting to keep the percentage of questionable outcomes low.

FUTURE DIRECTIONS

The IHP of Arkansas must continue to change and to explore new directions aimed at identifying and screening more infants more efficiently. One future direction will be in the area of program expansion. We visualize expansion in two areas—first, in the number of infants identified. By including more hospitals in the program, we will undoubtedly increase the number of infants screened and identified. In particular, our efforts will be focused on placing the high-risk register in the smaller rural hospitals. Most of the very sick infants born in these hospitals are transported to the ICNs of the larger Little Rock hospitals. These infants invariably are identified as being at risk for hearing loss while in these large ICNs. However, "healthy" infants who are born in rural hospitals and who are at risk for hearing loss (e.g., due to a family history of childhood hearing impairment) are not benefiting from our program. At the present time, we are relying on the conscientious efforts of the primary care physicians or public health medical staff in rural areas to refer these infants for testing. Of course, we are also relying on the parents to obtain appropriate medical intervention services for their infants. If we introduce the high-risk register directly into these rural hospitals, we can save precious time in the early identification process.

The second area of expansion considered will be an increase in the number of identified infants who receive the ABR screening. Recall that an attempt is made to screen all infants identified at risk while they are in the hospital. If they are released before we are able to screen them, their parents are encouraged to make an appointment for the screening at one of the ADH Hearing & Speech Clinics. With the present personnel and budget allocations for the IHP, increasing the number of screenings will be difficult indeed. One possible remedy is to locate alternative resources to fund these well-deserved activities (e.g., grants, contracts, private donations). Despite the perceived difficulties, it is a project to which we are truly dedicated, and we will begin to tackle it in the very near future.

We also anticipate a change in the approach the ADH will take toward early identification of hearing loss. The ADH may begin to play a consulting role in regard to statewide infant hearing programs. Those individuals interested in beginning infant hearing screening programs in their area could profit from the experience the ADH has gained while coordinating the prior efforts of the IHP. The ADH could constitute a valuable resource to these newly developing programs. Although the ADH will likely encourage other screening programs in the state, it would certainly discourage those programs to work solely for their own benefit. They would be urged to cooperate with the ADH, especially in the area of data organization and record keeping. Only in this way can a true and accurate picture of Arkansas' efforts for the early identification of hearing loss be maintained.

SUMMARY

The IHP is extremely critical for Arkansas due to the economic and health status of its residents. It is an ever-changing program—learning from its mistakes and building upon its strengths. For example, it has evolved from an all-volunteer program in one hospital using a high-risk register and telephone questionnaire to a relatively sophisticated state-wide program employing state-of-the-art ABR equipment. In its present form, the IHP is coordinated by the Arkansas Department of Health's Office of Hearing, Speech & Vision Services. It includes 16 Arkansas hospitals and is supported partially by federal funds (DHHS-Maternal & Child Health Block Grant). Health Department audiologists, using sophisticated ABR test equipment, screen the at-risk infants in both clinical and ICN settings. Despite the fact that the IHP has made these significant changes, two beliefs of the program remain unchanged. The first belief is that volunteers can play an important role in a program's success. Volunteers were the sole providers of the IHP for a number of years, and they continue to be instrumental in the program's growth. The second belief is that teamwork is essential. Audiologists must interact effectively with parents, physicians, nurses, hospital administrators, fellow audiologists, speech pathologists, and individuals or organizations interested in the early identification of hearing loss. All are integral parts of a team that must work in concert if an infant hearing screening program is to succeed.

The personnel currently involved with the IHP's functioning recognize that many individuals and organizations, past and present, have been instrumental in the program's success. Without the devotion and foresight of the founding council, the dedication and care of the numerous volunteers and organizations, or the continued support from professionals in the area of hearing and child welfare, the IHP's achievements would not have been possible. In fact, its very existence would be questionable. We commend and salute their hard work and generous efforts.

Although this report illustrates that great strides have been made in Arkansas in the area of early identification of infants with hearing loss, further distance must be traveled if we are to attain the year 2000 goal—*the identification of all infants who have a hearing loss by the age of 12 months* (U.S. DHHS 1990).

ACKNOWLEDGMENTS

I would like to thank Fred Beggs, Virginia Berry, and Lynn Coates for their indispensable help in reconstructing the early efforts of the IHP. In addition, I thank Kathy Caldwell and John Penn for their patient review of this manuscript.

The audiologists involved with the IHP wish to acknowledge the continued and past generosity of numerous organizations that have come to the aid of the program, specifically, the Arkansas Association for Hearing Impaired Children, the Arkansas Chapter of the Optimist Clubs of America, and the Telephone Pioneers of America. In addition, our deep appreciation goes to the other numerous volunteers who have given freely of their time to the program over the years.

REFERENCES

American Speech-Language-Hearing Association. 1974. Supplementary statement of Joint Committee on Infant Hearing Screening. *Asha* 16:160.

National Center for Health Statistics. 1990a. *Vital statistics of U.S., 1988.* Vol. 1, Natality, DHHS Pub. no. (PHS) 90-1100. Washington, D.C.: U.S. Government Printing Office.

National Center for Health Statistics. 1990b. *Advance report of final natality statistics, 1988.* Monthly Vital Statistics Report, vol. 39, no. 4 (Suppl.). Hyattsville, Md.: Public Health Service.

Raju, T.N.K. 1986. An epidemiologic study of very and very very low birthweight infants. In D. Vidyasagar (ed.), *Clinics in perinatology: The tiny baby.* Philadelphia: W.B. Saunders Co.

Reed, D.M., and Stanley, F.J. (eds.). 1977. *The epidemiology of prematurity.* Baltimore: Urban and Schwarzenberg.

U.S. Bureau of the Census. 1990. *Statistical abstracts of the U.S.,* (110th ed). Washington, D.C.: U.S. Government Printing Office.

U.S. Department of Health and Human Services, Public Health Service. 1990. *Healthy people 2000: National health promotion and disease prevention objectives.* Washington, D.C.: U.S. Government Printing Office.

Chapter 19

Screening the Preschool-Age Child

Thomas Mahoney

INTRODUCTION

Appropriate preschool hearing screening offers many challenges to health care professionals. By far, the most prominent of these challenges is how to gain access to a majority of preschool children so that successful screening and follow-up can significantly reduce the impact of hearing loss in the total population. This goal is, of course, more easily accomplished in countries that have a national health care system that encourages routine, preventive well-child visits at little or no direct cost to families. In the United States, however, preschool hearing screening must be addressed in a variety of settings that capture a large number of children, such as day-care centers, preschools, Head Starts, and primary care facilities. If a significant portion of the target population is to be addressed, there must be a coordinated public health effort to facilitate hearing screening services in all of these settings.

The mandatory child-find portion of Public Law 99-457 assures that increasingly more preschool children will be screened for hearing impairment. Recent expansions in Medicaid eligibility for children, and allowances for separate payment for early periodic screening and diagnostic treatment (EPSDT) screening services, should also begin to increase the number of preschool hearing screenings provided in the U.S.A.

Haggard (1990) recently summarized the ten Wilson-Jungner (1968) principles of screening: "The principles refer to the need for acceptable tests that will predict with reasonable accuracy during its asymptomatic stage the presence of a disease (or of an impairment that will lead to a disability) to the necessary availability of acceptable effective treatments, and to various other ethical and practical prerequisites for screening asymptomatic populations." He also urged consideration of the incidental harm done by the screening, and by the information (correct or otherwise) that screening provides. There should be agreed guidelines on whom to divulge the provisional and the final results to. All screening arrangements should be reviewed from time to time in the light of changes in demography, culture, health services, technologies, and the epidemiology of the target conditions. Because cases are not homogeneous, the balance of costs, benefits, and risks from screening, assessment, and treatments has to be worked out on a stratified basis, and the definition of the target group has to be revised so that this balance is favorable for all strata within it (Haggard 1990).

Other challenges more specific to preschool hearing screening center on what children should be screened, at what ages, and for what types of auditory problems. What procedures, strategies, and protocols, used with what equipment and personnel, will best provide a valid and cost-effective hearing screening program? Are there services available for diagnosis and treatment, and will the treatment provided make a difference in the short- and long-term well-being of the child?

RECOMMENDED GUIDELINES, STATEMENTS, AND PROTOCOLS

There have been several recommendations by professional associations and government agencies concerning hearing and middle ear screening in children. A brief review of several of the more pertinent recommendations is presented below.

1. U.S. Department of Health and Human Services, Public Health Service,
   "Protocols for Screening and Assessment of Preschool Children: Speech, Language, and Hearing" (1982).

These protocols were developed by a group of experts who met on several occasions at the invitation of the federal government. For 2- to 3-year-old children, the protocols include application of a risk register, three parental questions concerning auditory responses at home, pure-tone play audiometry, middle ear screening, and screening for speech and language development. For 3- to 6-year-olds, they recommended the risk register, identification audiometry incorporating the 1975 Guidelines of the American Speech-Language-Hearing Association (ASHA) and speech audiometry, pneumatic otoscopy, and tympanometry.

2. American Academy of Pediatrics Policy Statement
   "Middle Ear Disease and Language Development" (1984).

There is growing evidence demonstrating a correlation between middle ear disease with hearing impairment and delays in the development of speech, language and cognitive skills. A parent or other caretaker may be the first person to detect such early symptoms as irritability, decreased responsiveness and disturbed sleep. Middle ear disease may be so subtle that a full evaluation for this condition should combine pneumatic otoscopy, and possibly tympanometry, with a direct view of the tympanic membrane. This statement is not meant to be a recommendation for specific treatment methods. When a child has frequently recurring acute otitis media and/or middle ear effusion persisting for longer than three months, hearing should be assessed and the development of communicative skills must be monitored.

The committee feels it is important that the physician inform the parent that a child with middle ear disease may not hear normally. Although the child may withdraw socially and diminish experimentation with verbal communication, the parent should be encouraged to continue communicating by touching and seeking eye contact with the child when loudly and clearly speaking. Such measures, along with prompt restoration of hearing whenever possible, may help to diminish the likelihood that a child with middle ear disease will develop a communicative disorder. Middle ear disease can occur in the presence of sensory neural hearing loss. Any child whose parent expresses concern about whether the child hears should be considered for referral for behavioral audiometry without delay.

3. U.S. Preventive Services Task Force
"Screening for Hearing Impairment" (1989).

Hearing loss is one of 60 conditions listed in *A Guide to Preventative Services*, which was developed for presentation to the U.S. Department of Health and Human Services. It purports to be a product of over four years of effort by a panel of 20 experts in medicine and related fields. The section on hearing screening reads:

> *Recommendation: Screening should be performed on all neonates at high risk for hearing impairment (see Clinical Intervention). High-risk children not tested at birth should be screened before age 3, but there is insufficient evidence of accuracy to recommend routine audiologic testing of all children in this age group. There is also insufficient evidence of benefit to recommend for or against hearing screening of asymptomatic children beyond age 3. (P.193)*

4. American Public Health Association
"Children's Preschool Vision and Hearing Screening and Follow-Up" (1989).

> *Recognizing that the senses of vision and hearing play an important role in a child's educational and developmental progress, and are among the most prevalent chronic health problems in the preschool population; and that early identification of sensory problems through cost-effective screening programs can significantly reduce the impact of such disorders; and that most vision and hearing problems occur without pain, often unilaterally, and frequently are unnoticed by parents, children, or others; and that state and local health and education agencies have responsibilities in disease detection and can be effective in integrating screening, referral, and follow-up services into their health promotion and preventive programs; and that health agencies are an appropriate agency in which to develop coordinated screening services, especially as related to prevention and detection of disorders; therefore*

1. Encourages all state and territorial legislators to mandate preschool vision and hearing screening, referral and follow-up for treatment for all children, based on established standards;

2. Encourages state and local health departments in cooperation with agencies implementing early periodic screening, diagnosis, and treatment, PL 9414 and PL 99-457, to coordinate state-wide preschool vision and hearing screening, referral, and follow-up programs;

3. Encourages further research to develop appropriate and cost effective methods of earlier detection and treatment in young children; and

4. Encourages all primary health care providers to routinely conduct appropriate vision and hearing screening for all children under age six; and

5. Encourages the dissemination of information to the public about the importance of vision and hearing screening.

5. American Speech-Language-Hearing Association (ASHA) "Guidelines for Identification Audiometry" (1985) and "Guidelines for Screening for Hearing Impairments and Middle Ear Disorders" (1990).

The 1990 ASHA guidelines state that they "are not intended as a recommendation for or against mass screening for middle ear disorders or hearing loss." They also state that "it may be appropriate and beneficial to modify the procedures and pass-fail criteria for specific populations and purposes. This document is intended as 'guidelines' rather than a protocol that requires strict adherence." These ASHA guidelines will be reviewed in detail in the subsequent discussion.

PRESCHOOL HEARING SCREENING STRATEGIES

Appropriate preschool hearing screening requires the application of a wide variety of strategies to best suit diverse populations in diverse settings. Some factors influencing a decision on how to best screen a specific population are the age of the target group, the setting they are in, the ambient noise in the test environment, the time available, the equipment available, the qualifications and training of the personnel doing the screening, and the specific purpose of the screening effort. For example, most preschool screening protocols address children at a developmental age of 3 and older because the application of pure-tone audiometry is more difficult to administer before then. But what about the 2- to 3-year-old children who are still in the critical language development stage that requires normal hearing? Should we rely solely on parental complaints or on the observations of primary care providers as a check for possible hearing loss? Or are there procedures available to screen these children that are both reliable and valid, and can be delivered rapidly and simply at low cost to a large number of children?

The major purpose of hearing screening is to identify individuals with a high probability of hearing loss from a population that contains both normal hearing and hearing-impaired individuals. These individuals are then referred for diagnosis, which is the process of confirming the suspected impairment. The validity of hearing screening is poor if it misses many persons who ultimately are found with hearing loss (high false negative rate). This error is most serious because in "passing" the procedure persons with hearing loss are denied early intervention. A less serious but yet significant screening error is made by failing many individuals who are found upon diagnostic tests to have normal hearing (high false positive rate). This degrades the efficiency of the program, is costly, and may cause undue anxiety for families (Mahoney 1990).

Before suggesting specific preschool hearing screening strategies, it should be emphasized that screening is not a simple task to be dealt with by individuals who do not fully understand the necessity of applying rigid scientific principles to the endeavor. This is a critical first step that successful diagnosis and habilitation directly depend upon.

MIDDLE EAR SCREENING

Because middle ear disorders constitute one of the most prevalent chronic conditions in young children, and probably have a deleterious effect on speech and language development, it is important to consider middle ear screening in this paper. The use of acoustic immittance in a large-scale screening has historically been surrounded in considerable controversy (Bess 1980; Northern 1980). This is reported to be due to the use of overzealous pass-fail criteria, resulting in a large number of asymptomatic children referred for medical intervention, and the fact that many first-generation immittance instruments provided results in relatively arbitrary units (ASHA 1990).

In an attempt to avoid these problems, the 1990 ASHA screening guidelines include four sources of data: history, visual inspection, identification audiometry, and tympanometry (see also chapters 4 and 21). Briefly, a history of ear pain or ear discharge results in immediate medical referral. Similarly, if visual inspection finds a structural defect of ear, head, or neck, ear canal blood or effusion, occlusion, inflammation, excessive cerumen, a tumor, or foreign material, a direct medical referral is made. Tympanometry is not necessary when visual inspection indicates the need for medical referral. Also, the guidelines suggest tympanometry should not be performed unless ordered by a physician, when middle ear infection is present, or when a pressure equalization (PE) tube is in place.

Audiometric screening should be performed according to the 1985 ASHA guidelines (ASHA 1985), which recommend pure-tone pass-fail criteria of 20 dB HL at 1000, 2000, and 4000 Hz. Failures should be rescreened at a later date, and a second failure should mean referral for complete audiologic evaluation.

Low static immittance or a flat tympanogram associated with large volume is evidence of a tympanic membrane perforation and warrants immediate referral. Low static immittance by itself, with normal ear canal volume, may or may not be associated with middle ear disorders, and requires repeated observation. Only after two successive failures over a period of four to six weeks should medical referral be made.

Finally, abnormally wide tympanometric width, in the absence of other findings, may represent transient secretory otitis, and requires a failure at retest in four to six weeks for medical referral. Interim means and 90% ranges for static immittance, equivalent ear canal volume, and tympanometric width are presented in the guidelines for 3- to 5-year-old children. There are no established norms for younger children.

THE HIGH-RISK REGISTER

The 1990 position statement of the Joint Committee on Infant Hearing (Joint Committee on Infant Hearing 1991) is intended for neonates from 0 to 28 days and infants from 29 days to 2 years. It would seem reasonable, however, that many of the risk factors contained in the infant section could also offer the primary care provider a valuable screening tool for preschool children. Although, hopefully, most children with severe or profound congenital losses are detected by 2 years of age, risk factors such as parental concern, bacterial meningitis, head trauma, ototoxic drug administration, childhood neurogenic disorders, and childhood infectious diseases place a child of any age at risk for hearing loss.

PRIMARY CARE SCREENING

At the beginning of this chapter it was suggested that the major barrier to large-scale preschool hearing screening in the United States is lack of accessibility to the target population. Even though more children than ever are available in day-care centers, Head Starts, and preschools, the primary care physician's office is the one setting where most preschool children are available for early detection.

Speech and language development depends upon normal auditory function. Because hearing screening in physicians' offices is generally not accomplished, it would seem that assessment of early language development could offer an important hearing screening tool for the primary care provider. It is known, however, that developmental screening in general is infrequently used by pediatricians (Smith 1978), and that the most commonly used screening tool, the Denver Developmental Screening Test (DDST), is insensitive to language delay (Borowitz and Glascoe 1986). In a survey of 429 Colorado pediatricians and family practitioners, only 0.3% to 0.6% of children under three were ever referred to a speech-language pathologist (Walker et al. 1989).

In an attempt to improve this situation, Matkin (1984) recommended that primary care physicians use three simple questions as a basis for identifying preschool children who may be in need of referral for speech, language, and auditory evaluation. Matkin explained that delays in vocabulary, syntax, and phonological development are all sensitive indicators of even mild bilateral hearing loss, and that most parents are very accurate in making estimates of their child's communication development. The three questions to be included in each child's medical case history are:

1. How many different words do you estimate your child uses? Is it 100 words, 500 words, or . . . ?

2. What is the length of a typical sentence that your child uses? Is it two words, full sentences, single words, or . . . ?
3. How clear is your child's speech to a friend or neighbor? Would they understand 10%, 90%, 50%, or . . . ?

The parent's responses are then checked against guidelines that recommend a referral for hearing, speech, and language when there is a six-month delay in development.

Another instrument designed as a rapid means of screening language in children under 3 years of age is the Early Language Milestone Scale (ELM). Developed by Coplan (1983), the ELM was standardized on 191 high-risk children and has been shown to have a sensitivity and specificity rate of 97% and 93%, respectively (Coplan et al. 1982). The test takes only a few minutes to administer, and it can be immediately scored as "pass or fail." Northern and Downs (1991) reported an overall failure rate of 8% with the initial test and indicated that the best age range for ELM administration is from 24 to 30 months. A rescreen within one to two weeks is scheduled before referral is made for in-depth evaluation.

Rapid and efficient speech and language screenings in primary care offices are indeed attractive, especially when considering that they may be the only viable procedures for providing at least some sort of hearing screening in these settings. However, more clinical research is needed to better understand how effective these tools are in detecting preschool children who may have significant hearing loss.

Another option for primary care providers is the preschool child's localization and head-turning responses to soft, frequency-specific noisemakers. Although the intent is to screen for moderate-to-severe hearing losses, Northern and Downs (1991) indicated that experienced examiners can also use these techniques to identify unilateral or bilateral mild hearing loss due to middle ear effusion. They suggest noisemakers can be used with children 3 years of age, in accordance with expected auditory maturation responses, and as a screening technique only. Noisemakers have also been used successfully to screen the hearing of preschool children in the Tennessee Public Health Program (Casearella-Buchannan 1986) and in the countries of England, Israel, and Holland through their routine well-baby clinics.

A protocol for using a combination of the ELM and noisemakers for preschool children in primary care offices has been developed through a Robert Wood Johnson project in Colorado. This project reports screening more than 800 children under 31 months of age and has determined that such a screening protocol could be effectively incorporated into a busy office schedule (Walker et al. 1989; Northern et al. 1989).

VISUAL REINFORCEMENT AUDIOMETRY (VRA)

VRA can be used successfully from 6 to 24 months of age (Wilson and Thompson 1984). During this time the developmentally normal infant gives reliable and repeated head-turn localization responses to sound that are conditioned by visual reinforcers. After 24 months, the child becomes increasingly less under stimulus control by visual reinforcement alone, and to obtain an adequate number of responses to determine hearing status, the examiner must get the child more actively involved in the screening procedure.

Weber (1987) has developed a procedure for screening the hearing of infants and preschool children using a portable VRA system. Conventional VRA procedures and a special technique for 2½- to 5-year-old children called the "listening game" are described. In the listening game, the child becomes an active participant in the test, either by telling the examiner where the sound is coming from or by pointing to one of two sound field loudspeakers placed at a zero degree azimuth, 12 inches from each ear. If the child gets it right, an animal placed on the top of each loudspeaker is lit up by the examiner, effecting a reward for a correct response. Older toddlers may recognize they are being tested and refuse to play the game of identifying the animal that has made the sound. In this case, it is suggested to invite the child to make the animal light up by rubbing the belly of the animal as the sound is presented.

Weber reports on screening nearly 25,000 infants and preschoolers over a nine-year period, resulting in the medical follow-up of nearly 4,000 children and the identification of 30 with significant bilateral sensorineural hearing loss. Fifty-four percent were over 2 years of age.

IDENTIFICATION AUDIOMETRY

Identification audiometry using play, hand raising, or verbal responses is the most commonly used procedure to screen the hearing of preschool children. The previously discussed 1985 ASHA Guidelines for

Identification Audiometry (ASHA 1985) were written for children 3 years and older for the purpose of accomplishing rapid and efficient identification of hearing impairment in young children. The goal of identification audiometry is to identify children who have hearing impairments that may interfere with communication. ASHA states that when used with acoustic immittance measurements (ASHA 1990), the program will be most effective in identifying individuals in need of audiologic and/or otologic services.

Audiometric screening is recommended, under earphones, with a pass-fail criteria of 20 dB HL (ANSI S3.6-1969) at frequencies 1000, 2000, and 4000 Hz. Screening at 20 dB HL at 500 Hz may be included if acoustic immittance is not included in the program, and if ambient noise levels permit. Failure to respond at one or more frequencies in either ear is criterion for failure. Rescreening should be performed the same day, or no later than two weeks, for children failing the initial screening, and an audiologist should administer an audiologic evaluation to children failing the rescreening.

Procedurally, an audiologist should conduct or supervise the identification program. Support personnel may be used after appropriate training. Careful instructions are important, especially for young children. Ambient noise levels should not exceed 41.5 dB SPL at 500 Hz, 49.5 dB SPL at 1000 Hz, 54.5 dB SPL at 2000 Hz, and 62 dB SPL at 4000 Hz. Audiometers should meet ANSI 53.6-1969 specifications and be checked annually. Earphone output should be checked at least every three months, and biologic listening checks should be made daily.

Attempts to apply pure-tone screening procedures to 2- to 3-year-old children, even those incorporating "play" techniques, are often very frustrating. A number of these children will simply not wear earphones, and even if they do, they will not cooperate with a stranger to play a game. Northern and Downs (1991) remind us that the definition of screening as "rapid, simple measurements applied to large numbers of children" will be compromised at this age, in that attempting to gain voluntary responses from 2- to 3-year-olds will neither be rapid nor simple. If rapid hearing screening of a large number of 2- to 3-year-olds is required, some of the less-threatening techniques described earlier may be more appropriate. Acoustic immittance screening should be incorporated if detection of ear pathology with associated mild hearing loss is desired.

For developmentally normal children in the 3- to 4-year age range, play audiometric techniques are the method of choice. We find that placing blocks into a bucket is a pleasing task for most children. This technique is rapid and easy to set up to readminister to the next child. Peg boards, plastic rings on towers, or stacking blocks can also be used, and a variety of response methods should be available. The screener should demonstrate the procedure and teach the child to respond every time the tone is heard. The earphones of the audiometer can be placed on the table, and a 90 dB HL tone at 2000 Hz can be presented for this training. The screener demonstrates placing a block in the bucket each time the tone is presented, and the child is encouraged to "take a turn" after two demonstrations. The earphones can then be placed on the child's ears, and the screening can begin at 20 dB HL. Some children may require raising the level to about 50 dB at first, and sometimes it is necessary to "reshape" the child's behavior with the earphones on. In every case, simple praise for the appropriate response is a key to successful play audiometry. At 5 years of age and often earlier, conventional audiometric hand raising can be used to accomplish the screening task in one minute or less for each child, especially when whole groups are instructed at one time.

The Illinois Department of Health (1984) screens thousands of preschool children per year in a program that utilizes audiometric aides trained in administering play audiometry techniques. Their initial screening success rate is estimated at over 70% for 2- and 3-year-old children and well over 90% for 4- and 5-year-olds.

SUMMARY

This chapter reviews a variety of methods available to screen the hearing of 2- to 5-year-old preschool children. Although pure-tone procedures under earphones constitute the "best practice" in such screening and should be used whenever possible, many factors dictate the use of less-standardized techniques in certain circumstances. Accordingly, a variety of approaches have been presented for encouraging the screening of as many children as possible in the many diverse preschool settings.

As an audiologist working in a public health setting, the author realizes that it is not a lack of screening tools that prevents comprehensive preschool hearing screening in most communities. Rather, before such programs can emerge to the extent necessary to impact the target population, there is a need to address the problems surrounding the inaccessibility of these children; to increase the appreciation of the importance of normal hearing in childhood in the health care and lay community; and to initiate an aggressive public relations campaign that promotes the fact that prevention through early identification is a viable and worthwhile endeavor. Health care professionals in the public and the private sector, should assist this cause by appropriate, ongoing public health education.

REFERENCES

American Academy of Pediatrics. 1984. Policy statement. Middle ear disease and language development.

American National Standards Institute. 1970. *Specifications for audiometers ANSI S3.6-1969*. New York: American National Standards Institute.

American Public Health Association. 1989. Children's preschool vision and hearing screening and follow-up. *Resolution 8905*.

American Speech-Language-Hearing Association. 1985. Guidelines for identification audiometry. *Asha* 27:49-52.

American Speech-Language-Hearing Association. 1990. Guidelines for screening for hearing impairments and middle ear disorders. *Asha* 32(Suppl. 2):17-24.

Bess, F.H. 1980. Impedance screening in children: A need for more research. *Annals of Otology, Rhinology and Laryngology* 89:Suppl. 68.

Borowitz, K.C., and Glascoe, F.P. 1986. Sensitivity of the Denver developmental screening test in speech and language screening. *Pediatrics* 78:1075-1078.

Casearella-Buchannan, J.E. 1986. Finding ears that do not hear. *Journal of the Tennessee Medical Association*, January, 39.

Coplan, J. 1983. *The early language milestone (ELM) scale*. Tulsa: Modern Education Corp.

Coplan, J., Gleason, J., Ryan, R., Burke, B., and Williams, M. 1982. Validation of an early language milestone scale in a high risk population. *Pediatrics* 70:677-683.

Haggard, M.P. 1990. Hearing screening in children—state of the arts. *Archives of Disease in Childhood* 6:1193-1195.

Illinois Department of Public Health. 1984. *A manual for audiometrists*. Springfield.

Joint Committee on Infant Hearing. 1991. 1990 position statement. *Asha* 33 (Suppl. 5):3-6

Mahoney, T.M. 1990. Screening infants and children for hearing loss. In *Otolaryngology.* Philadelphia: Lippincott.

Matkin, N.D. 1984. Early recognition and referral of hearing-impaired children. *Pediatrics in Review* 6:151-156.

Northern, J.L. 1980. Impedance screening: an integral part of hearing screening. *Annals of Otology, Rhinology and Laryngology* 89:Suppl. 68.

Northern, J.L., Walker, D., Downs, M.P., and Guggenheim, S. 1989. Office screening for communicative disorders in young children. In M. Gottleib and J. Williams (eds.), *Developmental behavior disorders*, vol. 2 (pp. 218-281). New York: Plenum Publishing.

Northern, J., and Downs, M. 1991. Screening for hearing disorders. In *Hearing in children* (pp.231-283). 4th ed. Baltimore: Williams and Wilkins.

Smith, R.D. 1978. The use of developmental screening tests by primary-care pediatricians. *Journal of Pediatrics* 98:524-527.

U.S. Department of Health and Human Services. 1989. Protocols for screening and assessment of preschool children: speech, language, and hearing.

U.S. Preventive Services Task Force. 1989. Screening for hearing impairment. In *A guide to preventative services.* Baltimore: Williams and Wilkins.

Walker, D., Downs, M.P., Guggenheim, S., and Northern, J.L. 1989. Early language milestone and language screening of young children. *Pediatrics* 88: 284-288.

Weber, H. 1987. Ten years of searching for the hearing-impaired infant in rural Colorado. *Seminars in Hearing* 8:149-154.

Wilson, J.M.G., and Jungner, G. 1968. Principles and practice of screening for disease. Public Health Paper, no. 34. Geneva: WHO.

Wilson, W.R., and Thompson, G. 1984. Behavioral audiometry. In Jerger, J. (ed.), *Pediatric audiology* (pp. 1-44). San Diego: College Hill Press.

Chapter 20

Cheers for Ears:
A Community Immittance Screening
Program for Preschoolers

Nancy E. Harrison and Barbara J. Price

INTRODUCTION

The audiologic and medical communities in an adjacent two-county area of northwest Ohio have long been committed to the identification of middle ear disease and its related hearing and language problems in preschool and young school-age children. Historically, however, hearing screenings have been limited to the school-age children, kindergartners most consistently. This practice may be a common occurrence in many locations. Cheers for Ears, a project for community immittance screening of 2- to 5-year-old children, was created to meet the needs of northwest Ohio.

BACKGROUND/HISTORY

The Northwest Ohio Easter Seal Society has a history of interest and service to the hearing-impaired population of Wood and Lucas counties in Ohio—basically greater Toledo and its surrounding rural area. In 1983, Easter Seal invited audiologic representation on their board to provide professional guidance to their programming. They were already familiar with the screening process through an existing scoliosis program and were continually seeking new ways to provide direct services to clients.

In the spring of 1986, Easter Seal received a call from an inner-city service agency, which provided a child-care center, expressing the desire for immittance screening for the children at the center. These services were offered by a community hearing and speech center at a cost of $5 per child—a charge neither the child-care center nor the families could afford. Yet, the director of this agency was informed about preschoolers, language, and middle ear disease and wanted to explore the possibility of providing this screening to the children at the center.

A pilot study was proposed mainly to attempt to evaluate the need for immittance screening. Two centers were chosen for service: the inner-city center had requested the screening originally and a rural center. Results of this screening and support for the project as indicated through a questionnaire sent to child-care centers and preschools provided the impetus for the program initiation.

The goals for such a project were stated as follows: (1) early identification of hearing-related disorders and hearing loss; (2) public awareness of the importance of early identification of hearing problems; (3) public awareness of Easter Seal programs and services; (4) provision of cost-effective direct service; and (5) a program to meet public need.

In the Easter Seal tradition, the program would be created to utilize volunteers under professional supervision. The Junior League of Toledo was approached because the group was known to be supportive of hearing-related programs on both the local and the national levels. Junior League skills in implementation, funding, and coordination of volunteer programs were an additional incentive to this liaison.

A task force was created with personnel from both Easter Seal and Junior League, under the guidance of the audiologist from the Easter Seal board. In Ohio, state law mandates identification of at-risk children, a law enacted and shaped by the enactment of Public Law 99-457 (ODH 1988). Therefore, not only was there professional commitment to this program, but a legal justification as well. Four educational audiologists, who could conduct training and supervise the volunteers on site as part of their own job descriptions, including the audiologist on the task force, were available and interested in serving with the project. Preschools, day-care centers, and public libraries with preschool story hours were existing sites with the target population. Additionally, the Toledo area medical community was supportive of this type of program for early identification and intervention of middle ear pathology.

In view of all these considerations, the following objectives emerged: (1) public awareness of audiologic and medical services; (2) public education for day-care/preschool staff and parents; (3) identification of financial support; (4) volunteer development, training, and management; (5) identification of equipment needs; (6) development of specifications for volunteer training; (7) investigation of supervisory requirements as dictated by state/national guidelines (i.e., Ohio Board of Speech Pathology and Audiology and the American Speech-Language-Hearing Association); (8) identification of selection procedures for day-care/preschool sites; and (9) development of a feedback system with the medical and audiologic communities.

PROCEDURES

By fall 1987, the program was ready to begin. The Junior League provided volunteers and partial funding, while Easter Seal provided volunteers and funding and supervised community education. Audiologists provided guidance on equipment purchases, development of procedures and paperwork, volunteer training, and on-site supervision. After training, the volunteers were divided into teams of four plus an audiologist. Three teams with three immittance screeners could be mobilized, if needed, for large day-care centers. On-site, written parental permission was required, either through prior contact with the preschool/day-care facility or directly with the parents at drop-in library locations. Otoscopic examination was performed, followed by screening with a Maico 610 Immittance Screener. Because there was no mechanism for retesting available, a pass-fail criterion was used wherein a flat tympanogram constituted a failure. There was no at-risk category. All failures obtained by the volunteer screener were rescreened by the audiologist. If a flat, type B tympanogram was again obtained, a medical referral was made. Medical options for lower income families were offered. Accompanying the referral letter to the parents was a form for the physician to fill out and return to the Easter Seal office. At the preschool/day-care sites the audiologist had the opportunity to discuss outcomes with site staff and parents when they were available. At the library locations, parents were frequently available, and the medical and audiologic options could be discussed directly.

Table 1
Cheers for Ears Volunteer Training Sessions

Session I	Session II
A. Introductions/Background	A. Review
B. Anatomy of the Ear	B. Screening Guidelines
C. Otoscopic Inspection	C. Screening Results Interpretations
D. "Hands-On"- Otoscope	D. "Hands-On"-Screeners, Otoscope
E. Intro to Immittance Screeners	E. Techniques for Children
F. "Hands-On"-Screeners	F. Paperwork/Procedures
G. Questions/Comments	G. Team Leader Assignments

VOLUNTEER TRAINING

All volunteers were required to go through training each year. Volunteer training, which began as a three-session program with pre- and post-testing, was simplified to two sessions of three hours each. During the training, the audiologists provided background and rationale for middle ear screening as well as hands-on training with the project equipment (table 1). From 1987 to 1990, 45 volunteers were trained, representing approximately 25 active volunteers per year screening at 52 day-care and library sites.

CURRENT STATUS

In the 1990-91 screening year, additional volunteers were trained and utilized. This number of 23 to 25 represents a strong base of volunteers who have participated for more than one year. Many have been involved since the beginning of the project. Junior League, as is their custom after providing seed money and creative development, turned the project back to the community, Easter Seal, in this case. Volunteers now come from Quota Service Club, Junior League, and interested community participants, many of whom are retired preschool or kindergarten teachers.

Each year the program sites, procedures, and goals are evaluated. Because there was a continuing concern that the low-income children, who were initially targeted, were not being served, more library sites with more intensive neighborhood advertising were employed in 1990-91. Approximately 817 children were screened at 25 sites. A very

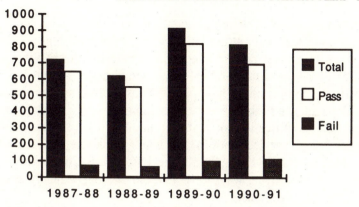

Figure 1. This figure illustrates the total number of children screened and the number that passed and failed the screening for each year since the project began.

consistent failure rate of 10% existed each year (figure 1). This year (1990-91) the failure rate jumped to 14% for reasons we are not able to explain as yet.

PROGRAM EVALUATION

The overall evaluation of the program by participants, both parents and preschool personnel, by volunteers, physician respondents, and participating audiologists has been good. The positive response from the volunteers, which has led to their return to the project year after year, may be due to a number of factors including: (1) the October through late April/early May schedule with holiday breaks; (2) the scheduling of volunteers well in advance; (3) the two- to three-hour screening "day"; (4) the streamlined, but effective, screening process; (5) the concern for volunteer safety in consideration of the screening locations; (6) the support of cooperative supervising audiologists; and (7) the Cheers for Ears T-shirts, tote bags, hand stamps, and coloring sheets that make the project fun for everyone.

FUTURE CONSIDERATIONS

Ongoing project evaluation has helped to create some considerations for future modifications of the project. In addition to the yearly search for ways to identify locations for screening of unserved low-income children, consideration has been made to expanding the age range of the children screened. The audiologic team has considered ways to include a pure-tone screening at the sites and has been working on a format to improve follow-up data sharing. An expanded information packet for day-care/preschool staff and parents is being created with information on specific symptoms of ear/hearing problems, normal speech and language development, and local agencies providing a variety of assistance in the event of identification of chronic middle ear problems. With the expansion of service options for young children and their families provided by Public Law 99-457, the Easter Seal Cheers for Ears team will also be exploring ways to tie into the existing or newly created case management programs.

DISCUSSION/CONCLUSION

The program is providing, free of charge, a service that no one else in the community has provided to date. Feedback about the educational component indicates that it is effective. Concerns still exist. How does the team best identify and access those disadvantaged low-income children needing, but not receiving, service? Physician response averages 36% (1990-91). How can that response mechanism be simplified? How can the project come more in line with new ASHA immittance screening guidelines (ASHA 1990)? (It should be noted that all but two of the physician response forms indicated middle ear pathology in some form, so the pass-fail criterion seems appropriate, if not optimum.)

SUMMARY

In conclusion, Cheers for Ears, the current immittance screening program operated through the efforts of community audiologists, volunteers, and the Easter Seal Society, provides a positive, flexible, cost-effective model for cooperative identification of preschoolers at risk for hearing-related disorders. Through the process of program creation, development, and implementation, some suggestions have emerged that may help community audiologists and others pursue similar projects. These suggestions are divided into two categories: necessities, which have been found to be vital for successful program development; and options, which may help share program success.

Necessities

1. Demonstrate community need
2. Define economic feasibility (funding options)
   a. Identify existing funds (use of monies already available)
   b. Explore availability of grant money (local, state, or federal)
3. Contact potential community agencies for economic support and personnel
4. Explore commitment of selected agency boards of directors and staff to proposed program
5. Identify project personnel requirements
   a. Pursue availability of current agency staff
   b. Confirm volunteer base
6. Explore interest, commitment, and availability of area audiologists
   a. Provide input on project development
   b. Train volunteers
   c. Supervise project activities
   d. Participate in agency committees

Options

1. Consider audiologic representation on agency boards of directors
2. Seek medical community consultation/support of project concept and development
3. Pursue public school staff involvement
   a. Seek cooperative agreement from school administration
   b. Obtain commitment from educational audiologists

The process of program conceptualization and implementation has proven to be as valuable as the resultant screening process. Community awareness has increased with respect to middle ear disorders and related problems with respect to the role of the audiologist in the identification process. Perhaps more important Cheers for Ears has demonstrated the potential for collaborative community effort in northwest Ohio.

REFERENCES

American Speech-Language-Hearing Association. 1990. Guidelines for screening for hearing impairments and middle-ear disorders. *Asha* 32(4)(Suppl. 2):17-24.

Ohio Board of Speech Pathology and Audiology. *Laws and regulations governing the Ohio board of speech pathology and audiology.* Columbus, Ohio: Board Publications.

Ohio Department of Health. 1988. *Policies for hearing conservation programs for children: Requirements and recommendations.* Columbus, Ohio: ODH Press.

PART IV.

Screening School-Age Children for Auditory Function

Chapter 21

Screening School-Age Children

Jackson Roush

INTRODUCTION

Hearing screening in the school-age population has long been regarded as a necessary and worthwhile endeavor. From its inception nearly 70 years ago, hearing screening in the schools has progressed from live voice "whisper" tests to the use of phonographic recordings of speech stimuli (figure 1) to electrically generated pure tones. By the

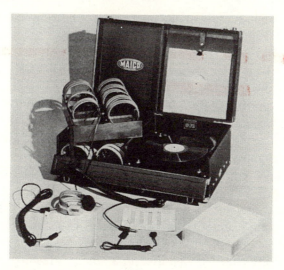

Figure 1. The Maico RS Screening Audiometer (from Watson and Tolan 1949). Group speech tests, popular in the 1940s, were eventually replaced by the pure-tone "sweep check." Although more time consuming, individually administered pure-tone tests proved to be more accurate and cost-effective.

1960s, all states were providing hearing screening in some form. More recently, many programs have added acoustic immittance measures to their screening protocols.

Considering the long history of screening in the school-age population, one would expect to find consistent and well-standardized test procedures. Instead, nationwide surveys have repeatedly shown substantial disagreement on the philosophical as well as procedural aspects of school screening. In an effort to delineate some of the key issues regarding the screening of school-age children, this chapter will examine (1) the prevalence and impact of hearing loss and middle ear disease in the school-age population; (2) the characteristics of existing screening protocols and research comparing their relative performance; and (3) the areas of agreement and disagreement related to hearing and immittance screening in the school-age population. Research needs and programmatic issues will also be addressed.

HEARING LOSS AND MIDDLE EAR DISEASE IN THE SCHOOL-AGE CHILD: PREVALENCE AND IMPACT

It is difficult to estimate the prevalence of hearing impairment in the school-age population. Estimates are affected by many variables including age, race, test environment, and seasonal variation. The audiometric level used to define *normal hearing* is also an important variable. Using 15 dB HL as the normal cutoff, Kessner et al. (1974) found that approximately 7% of the 4- to 11-year-old children they studied had significant hearing loss in one or both ears. Other investigators, using different screening criteria, have reported prevalence estimates ranging from 0.5% to 21% (Connor 1961). More recent estimates have put the incidence of hearing loss in the school-age population at 5% to 10% (Silverman et al. 1978; Eagles et al. 1967). In terms of total numbers, Bess and Humes (1990) note that there are over a million young people in the United States under the age of 18 years with significant hearing loss in one or both ears.

Most of the children identified in a school screening program have hearing impairments secondary to middle ear dysfunction. Otitis media with effusion (OME) is among the most common diseases affecting young children. Howie (1975) reported that nearly all children have had at least one occurrence of OME by the age of 6 years, with nearly three-fourths experiencing their first episode before the age of 2 years.

The prevalence is lower in school-age children; however, Lous and Fiellau-Nikolajsen (1981) reported that nearly one-third of the 7-year-old Swedish children they studied experienced at least one episode of OME during the school year. The prevalence of middle ear disease has been shown to decline substantially above that age, dropping to around 15% by age 11 (Kessner et al. 1974).

In addition to age, increased risk of otitis media has been associated with a number of other factors including race and socioeconomic status. Teele et al. (1980), in a study of over 2,500 preschool-age children in Boston, reported that Hispanic youngsters had the highest incidence of acute otitis media followed by white and then African-American children. Other groups at increased risk for OME include children of low socioeconomic status, Eskimos, American Indians, and children with Down syndrome or cleft palates (Northern and Downs 1991).

The effects of the mild conductive hearing loss that typically accompanies otitis media are uncertain; however, several studies have implicated early persistent OME as a causal factor in speech and language disorders, learning disabilities, and academic difficulties (Silva et al. 1982; Teele et al. 1984; 1989). In a recent review of the literature, Roberts and Roush (1992) noted that children with histories of recurrent OME have also been shown to score lower on standardized tests of speech production and speech discrimination as well as receptive and expressive language, intelligence, and academic achievement (Teele et al. 1984; 1990; Friel-Patti and Finitzo-Hieber 1990). In addition, children with OME histories have been described as exhibiting more attention and behavioral problems in school as well as greater need for school support services (Silva et al. 1982; Roberts et al. 1989). But despite this growing body of evidence, other studies have not supported a relationship between OME and later developmental problems (Fischler et al. 1985; Roberts et al. 1986). Furthermore, among those studies that *have* demonstrated a relationship, serious concerns have been raised about their validity (Paradise and Rogers 1986; Ruben et al. 1989). The effects of OME and associated hearing loss on development in young children remain unclear; however, there is convincing evidence that at least some children experience developmental delays as a result of OME, particularly in cases where the disease is chronic.

The developmental implications of sensorineural hearing loss in young children are more clearly established. There is a large body of literature documenting the effects of severe-to-profound hearing loss on speech and language development (e.g., Kretschmer and Kretschmer 1978). Although most children with severe-to-profound hearing losses would be identified well before school age, those with milder degrees of sensorineural loss may escape early detection. Blair et al. (1985) showed that even mild sensorineural hearing loss can result in academic delays and that those delays become progressively more severe as the child proceeds through school. A study by Davis (1974) showed that school-age children with mild-to-moderate sensorineural hearing losses experience difficulty acquiring basic concepts essential to understanding instructions and verbal directions. Seventy-five percent of the young children studied with hearing impairment scored below the tenth percentile in their knowledge of concepts related to time, quantity, and space.

In summary, hearing loss and middle ear disease affect a large number of young school-age children. Undetected hearing impairments can have serious consequences for speech-language acquisition and academic performance. Effective screening programs are needed to identify hearing loss and middle ear dysfunction in their early stages so that appropriate intervention can be undertaken in time to prevent or minimize the developmental delays associated with those conditions.

SCREENING FOR HEARING LOSS

PURE-TONE SCREENING PROCEDURES

In an effort to achieve greater standardization of pure-tone screening procedures, a monograph by Darley (1961) was published as a supplement to the *Journal of Speech and Hearing Disorders*. The document was revised and updated in 1974 and formed the basis of ASHA's first Guidelines for Identification Audiometry (ASHA 1975). These guidelines, which were later revised (ASHA 1985; 1990),[1] now recommend individual, manually administered pure-tone screening at 20

---

[1] The recently revised Guidelines for Screening for Hearing Impairments and Middle Ear Disorders (ASHA 1990) incorporate the ASHA Guidelines for Identification Audiometry (ASHA 1985).

dB HL for the frequencies 1000, 2000, and 4000 Hz.[2] Failure to respond at one or more frequencies in either ear constitutes a fail. Rescreening is then required, preferably on the same day but always within two weeks. The guidelines recommend that an audiologist evaluate the hearing of all children who fail the rescreening.

EVALUATING PURE-TONE SCREENING PROCEDURES

Considering the long history of hearing screening in the school-age population and the substantial resources expended each year to support this activity, relatively little research has been undertaken to examine the validity and predictive value of these procedures. Melnick, Eagles, and Levine (1964) evaluated the procedures recommended by Darley (1961); however, since testing was done in a sound-treated environment, results were difficult to generalize to most school-based screening programs. Recognizing this, Wilson and Walton (1974) evaluated pure-tone screening in a group of more than 1000 5- to 10-year-old children who were screened under conditions typical of most school environments. Their procedures followed ASHA's 1975 Guidelines for Identification Audiometry, which are similar to ASHA's current protocol[3] (ASHA 1985). Wilson and Walton reported that the procedure was approximately 95% accurate when compared to the results of a threshold test; however, as Roeser and Northern (1988) point out, quite a different picture emerges when the data are examined in terms of sensitivity and specificity. Using Wilson and Walton's data, Roeser and Northern noted that 97% of the children with normal hearing were correctly identified, a finding that indicates excellent specificity. In contrast, when the data were examined in terms of sensitivity, only 63% of the children with hearing losses were correctly identified; that is, over one-third of the children with significant hearing losses were missed. This is an alarming observation in view of the widespread application of ASHA's pure-tone screening procedures. It is clear that further research is needed even for pure-tone screening, the most basic and familiar of all identification procedures. In addition to measures of sensitivity and specificity, it is

---

[2] The inclusion of 500 Hz is recommended if acoustic immittance measures are not included and if ambient noise levels permit.

[3] Among other minor differences, the 1975 guidelines permitted increasing the intensity to 25 dB HL at 4000 Hz.

important for future research to examine the positive and negative predictive value of these procedures as applied to various school-age populations.

SCREENING FOR MIDDLE EAR DYSFUNCTION

ACOUSTIC IMMITTANCE SCREENING PROCEDURES

Several studies have shown that over half the children with middle ear dysfunction will be missed on the basis of audiometric screening alone (e.g., Roberts 1972). Consequently, many programs now employ acoustic immittance measures to screen for undetected middle ear disorders. Immittance screening generally involves several different measurements, the specific features of which vary according to the screening protocol adopted. Four of the most familiar procedures are summarized below.

ASHA Guidelines. In 1979, the ASHA Subcommittee on Impedance Measurements developed a set of guidelines for screening programs electing to include acoustic immittance measures (ASHA 1979). This protocol recommended a combination of tympanometry and acoustic reflex measures, which resulted in three possible outcomes: "Pass" (no additional follow-up), "At Risk" (scheduled for rescreening), or "Fail" (medical referral). An individual was passed if the tympanometric peak pressure was between +100 and −200 mm/H₂0 and an acoustic reflex was present. If a peak was identifiable but outside this range and the acoustic reflex was present, or if peak pressure was within this range but the acoustic reflex absent, the individual was considered to be "at risk" and rescreening was performed in three to five weeks at which time the individual was reclassified as either a pass or fail. Immediate medical referral was recommended if tympanometric peak pressure was outside the +100 to −200 range and the acoustic reflex absent.

Nashville Symposium Guidelines. The Nashville guidelines, which emerged from a national symposium at Vanderbilt University (Harford et al. 1978), recommended similar tympanometric and acoustic reflex criteria; however, they differed from the original ASHA guidelines with respect to referral criteria. In contrast to the 1979 ASHA protocol, which in some cases recommended medical referral on the basis of initial immittance findings, the Nashville guidelines recommend rescreening all individuals with abnormal tympanometric results four to six weeks after the initial test is failed. Those children who are again classified as being at risk are scheduled for periodic monitoring rather than medical referral.

Hirtshals Procedure. Lous (1983) described an immittance screening protocol used in Denmark that employs tympanometry without the acoustic reflex. Children who fail an initial screening are retested four to six weeks later; only those with flat tympanograms are referred. A third screening is then provided after another four- to six-week interval, and children with flat tympanograms or with peaks more negative than −200 daPa are referred for medical management.

ASHA's Revised Screening Protocol. ASHA recently adopted a new set of guidelines (ASHA 1990) combining pure-tone and immittance measures. Revisions to the immittance portion of the protocol were made in an effort to address problems with excessive overreferrals as well as the need to consider advances in acoustic immittance instrumentation and standards (ANSI 1988). The new protocol consists of four components: history, visual inspection, identification audiometry (pure-tone screening), and tympanometry (see chapter 4 for further discussion of these guidelines). The revised guidelines for pure-tone screening are the same as those established in the ASHA Guidelines for Identification Audiometry (ASHA 1985), described earlier. The three acoustic immittance measurements contained within the new set of guidelines are static admittance, equivalent ear canal volume, and tympanometric width (gradient). The new guidelines do not include measures of tympanometric peak pressure and acoustic reflex, citing evidence that these measures contribute little to the sensitivity of immittance screening while substantially lowering specificity. Immediate medical referral is never recommended on the basis of initial immittance findings alone except when there is evidence of an abnormally large ear canal volume accompanied by low static admittance, i.e., when there is reason to suspect a perforation of the tympanic membrane. When tympanometric results for static admittance and/or gradient are abnormal, rescreening is done after four to six weeks. If results are again abnormal, a medical referral is advised.

EVALUATION OF MIDDLE EAR SCREENING PROTOCOLS

Several studies have sought to evaluate the relative performance of these protocols. Comparison of studies is complicated by numerous variables including subject selection procedures, pass-fail criteria, and selection of a gold standard. In general, studies have reported an excessive number of false positive medical referrals, although some have also reported low sensitivity. Using the original ASHA guidelines (ASHA 1979), Lucker (1980) in a school-age population, and Roush and Tait (1985) in a preschool-age sample, predicted an overreferral rate in excess of 50% using the recommended criteria. Both studies predicted a significant reduction in the number of false positives by rescreening all ears prior to medical referral. Queen et al. (1981) also reported a substantial reduction in overreferrals by rescreening combined with modified use of the acoustic reflex. Schow et al. (1981) reported use of the ASHA protocol with a group of children seen for medical examinations in a pediatric office. In their study, sensitivity was calculated at 89%, with specificity relatively lower at only 81%.

Lous compared the ASHA and Nashville protocols to the Hirtshals procedure. This procedure resulted in relatively low sensitivity (80%) but excellent specificity (95%). Sensitivity was reported at 83% and 90% for the ASHA and Nashville protocols, respectively; specificity was much lower at 71% and 67% for the two protocols.

Recognizing the overreferral problems associated with the original ASHA immittance screening protocol, ASHA's revised guidelines (1990) call for the elimination of tympanometric peak pressure and acoustic reflex. To date, there are no published reports on the application of the revised protocol in its entirety; however, Roush, Drake, and Sexton (1992) recently compared the tympanometric measures contained within ASHA's 1990 guidelines to a more traditional procedure consisting of tympanometric peak pressure and acoustic reflexes. In an unselected sample of 3- and 4-year-old children, using pneumatic otoscopy as the standard, they found that the immittance measures contained within the revised ASHA procedure achieved a moderate level of sensitivity (84%) but not as high as that achieved using the more traditional procedure (95%). Specificity, on the other hand, was much higher using ASHA's revised immittance protocol. With regard to predictive value, normal tympanometric results were highly predictive of normal middle ear function for both protocols. In contrast, the predictive value of a positive (abnormal) outcome was much lower for both procedures. The positive predictive value for the traditional procedure was 27%, meaning that only about one-fourth of the subjects who failed the screen were classified otologically as needing medical follow-up. The positive predictive value of the revised ASHA immittance measures, although considerably higher (69%), was still somewhat low for routine screening purposes. These findings underscore the need to consider immittance findings in the context of hearing levels and other relevant data, a point also emphasized in the revised ASHA protocol (1990).

PURE-TONE AND MIDDLE EAR SCREENING PRACTICES

Several nationwide surveys have examined the procedural aspects of school-age screening, and virtually every study has shown that few programs adhere to a specific set of guidelines, even within a state. Connor (1961), in an effort to estimate the prevalence of hearing loss in young children, reviewed 31 articles published from 1926 to 1960. Although his review was not intended to examine screening protocols, he noted that differences in instrumentation, test frequencies, ambient noise levels, and examination procedures made comparison of studies nearly impossible. The first attempt to examine school-based screening practices in the U.S. was reported by Murphy (1972) in a study conducted by the Office of Demographic Studies at Gallaudet College. This report found widespread lack of uniformity for nearly every procedure examined. Little had changed by the early 1980s when Rosenberg and Rosenberg (1982) attempted a similar but more detailed survey of screening practices. Their findings, which they characterized as "a chaotic myriad of standards, regulations, guidelines, techniques, and recommendations," revealed that states differed with respect to legislative mandates and regulations, as well as grade levels screened, presentation levels, test frequencies, and inclusion of tympanometry. There was also considerable variation in the treatment of various "special populations." Similar observations were reported by Wall et al. (1985), who surveyed school nurses, speech-language pathologists, and audiologists. In addition to differences in pure-tone procedures, they noted that fewer than one-third of the programs included acoustic immittance measures, even though most indicated that identification of middle ear disorders was among their primary goals. Recently, Roush and Davidson (1991) conducted a nationwide survey aimed at determining whether the recently revised ASHA protocol (ASHA 1990) had affected screening practices in the schools. The study also sought to determine how recent changes in federal law (Public Law 99-457) were affecting educational audiology practices. Preliminary data based on responses from 30 states revealed significant disparities along several dimensions including screening personnel, screening levels, inclusion of acoustic immittance measures, and referral criteria. When asked to describe their greatest frustration, most respondents identified problems related to providing appropriate follow-up services after hearing loss or middle ear dysfunction had been identified.

IMPLEMENTATION OF SCREENING PROGRAMS: AREAS OF AGREEMENT AND DISAGREEMENT

PURE-TONE SCREENING

There appears to be general agreement that mass screening for hearing loss is justified and that screening efforts should be concentrated at the early elementary levels. As shown in figure 2, nearly all of the programs surveyed by Roush and Davidson provided pure-tone hearing screening at kindergarten and first grade; above the first grade, screening occurs primarily on alternate years. Very few programs conduct pure-tone screening at the secondary level. Past surveys also reveal general agreement regarding the selection of the frequencies to be screened (1000, 2000, and 4000 Hz), the failure criterion (any frequency, either ear), and the importance of rescreening all who fail initially. There is considerably less agreement regarding the selection of screening levels. Although few programs attempt to screen below 20 dB HL, many appear to screen at higher levels, presumably to compensate for excessive ambient noise levels.

Surprisingly, there has been minimal research on the validity and predictive accuracy of pure-tone screening. Additional research is needed to address these issues. Particularly disturbing is the apparently low sensitivity of pure-tone screening in the schools. It seems inconceivable that such a serious problem could be neglected for so long yet, as shown by Roeser and Northern (1988), the limited data currently available seem to support this conclusion.

Other issues needing further study are how often to screen and at what ages. ASHA recommends annual hearing screening of children at developmental ages of 3 to 8 years, and any high-risk children above this age range (ASHA 1985). Examples of high-risk conditions cited in the guidelines are children in special education or those who repeated a grade; those new to the school system; those who failed a threshold test during the past year; those with speech-language or other communicative disorders; those engaged in noisy activities; and those with a history of chronic middle ear disease. There is evidence that some of these conditions place a school-age child at increased risk for hearing loss; however, comparative data for these high-risk groups are lacking (Roush 1990). Further research is needed to determine if the added expense of providing annual screening of these special populations is justified.

ACOUSTIC IMMITTANCE SCREENING

With regard to acoustic immittance screening, there are few areas of agreement and numerous issues that remain controversial or unresolved. Figure 2, from Roush and Davidson (1991), indicates that acoustic immittance screening is concentrated at the early elementary levels. Beyond this, there is little agreement regarding acoustic immittance screening. The surveys of Rosenberg and Rosenberg (1982), Wall et al. (1985), and Roush and Davidson (1991) reveal considerable disagreement with regard to the inclusion of acoustic immittance measures and, if included, the specific measurements and pass-fail criteria applied. The consensus of "expert opinion" (e.g., Bluestone et al. 1986) is that acoustic immittance screening should be limited to "special populations" known to be at high risk. This would include children with cleft palates, Down syndrome, and craniofacial anomalies as well as those from high-risk ethnic groups such as American Indians and Alaskan Eskimos.

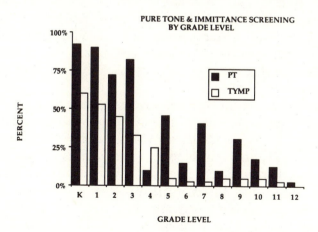

Figure 2. Percentage of programs conducting pure-tone and acoustic immittance screening, by grade level (from Roush and Davidson 1991).

Programs electing to use a protocol combining pure-tone and immittance screening now have a new set of guidelines to consider (ASHA 1990). Critical evaluation of these new guidelines is needed to establish their sensitivity, specificity, and predictive value. The visual inspection criteria, in particular, will require careful appraisal. Applied successfully, routine otoscopy could expedite medical management. But applied improperly, the visual inspection criteria could result in a new source of overreferrals. The revised tympanometric criteria also needs careful study. Rescreening, combined with the elimination of tympanometric peak pressure and acoustic reflex, should reduce the number of false positive medical referrals but possibly at the expense of lower sensitivity. Additional research is needed to determine what specific measure or combination of measures results in the best overall screening protocol.

CONCLUSIONS

Beginning in the early part of this century, the school-age population was the first to undergo widespread, systematic attempts at auditory screening. Pure-tone and immittance screening now involves millions of children each year at substantial cost to our educational and health care institutions. Considering the long and enduring history of school-age screening, one would expect to find specific and well-established protocols. Instead, we are faced with a litany of procedural inconsistencies and philosophical contradictions. Especially distressing is the issue of follow-up. Virtually every set of guidelines and every author who has written on the subject have emphasized the importance of appropriate management following identification, yet lack of follow-up remains a major frustration.

Improving the quality of our screening programs will require continued research as well as interdisciplinary communication and collaboration. Screening guidelines must consider the role of each discipline represented: audiologists, school nurses, physicians, and administrators. In reviewing the status of hearing screening over 15 years ago, Bess, Baker, and Mencher (1976) wrote: "We have convinced ourselves of the necessity and educated ourselves relative to the methodology, but we have not done so for other professional groups." Regrettably, the current state of affairs indicates that little has changed in the ensuing years. Moreover, the extent to which we have convinced and educated ourselves must be questioned, in view of the perpetual difficulties that seem to plague our screening and follow-up efforts.

Recent federal legislation, reflecting changes in public and professional views of "best practice," puts substantial emphasis on the importance of early identification. Hopefully, the climate is right for some new initiatives aimed at bringing greater uniformity to our screening practices and a broader, more comprehensive approach to our identification efforts. Pure-tone and immittance testing will remain essential, but screening the school-age child will not accomplish its intended purpose unless there is concurrent follow-up to address educational and developmental needs as well as those related to medical management.

SUMMARY

Screening for hearing loss in the school-age population has occurred for most of this century. Still, there remains substantial variability in the selection of screening practices and procedures. Surprisingly, minimal research has been done to evaluate the accuracy of mass pure-tone screening. The results of at least one study suggest high specificity but low sensitivity. That is, conventional pure-tone screening procedures, although accurate in the classification of children with normal hearing, may be missing a significant number of children with hearing losses.

In recent years many programs have added acoustic immittance measures to screen for middle ear dysfunction, but here, too, there has been considerable disagreement regarding methodology and referral criteria. In general, immittance screening has resulted in fairly high sensitivity but low specificity. That is, most immittance screening procedures have been reasonably accurate in identifying children with middle ear dysfunction but largely inaccurate with regard to classification of nondiseased ears.

For both pure-tone and immittance measures, a renewed commitment is needed to determine the protocols best suited for screening purposes. Equally important is a commitment to appropriate intervention and follow-up after hearing loss or middle ear dysfunction has been identified.

REFERENCES

American National Standards Institute. 1988. American National Standard specifications for instruments to measure aural acoustic impedance and admittance (aural acoustic immittance). ANSI S3.39-1987. New York: American National Standards Institute.

American Speech-Language-Hearing Association. 1975. Guidelines for identification audiometry. *Asha* 17:94-99.

American Speech-Language-Hearing Association. 1979. Guidelines for acoustic immittance screening of middle ear function. *Asha* 21:550-558.

American Speech-Language-Hearing Association. 1985. Guidelines for identification audiometry. *Asha* 27(5):49-52.

American Speech-Language-Hearing Association. 1990. Guidelines for screening for hearing impairments and middle ear disorders. *Asha* 32 (Suppl. 2):17-24.

Bess, F., Baker, C., and Mencher, G. 1976. The pediatrician's view of neonatal auditory screening. In G.T. Mencher (ed.), *Early identification of hearing loss*. Basel, Switzerland: S. Karger, A.G.

Bess, F., and Humes, L. 1990. *Audiology: The fundamentals*. Baltimore: Williams and Wilkins.

Blair, J., Peterson, M., and Viehweg, S. 1985. The effects of mild sensorineural hearing loss on the academic performance of young school-age children. *Volta Review* 87(2):87-93.

Bluestone, C., Fria, T., Arjona, S., et al. 1986. Controversies in screening for middle ear disease and hearing loss in children. *Pediatrics* 77(1):57-70.

Connor, L.E. 1961. Determining the prevalence of hearing impaired children. *Exceptional Child* 27:337-344.

Darley, F. 1961. Identification audiometry. *Journal of Speech and Hearing Disorders* Monograph Suppl. no. 9

Davis, J. 1974. Performance of young hearing impaired children on a test of basic concepts. *Journal of Speech and Hearing Research* 17:(3):342-351.

Eagles, E.L., Wishik, S.M., Doerfler, L.G., Melnick, W., and Levine, H.S. 1967. Hearing sensitivity and ear disease in children: A prospective study. *Laryngoscope* (monograph)1-274.

Education of the Handicapped Act Amendments of 1986 (P.L. 99-457), 20 U.S.C. Secs. 1400-1485.

Fischler, R., Todd, N., and Feldman, C. 1985. Otitis media and language performance in a cohort of Apache Indian children. *American Journal of Diseases of Children* 139:355-360.

Friel-Patti, S., and Finitzo-Hieber, T. 1990. Language learning in a prospective study of otitis media with effusion in the first two years of life. *Journal of Speech and Hearing Research* 33:188-194.

Harford, E.R., Bess, F.H., Bluestone, C.D., and Klein, J.O. (eds.). 1978. *Impedance screening for middle ear disease in children*. New York: Grune and Stratton.

Howie, V.M. 1975. Natural history of Otitis Media. *Annals of Otology, Rhinology and Laryngology*. Suppl. 19:67-72.

Kessner, D.M., Snow, C., and Singer, J. 1974. Assessment of medical care in children. In Contrasts in Health Status. Washington, D.C.: Institute of Medicine, *National Academy of Sciences* Vol 3.

Kretschmer, R.R., and Kretschmer, L.W. 1978. *Language development and intervention with the hearing impaired*. Baltimore: University Park Press.

Lous, J. 1983. Three impedance screening programs on a cohort of seven-year-old children. *Scandinavian Audiology* Suppl. 17:60-64.

Lous, J., and Fiellau-Nikolajsen, M. 1981. Epidemiology of middle ear effusion and tubal dysfunction: A one year prospective study comprising monthly tympanometry in 387 nonselected seven year old children. *International Journal of Pediatric Otorhinolaryngology* 3:303.

Lucker, J.R. 1980. Application of pass-fail criteria to middle-ear screening results. *Asha* 22:839-840.

Melnick, W., Eagles, E.L., and Levine, H.S. 1964. Evaluation of a recommended program of identification audiometry with school-age children. *Journal for Speech and Hearing Disorders* 29:3-13.

Murphy, N.J. 1972. National survey of state identification audiometry programs and special education services for hearing impaired children and youths. United States: Series C, no. 1, *Annual survey of hearing impaired children and youth*. Washington, D.C.: Office of Demographic Studies, Gallaudet College.

Northern, J., and Downs, M. 1991. *Hearing in children*. Baltimore: Williams and Wilkins.

Paradise, J.L., and Rogers, K.D. 1986. On otitis media, child development, and tympanostomy tubes: New answers or old questions? *Pediatrics* 77:88-92.

Queen, S., Moses., F, and Wood, S. 1981. The use of immittance screening by the Kansas City, Missouri, Public School District. *Seminars in Speech, Language, and Hearing* 2:119.

Roberts, J. 1972. Hearing sensitivity and related medical findings among children in the United States. *Transactions of the American Academy of Ophthalmology and Otolaryngology* 76:355-359.

Roberts, J.E., and Roush, J. 1992. Otitis media. In M. Levine, W. Carey, and A. Crocker (eds.), *Developmental behavioral pediatrics* 2d ed. Philadelphia: W.B. Saunders Co.

Roberts, J.E., Sanyal, M.A., Burchinal, M.R., Collier, A.M., Ramey, C.T., and Henderson, F.W. 1986. Otitis media in early childhood and its relationship to later verbal and academic performance. *Pediatrics* 78:423-430.

Roberts, J.E., Burchinal, M.R., Collier, A.M., Ramey, C.T., Koch, M.A., and Henderson, F.W. 1989. Otitis media in early childhood and cognitive, academic, and classroom performance of the school-aged child. *Pediatrics* 83:477-485.

Roeser, R.J., and Northern, J.L. 1988. Screening for hearing loss and middle ear disorders. In R.J. Roeser, and M.P. Downs (eds.), *Auditory disorders in school children*. New York: Thieme-Stratton.

Rosenberg, P., and Rosenberg, J. 1982. Hearing screening. In N.J. Lass, L.V. McReynolds, J.L. Northern, and D.E. Yoder (eds.), *Speech, language, and hearing*. Philadelphia: W.B Saunders.

Roush, J. 1990. Identification of hearing loss and middle ear disease in pre-school and school-age children. *Seminars in Hearing* 11(4):357-371.

Roush, J., and Tait, C. 1985. Pure tone and acoustic immittance screening of preschool-age children: An examination of referral criteria. *Ear and Hearing* 6(5):245-249.

Roush, J., and Davidson, D. 1991. A nationwide survey of hearing and immittance screening practices (in preparation).

Roush, J., Drake, A., and Sexton, J. 1992. Identification of middle ear dysfunction in young children: A comparison of tympanometric screening procedures. *Ear and Hearing* 13(2):63-69.

Ruben, J.R., Bagger-Sjorback, D., Downs, M.P., Gravel, J.S., Karakashian, M., Klein, J.O., Morizono, T., and Paparella, M.M. 1989. Complications and sequelae. *Annals of Otology, Rhinology and Laryngology* 98 (Suppl. 139):46-55.

Schow, R.L., Pederson, J.K., Nerbonne, M.A., and Boe, R. 1981. Comparison of ASHA's immittance guidelines and standard medical diagnostic procedures. *Ear and Hearing* 2(6):251-255.

Silva, P., Kirkland, C., Simpson, A., Steward, I., and Williams, S. 1982. Some developmental and behavioral problems associated with bilateral otitis media with effusion. *Journal of Learning Disabilities* 15:417-421.

Silverman, S.R., Lane, H.S., and Calvert, D.L. 1978. Early and elementary education.In H. Davis and S.R. Silverman (eds.), *Hearing and deafness*. 4th ed. Baltimore: Holt, Rinehart and Winston.

Teele, D.W., Klein, J.O., and Rosner, B. 1980. Epidemiology of otitis media in children. *Annals of Otology, Rhinology and Laryngology* 89(Suppl. 68):5-6.

Teele, D.W., Klein, J.O., Rosner, B.A., and the Greater Boston Otitis Media Study Group.1984. Otitis media with effusion during the first three years of life and development of speech and language. *Pediatrics* 74:282-287.

Teele, D.W., Klein, J.O., Rosner, B.A., and the Greater Boston Otitis Media Study Group. 1989. Epidemiology of otitis media during the first seven years of life in children in greater Boston: A prospective cohort study. *Journal of Infectious Diseases* 160:83-94.

Teele, D.W., Klein, J.O., Chase, C., Menyuk, P., Rosner, B.A., and the Greater Boston Otitis Media Study Group. 1990. Otitis media in infancy and intellectual ability, school achievement, speech, and language at age 7 years. *Journal of Infectious Diseases* 162:685-694.

Wall, G.L., Naples, G.M., Buhrer, K., and Capodanno, C. 1985. A survey of audiological services within the school system. *Asha* 27:1, 31-34.

Watson, L.A., and Tolan, T. 1949. *Hearing tests and hearing instruments.* Baltimore: Williams and Wilkins.

Wilson, W.R., and Walton, W.K. 1974. Identification audiometry accuracy: evaluation of a recommended program for school-age children. *Language, Speech, and Hearing Services in the Schools* 5:8-12.

Chapter 22

Sensitivity, Specificity, and Predictive Value of Immittance Measures in the Identification of Middle Ear Effusion

Robert J. Nozza, Charles D. Bluestone, and David Kardatzke

INTRODUCTION

Acoustic immittance has been used for the identification of middle ear disease for many years. Although there are data in the literature regarding the relationship between acoustic immittance variables and the presence of middle ear effusion (MEE) (Orchik et al. 1980; Paradise et al. 1976), recent standards for aural acoustic immittance testing (ANSI 1987) have made obsolete the measures (in arbitrary "compliance" units) provided by impedance meters such as the Madsen ZO-73. There is a need for data on the relationship between immittance variables, measured under current standards, and the status of the middle ear as a function of age. Koebsell and Margolis (1986) and Margolis and Heller (1987) have provided some data on acoustic admittance and middle ear function in preschool children with normal middle ear function and normal hearing, and have noted the lack of acoustic admittance data for ears with middle ear disease. The studies described in this report were designed to provide data on the relationship between aural acoustic admittance variables, determined using an instrument that is in compliance with the current standard (ANSI 1987), and middle ear function in children. The data from our studies have relevance to the identification and diagnosis of otitis media with effusion (OME) in both screening and clinical programs.

EXPERIMENTAL SAMPLE: SURGERY GROUP

In the first study, we sought to determine the relationship between the presence or absence of MEE, as determined by a surgeon at the time of myringotomy and tube (M&T) placement, and tympanometric variables, otoscopic diagnosis, and various combinations of the two. There is general agreement that a finding at the time of middle ear surgery is the gold standard for diagnosis of middle ear effusion. There are some flaws in that notion, however. For example, children who are appropriate candidates for M&T surgery may or may not be representative of the group of children on whom given diagnostic or screening tests will be used in a given setting. Also, determination of the presence or absence of MEE during surgery can be subjective and may vary between surgeons. Nevertheless, findings at time of M&T surgery are still widely regarded as the standard against which other tests must be validated.

METHODS

Subjects were young children with history of chronic or recurrent OM who were referred for M&T surgery. For aural acoustic admittance measures, we used a GSI-33 Middle Ear Analyzer, which complies with the new ANSI standard for aural acoustic immittance testing. The admittance test parameters used in the study of surgical patients are described in table 1. Admittance measurements were made by an audiologist. A validated otoscopist, a pediatric nurse practitioner with

Table 1
Tympanometric Protocol

Instrument:	GSI-33, Version I
Probe Tone:	226 Hz
Pressure Sweep:	+400 to −600 daPa
Ear Canal Volume:	Estimated at +400 daPa
Pump Speed:	600/200 daPa/s
Mode:	Diagnostic
Reflex:	1000 Hz, 100 dB HL, IPSI

daPa: dekapascal, daPa/s: dekapascal per second, dB: decibel, GSI-33: Middle Ear Analyzer (Lucas-Grason Stadler, Inc.), HL: hearing level, Hz: hertz (cycles per second), IPSI: ipsilateral.

more than 20 years of experience in OM clinical research studies, used pneumatic otoscopy to make a diagnosis of presence or absence of effusion for each ear. The admittance tests and the otoscopy were done in the same-day surgery examination rooms immediately before the children were moved to the operating room waiting area. The otoscopist was unaware of the tympanometric findings and simply recorded her diagnosis on a data form. During the surgery, one of the two participating surgeons attempted to suction fluid from the middle ear. If any effusion could be drawn, the ear was scored positive for MEE. The surgeon was unaware of the tympanometric and otoscopic findings.

RESULTS

One hundred seventy-one children between 1 year and 12 years of age (mean=4 years) were evaluated. Of those children, 249 ears provided valid otoscopic and acoustic admittance measures and were also examined surgically. One hundred thirty-seven ears had evidence of effusion at the time of surgery, and 112 ears were found to be free of

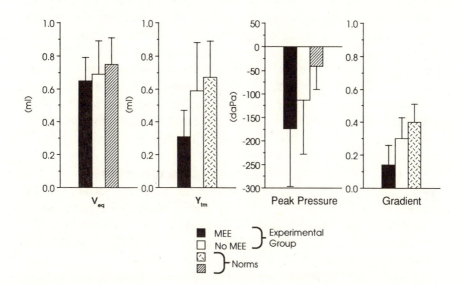

Figure 1. Data from ears with and ears without middle ear effusion (MEE) from children undergoing myringotomy and tubes (M&T) surgery, along with normative data for acoustic admittance (Y_{tm}) and gradient (Gr) (Koebsell and Margolis 1986) and for equivalent ear canal volume (V_{eq}) and tympanometric peak pressure (TPP) (Margolis and Heller 1987).

effusion, yielding a prevalence of MEE of 55%. For purposes of this report, we will focus on the data from the acoustic admittance tests. It is likely that in most screening applications validated pneumatic otoscopy will not be available.

A descriptive analysis of the data is presented in figure 1, using the ear rather than the child as the unit of analysis. Measures on two ears from the same child are not independent, so an analysis by ears should be considered with some caution. In the literature the relationship between tympanometry and MEE is based on analysis by ears. However, in a screening setting, performance with the child as the unit of analysis would be more appropriate (Rockette and Casselbrant 1988). There are three groups for each measure. The measures are equivalent ear canal volume (V_{eq}), peak compensated static acoustic admittance (Y_{tm}), tympanometric peak pressure (TPP), and gradient (Gr), a ratio as used by Paradise et al. (1976), after Brooks (1969), and as computed by the GSI-33. The groups are those with MEE and those without MEE from our surgery group and normative data taken from either Koebsell and Margolis (1986) or Margolis and Heller (1987), depending on which study used parameters most similar to those used in the present investigation. For tympanograms scored as "no peak" (i.e., "flat"; N = 17) by the GSI-33, Y_{tm} and Gr were assigned a value of zero (0). Flat tympanograms were excluded from the descriptive statistics for TPP. Except for V_{eq}, the measures of both our groups with and without MEE differ somewhat from the norms. This illustrates that ears with no MEE in children with history of chronic or recurrent OME, as a group, differ from ears with no MEE in children with documented normal middle ear function and normal hearing.

A test of the acoustic reflex (AR) that was considered valid was made on 218 (87.5%) of the 249 ears in the sample. That is, AR was listed as "could not test" (CNT) for 31 ears. Of the 218 ears for which a valid test of the AR was made, 124 had MEE and 94 had no MEE. Of the 124 ears with MEE, 18 (15%) had a measurable AR, whereas of the 94 ears without MEE, 61 (65%) had a measurable AR.

Discriminant analyses were performed to determine which variables contributed most to correct prediction of middle ear status. Otoscopy combined with Y_{tm} and otoscopy combined with Gr had the greatest accuracy. However, AR combined with Y_{tm} and AR combined with Gr are also reasonably accurate. To display the sensitivity and specificity of

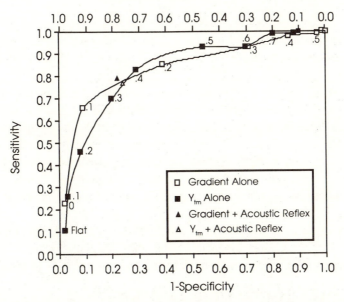

Figure 2. Receiver operating characteristic (ROC) space illustrating performance of acoustic admittance variables in identification of middle ear effusion (MEE). ROC curves are for gradient (Gr) and for acoustic admittance (Y_{tm}).

some of the measures that performed well, we plotted them in a receiver operating characteristic (ROC) space (figure 2). Complete ROC curves for the tympanometric variables Gr and Y_{tm} are shown, along with points representing the best performance attainable by combining AR with Gr and with Y_{tm}. For Gr and AR, MEE was classified with the greatest accuracy if Gr ≤ .1 or if Gr = .2 with an absent AR. This rule yielded 78% sensitivity and 79% specificity. Ten ears with Gr = .2, and thus requiring AR for classification, had AR as CNT and, therefore, could not be classified by that rule. In a similar way, the rule that classifies ears as having MEE by "no peak" or Y_{tm} ≤ .2 OR Y_{tm} = .3, .4, or .5 with absent AR had sensitivity of 77% and specificity of 76%. Again, ten ears were left unclassified using that rule.

The AR test alone was highly sensitive. However, for 31 ears AR could not be tested. If we disregard the 31 ears that could not be tested, AR had sensitivity of 86% (106/124) and specificity of 65% (61/94). If we compute the test characteristics based on the 249 ears that were tested validly by tympanometry and otoscopy, that is, we consider the missing

AR data as errors, performance of the AR is much poorer. In the analysis that includes all ears, if ears that are CNT are counted as errors, the AR alone had sensitivity of 77% (106/137) and specificity of 55% (61/112).

Each point on the ROC curve for Gr represents a different cutoff value for separating ears with and ears without MEE. A rule that labeled an ear with MEE when Gr ≤ .1 had sensitivity of 66% and specificity of 91% (figure 2). With a cutoff of ≤ .2, sensitivity increased to 85% but specificity dropped to 62%. Similar relationships were seen for the Y_{tm} ROC curve. TPP was not very useful, either alone or in combination with other variables, for identifying MEE and is not included in the figure.

Many criteria employed with our data set gave similar results. However, the best performance, even with validated otoscopy incorporated into the criteria, was 81% for sensitivity and 85% specificity.

"NORMATIVE" SAMPLE: OUTPATIENT GROUP

To investigate the performance of some admittance criteria on a different population, we examined data that had been collected on a group of children who were unselected with respect to OM history. These children were outpatients in our hospital's allergy clinic and were undergoing allergy treatment or evaluation.

METHODS

We used an admittance test protocol similar to that used with the surgery group, except that the automatic screening mode was employed. This permitted the AR activating stimulus to reach levels as high as 105 dB HL. Also, there was no M&T surgery for validation of middle ear status for obvious reasons. Rather, the validated otoscopist's diagnosis was used as the standard. While this method of diagnosis is less valid than findings at surgery, it is the only reasonable alternative in cases where surgery is not indicated. The comparisons between the data from the surgery group and those from our outpatients should be considered with this methodological difference in mind.

RESULTS

Seventy-seven outpatients, 3 to 16 years of age (mean=9), were examined otoscopically. Of the 154 ears, 144 could be evaluated by both otoscopy and tympanometry. One hundred thirty-five ears were considered free of effusion by otoscopy, and 9 ears were considered to have OM, including 2 with acute infections and 7 with OME. Of those with OME, 4 had otoscopic evidence of a fluid level or bubbles and 3 did not. Prevalence of MEE in this group was 7%. Sixty-eight of the children were effusion free bilaterally by otoscopy. Of the 136 ears among the bilaterally effusion-free children, 130 yielded valid tympanograms. The data from the 130 effusion-free ears from this group were viewed as a normal subsample and are shown in comparison to the normative data in table 2. Agreement between data sets is quite good,

Table 2

Descriptive Statistics for Tympanometric Variables for Ears with No MEE

	Experimental	Normative Data	
	Outpatient Group	Koebsell/ Margolis[■]	Margolis/ Heller[•]
V_{eq} (ml)		N/A	
M	0.90		0.74
5% to 95% Range	0.60 to 1.35		0.42 to 0.97
N	130		92
Y_{tm} (mmho)			
M	0.78	0.67	0.50
5% to 95% Range	0.40 to 1.39	N/A	0.22 to 0.81
N	130	60	92
TPP (daPa)		N/A	
M	−34		−30
5% to 95% Range	−207 to +15		−139 to +11
N	130		92
Gr			N/A
M	.45	.40	
5% to 95% Range	0.30 to 0.60	0.25 to 0.59	
N	130	60	

[■] Koebsell and Margolis (1986): +400 to −400 daPa; 2.8- to 5.8-year-olds.
[•] Margolis and Heller (1987): +200 to −300 daPa; 3.7- to 5.8-years-olds.
daPa: dekapascal, Gr: gradient, M: mean, ml: milliliter, mmho: millimho, N: sample size, N/A: not available from report, TPP: tympanometric peak pressure, V_{eq}: equivalent ear canal volume, Y_{tm}: acoustic admittance.

especially considering that the age range for the outpatient group was broader than for the group comprising the norms (Koebsell and Margolis 1986; Margolis and Heller 1987) and the instrument settings (such as ear canal pressure at which V_{eq} is estimated) varied across the different studies. The 9 ears with OM by otoscopy were too few and too variable with respect to admittance findings to be characterized meaningfully as a group.

TEST PERFORMANCE VERSUS SUBJECT GROUP

It is important to remember that the prevalence of disease and the nature of disease in the target population can influence outcome of the test with respect to predictive values and with respect to choices of screening criteria. (See chapters 1 and 6). In the surgery group, there were ears with and without MEE. To illustrate the difference between ears of children with chronic or recurrent OM and those of children more representative of the general population, the distributions of Gr for ears with and without MEE are shown in figure 3. The curve on the left is for the ears with MEE of the surgery group; the second curve is for the ears with no MEE from the same group; the curve on the right is for

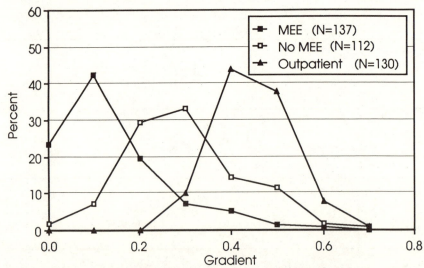

Figure 3. Distribution of gradient (Gr) values for ears of three subject groups: (1) ears with middle ear effusion (MEE) from the group of children undergoing myringotomy and tube (M&T) surgery; (2) ears with no MEE from the same group; (3) ears with no MEE from children attending outpatient allergy clinic (unselected re: OM history).

the 130 ears with no MEE of the bilaterally effusion-free patients in the outpatient group. The distributions are different for all three groups, which include ears diagnosed as having no MEE from two different populations.

To demonstrate the effects of both the different prevalences of disease (55% versus 7% in our studies) and possibly different disease processes or disease states in our two populations on performance of our test, we applied a simple diagnostic criterion to the data from both subject samples. We chose to call the test positive for MEE if the Gr ≤ .2. According to Koebsell and Margolis (1986), this value is just outside the 90% range of normal values for children, which is the same criterion used for selecting cutoffs for other variables in the current ASHA guidelines (ASHA 1990). Figure 4 illustrates, by way of 2X2 matrices, the sensitivity, specificity, and predictive values for that diagnostic criterion on the two different subject groups. Not only are predictive values different, an outcome that is anticipated based on the difference in prevalence of MEE in the two groups, but also specificity is quite different. Sensitivity estimate in the outpatient group is based on too few data to be reliable. In theory, the test characteristics sensitivity and specificity should not be influenced by disease prevalence, so the difference seen in specificity must be due to a difference in the status of

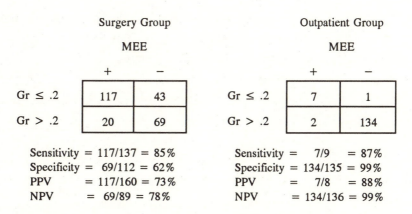

Figure 4. Sensitivity, specificity, positive predictive value (PPV), and negative predictive value (NPV) of tympanometric criterion whereby gradient (Gr) ≤.2 is positive for middle ear effusion (MEE).

the ears with no MEE in the two subject groups (see figure 3), or other factors. This finding is important and brings attention to one of the problems associated with developing diagnostic criteria on one population and applying them indiscriminantly to other populations that may or may not be well represented by the group on which the criteria were developed. To further illustrate the point, a similar analysis was done using a criterion recommended in the ASHA guidelines (ASHA 1990). The guidelines state that ears with acoustic admittance values outside the 90% range of normal values should be pursued according to the recommended retest and/or follow-up protocol. According to the data presented in the guidelines, that would mean Y_{tm} values $< .2$ mmho should be followed or referred. Figure 5 illustrates clearly the difference in the performance of that criterion based on the two different subject groups from the present investigation.

Our data suggest that by establishing criteria on the group with chronic or recurrent OM, we may be underestimating the predictive ability of acoustic admittance to identify MEE in the general population. However, more data on children from the general population or from high-risk groups for whom screening might be recommended are needed before such a conclusion can be drawn.

	Surgery Group				Outpatient Group		
	MEE				MEE		
	+	−			+	−	
$Y_{tm} < .2$	35	3		$Y_{tm} < .2$	6	0	
$Y_{tm} \geq .2$	102	109		$Y_{tm} \geq .2$	3	135	

Sensitivity = 35/137 = 26%
Specificity = 109/112 = 97%
PPV   = 35/38 = 92%
NPV   = 109/211 = 52%

Sensitivity = 6/9 = 67%
Specificity = 135/135 = 100%
PPV   = 6/6 = 100%
NPV   = 135/138 = 98%

Figure 5. Sensitivity, specificity, positive predictive value (PPV), and negative predictive value (NPV) of the tympanometric criterion whereby acoustic admittance (Y_{tm}) $<.2$ [as per American Speech-Language-Hearing Association (ASHA) guidelines] is positive for middle ear effusion (MEE).

Tympanometric Width: Preliminary Data

According to the ASHA guidelines (ASHA 1990), the recommended gradient measure is tympanometric width (TW), the pressure interval (in daPa) at half the Y_{tm} of the tympanogram, rather than the ratio (Gr) as computed by the GSI-33 used in our studies. Based on normative studies, it has been suggested that TW might be a better measure to use for identifying ears outside a normal range (Koebsell and Margolis 1986; Margolis and Heller 1987). To explore that possibility with our data set, we measured TW using a computer-based optical digitization system. The system is used by our Ear, Nose, and Throat Laboratory for digitization of shape and size of anatomic structures in slide preparations. To date, we have made measurements and analyzed 231 (taken sequentially) of the 249 tympanograms from the surgery group and the tympanograms from the "normative" sample taken from the outpatient allergy clinic. Software was written to measure TW and other variables on the digitized data set. There was good agreement in Y_{tm}, Gr, and TPP between the digitized data and the original values produced by the GSI-33. No differences were statistically significant. Table 3 has the means and standard deviations of the TW measures for both our subject groups as well as the norms as published in the ASHA guidelines for screening (ASHA 1990). The data from our "normative" group compare quite favorably with those

Table 3

Means, Standard Deviations, 90% Range, and Sample Sizes for Tympanometric Width (TW) Estimates from the Present Experiment and from Published Norms

	Typanometric Width (daPa)			
	Surgery		Outpatient	Norms*
	MEE	No MEE	No MEE	No MEE
M	377	215	104	100
(s.d.)	(119)	(90)	(32)	(28)
5% to 95%	147 to 542	84 to 393	60 to 168	60 to 150
N	123	108	130	92

* ASHA guidelines (1990).
daPa: dekapascal, M: mean, MEE: middle ear effusion, N: sample size, s.d.: standard deviation.

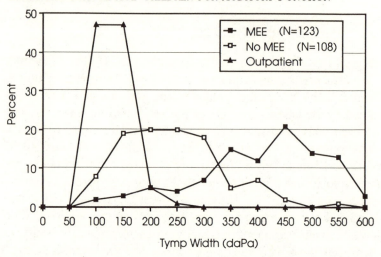

Figure 6. Distributions of tympanometric width (TW) on subset (231 of 249) of ears from surgery group and on "normative" group of outpatients (No MEE).

published previously. Figure 6 has the distributions for TW for the outpatient group and for the 231 tympanograms from the surgery group for which we have made measurements. Again, the trend is clear. There are three distinct distributions. Ninety-four percent of the ears in our normal group had TW ≤ 150 daPa, the 95% point according to Koebsell and Margolis (1986). That point also separates the outpatients with no MEE from the group of ears with MEE from our surgery group. However, the ears of children with history of chronic or recurrent OM, but with no MEE at the time of testing (distribution in center), are difficult to categorize using TW (as they were with the other admittance variables). Preliminary analysis of the ears of the surgery group revealed that a cutoff of TW ≥ 300 daPa had sensitivity of 85% and specificity of 78%, better performance than the best cutoff using Gr or Y_{tm}. The fact that TW is virtually a continuous variable and, as such, permits much better definition of the ROC curve than does Gr or Y_{tm} may provide a better opportunity to find the optimal cutoff. Work is in progress to analyze the complete data set to determine the performance of TW relative to Gr, Y_{tm}, and other variables. However, based on our findings with other variables, we expect that the best cutoff using TW based on data from the surgery group will not be the best for all other groups.

CONCLUSION

It is necessary to develop reasonably standardized criteria for protocols both for screening and for diagnosis of MEE. Simple and objective methods, such as aural acoustic admittance measures, are highly attractive for identifying ears with MEE and are often incorporated into screening protocols as well as into diagnostic decision making in research studies and in the clinic. We have examined the ability of aural acoustic admittance measures to identify ears with MEE and without MEE in two subject groups. One group, with a high prevalence of MEE, was comprised of children who had history of chronic or recurrent OM and who were scheduled for M&T surgery. The second group, with a much lower prevalence of OM, was comprised of children more representative of those in the general population. The data have relevance to the question of screening for MEE using acoustic admittance measures. Most notably, the ability of admittance test criteria to identify ears with MEE varied with the subject population under study. Performance of the admittance test variables was much better in our group representing the general population than in our group undergoing M&T surgery. Prevalence of disease and possibly different states of disease in ears labeled as having no MEE in the two different groups probably account for the differences in test performance. This serves to remind us that, to have an effective screening instrument, characteristics (such as prevalence of disease and nature of the disease) of the population to be screened must be known. Criteria developed on one group may or may not be applicable to another group. In our studies, criteria developed on the surgery group appeared to perform better when applied to the outpatient group. However, this relationship cannot be assumed to pertain to all groups on whom the test might be used and, in fact, could be quite the opposite. For example, criteria developed on a group more like our outpatient group might fare quite poorly if applied to a high-risk group similar to those in our surgery group.

Preliminary data from children with and without MEE are consistent with suggestions that TW may be a better indicator than other single acoustic admittance variables for identification of MEE (Koebsell and Margolis 1986). Further analyses are under way to investigate the value of TW in the identification of MEE in children.

SUMMARY

Tympanometry commonly is used in screening for and diagnosing middle ear disease. New standards for acoustic immittance testing have been developed, and normative data are being gathered as part of the process that must be completed before new acoustic immittance measures can be used in the clinical setting. While there are data available on the performance of acoustic immittance variables relative to normally functioning ears in children, there are no data on the performance of the same variables in ears with documented middle ear disease. We did two studies to provide data on the relationship between acoustic immittance measures that conform with the new standard (ANSI S3.39-1987) and middle ear condition.

In the first study, a group of children with history of chronic or recurrent OME was tested using acoustic immittance and pneumatic otoscopy immediately prior to going into the operating room for M&T surgery. The acoustic immittance and otoscopic findings were analyzed using the surgeon's findings (effusion versus no effusion) as the gold standard. A second group of children, unselected with respect to OME history, was also tested using acoustic immittance measures and validated otoscopy, with otoscopy used as the gold standard. This group was comprised of children coming to an outpatient allergy clinic.

The results revealed that Y_{tm}, Gr, and TW are much better than AR and TPP at separating ears with MEE from ears without MEE in the group of children with history of chronic or recurrent OME (the surgery group). The best diagnostic criteria developed on the data from the surgery group also fared quite well in ears from a group of children more representative of the general population (outpatient group). However, because the prevalence of disease was different in the two groups, the predictive values of the different test criteria were different in the two groups. In addition, the distributions of the values of Y_{tm}, Gr, and TW for ears with no MEE were different in the two subject groups. Therefore, the optimal cutoff point for separating ears with MEE from ears without MEE, for each of the different immittance variables, would be different depending on which subject group was being tested. Clearly, disease prevalence and population characteristics make a difference in the performance of a screening test, and our data support the proposition that screening test criteria developed on one group should not be used on a second population or on a subpopulation without first determining that differences in population characteristics will not affect the distribution of values on the test measure or the test characteristics.

ACKNOWLEDGMENTS

The authors would like to thank the following people for their contributions to this project: Tammy Sobek, M.A., for performing the acoustic admittance tests; Ruth Bachman, R.N., for performing the otoscopic examinations; Herman Felder, M.D., for performing many of the surgeries; Doug Swarts, Ph.D., who gave us access to and performed the programming of the system for digitization of the tympanograms; Michele Chirdon, B.A., for digitizing the tympanograms; Eric Jablonowski for assistance in preparing the figures; and Donna M. Schuster for preparation of the manuscript. This work was supported, in part, by NIH grant NS16337.

REFERENCES

American National Standards Institute. 1988. American National Standard specifications for instruments to measure aural acoustic impedance and admittance (aural acoustic immittance). ANSI S3.39-1987. New York: American National Standards Institute.

American Speech-Language-Hearing Association. 1990. Guidelines for screening for hearing impairments and middle ear disorders. *Asha* 32(Suppl. 2):17-24.

Brooks, D.N. 1969. The use of the electro-acoustic impedance bridge in the assessment of middle ear function. *International Audiology* 8:563-569.

Koebsell, K.A., and Margolis, R.H. 1986. Typanometric gradient measured from normal preschool children. *Audiology* 25:149-157.

Margolis, R.H., and Heller, J.W. 1987. Screening tympanometry: Criteria for medical referral. *Audiology* 26:197-208.

Orchik, D.J., Morff, R., and Dunn, J.W. 1980. Middle ear status at myringotomy and its relationship to middle ear immittance measurements. *Ear and Hearing* 1:324-328.

Paradise, J.D., Smith, C.G., and Bluestone, C.D. 1976. Tympanometric detection of middle ear effusion in infants and young children. *Pediatrics* 58:198-210.

Rockette, H., and Casselbrant, M. 1988. Screening and diagnosis: Methodologic issues in screening for otitis media. In D. Lim, C. Bluestone, J. Klein, and J. Nelson (eds.), *Recent advances in otitis media with effusion* (pp. 42-44). Toronto: B.C. Decker.

Chapter 23

Hearing Screening in Montana: A Public/Private Partnership

Michael K. Wynne, Mary Jo Grote, Susan A.W. Toth, and Merle DeVoe

INTRODUCTION

Since its introduction on July 1, 1986, the Rural Speech and Hearing Outreach Program sponsored by the US WEST Foundation in conjunction with the Montana Educational Hearing Conservation Program has provided hearing screenings to over a quarter of a million people in Montana. In addition, this program has provided comprehensive diagnostic and rehabilitation services to those children who have been identified as being at risk for or having communication difficulties due to a hearing loss or central auditory processing deficits. Finally, the program has designed and implemented a hearing conservation program for migrant workers and their families, one of the few audiologic programs that focuses on this special population in the United States. As a result of these services in Montana, and similar services sponsored by the US WEST Foundation in other states, the Rural Speech and Hearing Outreach Program received awards and recognition from the National Council of Communicative Disorders, the Alexander Graham Bell Association of the Deaf, and the Bellringer Award Foundation, as well as several official accolades from state organizations from Arizona to Montana. Still, the value of the program extends well beyond the plaques and speeches presented at awards ceremonies. The real value of the Rural Speech and Hearing Outreach Program lies in the nature, extent, and quality of the audiologic services provided to hearing-impaired children and adults. In Montana, the Rural Speech and Hearing Outreach Program is considered an integral component of a comprehensive educational hearing conservation program for children from birth to 21 years of age. This program illustrates that an exemplary public/private sector model can be developed and successfully implemented to provide extensive outreach hearing services throughout a large, predominantly rural state. In addition, this model provides a clear illustration of the mechanisms that successfully integrate the resources and services offered by other agencies to deliver a comprehensive auditory health care program to the citizens in Montana.

GEOGRAPHY AND HISTORY

Montana, the northernmost mountain state among the contiguous 48 states, ranks fourth in area (145,587 square miles) yet ranks only forty-fourth in population (768,000). The widespread distribution of the population across such a vast area creates a significant challenge for audiologists attempting to meet the hearing health needs of Montanans. During the 1960s, the state's Department of Health determined that special services were needed to identify children and adults who suffered from hearing loss. Additional special services were also needed to provide these individuals with a full range of audiologic services to meet their hearing needs. Finally, these special services were needed at reasonable costs to these consumers. The department established two centers for the clinical evaluation of hearing, one in central Montana and one in eastern Montana. In addition, the Department of Health coordinated efforts with the University of Montana to develop a center at the university in western Montana. The audiologist at each site was responsible for developing guidelines for pure-tone hearing screening, providing hearing screening where possible, and investigating the need for continued and expanded service for the identification of children and adults considered to be at risk for hearing loss. The field pure-tone screening delivery model generally followed a two-tiered pattern of screening. During the day, the audiologist would screen the hearing status of children at their schools. Then in the evening, the audiologist would provide an adult hearing screening clinic at a central community site.

The need for continued or expanded services immediately became evident. The audiologists received requests to provide hearing screenings and follow-up services from school administrators, county health departments, senior citizen centers, nursing homes, industry, and preschool operators. These requests were generally handled on a "first-come, first-served basis," and waiting lists soon extended into the following year. The field personnel constantly traveled large distances to provide the hearing screenings. In many instances, those individuals who were identified as being at risk were required to travel large distances for the hearing evaluations.

By 1972, the program attempted to decentralize the services by creating more regionally based audiologic centers. The personnel from each center would serve a five- to nine-county area, depending on the population distribution and the location of population centers within the state. The program attempted to provide one audiologist for each 10,000 children residing in each area. The centers were funded initially by the various public schools requesting additional assistance, the Office of Public Instruction, and the Commission on Aging and Vocational Rehabilitation. With this cooperative funding, the centers were designed to provide comprehensive audiologic services across the age spectrum. The Department of Health, the Easter Seal Society, and county health departments provided the administration, management, and staffing of each center. These agencies asked the personnel within each center to serve as liaisons between all agencies by developing careful linkages with the public school administrators, the local physicians, and area politicians. By 1980, 13 regional centers had been established throughout the state of Montana. These regional centers are illustrated in figure 1.

As this program developed, funding levels began to shift, and it was not long before the funding for each center was allocated through the special education funds from the Office of Public Instruction. The legislature responded to this change in funding levels and provided a line item appropriation for a Hearing Conservation Program, funneling the funds through the state Board of Public Education. This action coupled with the emergence of private practice audiologists caused the audiologic services to the adult and geriatric populations to diminish and consequently cease to exist as part of the program mission. By 1985, the program's primary mission changed to provide audiologic services to only those children allowed by Montana law. The state Board of Public

Bid Areas
Educational Hearing Conservation Program for
MONTANA

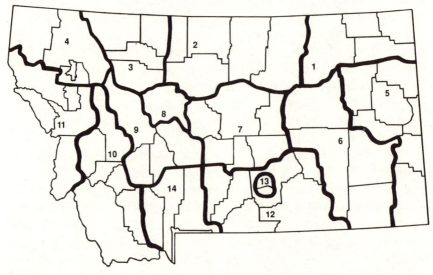

Figure 1. Regional audiologic centers in Montana's Educational Hearing Conservation Program.

Education interpreted "those children allowed by Montana law" to mean that audiologic services would be available to all children in Montana from birth through age 21 years, including those children who attended private and public schools and other institutions. The Board also defined audiologic services as comprehensive audiologic services, which included the identification and evaluation of hearing loss, aural habilitation, the issue and fit of hearing aids and assistive listening devices as appropriate, hearing aid orientation and monitoring, and other case management responsibilities, such as participation in the educational planning for hearing-impaired children. Furthermore, these services were to be made available throughout each year in order to improve the continuity of the audiologic services available for hearing-impaired children and their families. Several sets of guidelines to provide these services were developed in the early 1980s, and the program went through a comprehensive evaluation during the 1985-86 academic year (Johnson, Bain, Goldberg, and Wynne 1986).

The Educational Hearing Conservation Program received its highest level of funding ($740,000) in 1983-84. At that time, the 13 audiology centers were fully equipped, staffed, and operational to serve the school-age population. The global intent of the program was to provide as much audiologic service for children at the local level as possible and from every perspective; this amount of funding was deemed adequate for this purpose. Each center was staffed with between 0.8 and 2.0 full-time equivalent (FTE) audiologists, between 1.0 and 2.0 FTE audiometric technicians, and between 0.5 and 1.0 FTE clerical staff. In certain instances, the center was developed through a subcontract with a private practice audiologist.

In 1985, the Educational Hearing Conservation Program's appropriation was reduced by approximately $70,000. This action reduced the extent of the program, closed one of the centers, and reduced personnel by two audiologists, three technicians, and one secretary. Even with this 9% cut, the program remained relatively intact and was implemented successfully. The following year, the program's funding level was cut to $490,000, resulting in a dramatic change in the service delivery model. Additional financial constraints were added in 1987 when the Montana legislature voted to reduce the program to $310,000. At that time, a new model was needed to ensure that at least some audiologic services could be provided in the rubric of a statewide hearing conservation program. It was recognized that the availability and the extent of the services would be diminished but still remain adequate to serve the hearing health needs of the children.

During this same period, Dr. Peter Ramig at the University of Colorado and Dr. Tom Longhurst at Idaho State University initiated a speech, language, and hearing outreach pilot program with funding from the US WEST Foundation. Recognizing the need to identify communicative disorders in rural communities, the US WEST Foundation provided grants to these two universities to provide a statewide screening program. Dr. Ramig designed a program to identify speech and language problems in children throughout Colorado while Dr. Longhurst developed a program to screen hearing in preschool children and adults across southern and central Idaho. Both programs operated from a centralized base. Two professionals would travel to a particular location within the state to provide speech-language and hearing screenings. Those individuals who were identified as being at risk for a communicative disorder were referred to local speech-language pathologists and audiologists. Both programs were successful, and the US WEST Foundation was looking to expand the program to the other six states within its service region. The funding crisis in Montana presented a perfect opportunity to expand the Foundation's Rural Speech and Hearing Outreach Program (SHOP) to Montana.

PROGRAM DEVELOPMENT

With the infusion of funds from the US WEST Foundation, the service delivery model of Montana's Educational Hearing Conservation Program (HCP) was transformed noticeably. First, the goals and missions of Montana's HCP and the Rural Speech and Hearing Outreach Program were successfully integrated to provide a unified service delivery model. This new program required that the audiologists extend the school-age program in order to truly provide comprehensive audiologic services for children between birth and 5 years of age. The infant and preschool population was designated a specific target group, and a renewed emphasis on the early identification of hearing loss was required for all program personnel. In addition, by integrating a screening program for preschool children with the public school's hearing conservation program, additional medical and audiologic follow-up services were now available for all children. As a consequence, every child within Montana was eligible to receive state support for hearing evaluations and aural habilitation services once the child was determined to be at risk for a hearing loss.

Second, the identification and education components of the program were once again expanded to serve hearing-impaired adults. Therefore, the program needed to identify and acquire locations accessible to older adults to conduct the additional pure-tone screenings and self-assessment interviews. The program provided funding for all audiologists to participate in health fairs and to visit senior citizen centers. In addition, the program needed a mechanism to ensure that each service provider referred those individuals who were identified as being at risk for significant hearing loss to all audiologists in the region, regardless of whether the audiologist worked in a private practice or in a nonprofit setting.

Third, the program needed to develop new funding strategies for the existing centers. As the US WEST Foundation could provide grants only to government agencies and nonprofit organizations holding 501(c)(3) tax status, those centers that had been previously staffed by private practice audiologists needed new contract providers. The new contract provider could then subcontract with a private practice audiologist to provide the audiologic services within their region or area, if needed.

Finally, a new administrative model was needed to coordinate the communication between the program managers, contract providers, service providers, school personnel, agency personnel, audiologists, speech-language pathologists, audiologic technicians, and the citizens of Montana. The administrative model was required to include the following criteria:

1. It would ensure that all parties involved were profiting from the program and that these benefits were easily recognized.
2. It would ensure that the contract providers needed to provide only minimal supervision as indirect cost funds were extremely limited.
3. It would ensure nearly total autonomy for the audiologists who were providing the comprehensive audiologic services.
4. It would ensure that each and every activity addressing the hearing health needs of Montana children fell within the public policy of the Office of Public Instruction.
5. It would ensure that the program would meet the goals delineated in the grant application to the US WEST Foundation and that the Foundation would be recognized for its generous contribution to the program.

Thus, the program administrators would be required to gather all of the resources in a given region, direct the allocation of these resources to provide a given activity, guide each participant in the program along the least resistive path, assist these participants in overcoming obstacles, and focus all elements of the program to produce the greatest effect while protecting the availability of the resources within the region. The loss of any element in the model presented above would greatly diminish the overall program.

PROGRAM ADMINISTRATION

The organizational chart for the Educational Hearing Conservation Program and the Rural Speech and Hearing Outreach Program in

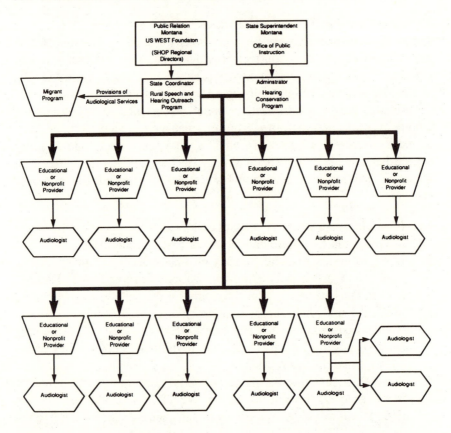

Figure 2. Organizational chart for the Educational Hearing Conservation Program and the Rural Speech and Hearing Outreach Program in Montana.

Montana is presented in figure 2. Initially, the program was designed so that audiologists in the field would respond to each program individually. That is, during the field screenings, the audiologist would don the Hearing Conservation Program hat to manage the hearing health needs of the school-age children. Once work within the public schools was completed, the audiologist would don the Rural Speech and Hearing Outreach Program hat by remaining in the community to provide audiologic services to preschool children and hearing screening for adults under the US WEST program. Fortunately, the audiologists working for the contract providers had integrated the two programs together in the beginning stages and immediately communicated their concern and objection to two separate and distinct programs. Consequently, they adopted a simpler service delivery model during which they simply wore one hat for all services provided and gave credit to all agencies who contributed for these services.

On the surface, the organizational chart fails to illustrate the diversity that was exhibited at the level of the contract providers. Figures 3 through 5 illustrate the various models of service delivery provided by the contract providers. In figure 3, both state funds and US WEST Foundation grants were awarded to a school district or special education cooperative serving as the contract provider. In addition to this funding, the contract providers would, in some instances, provide additional funding from their own resources to provide comprehensive audiologic services to the children within the region. In this case, each contract provider hired an educational audiologist to manage the hearing conservation program. Although appearing similar, the model presented in figure 4 differs slightly. In this case, the school district or special

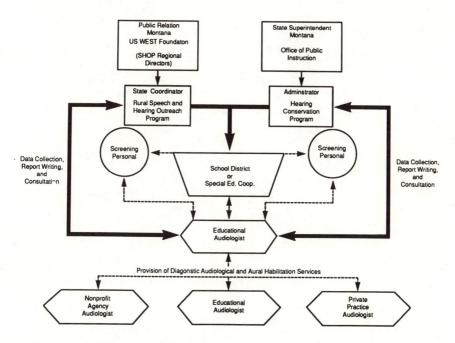

Figure 3. Traditional service delivery model using a school district or special education cooperative as the contract provider and an educational audiologist as the service provider.

education cooperative would subcontract the hearing conservation program to one or more private practice audiologists. These private practice audiologists would in turn develop and implement the hearing conservation program in their contracted areas. Finally, in those cases in which the contract was awarded to a nonprofit agency (as illustrated in figure 5), the nonprofit agency would contract with a private practice audiologist to develop and implement the hearing conservation program in their areas.

As one might imagine, the situations described above would be ideal if there was only one audiologist within a specific contracted area, and particularly if the service provider was a private practice audiologist. In some instances, this was indeed the case. For example, many hearing-impaired children and adults in certain regions within the state of Montana do not have readily accessible audiologic services. Under the umbrella of this program, private practice audiologists often traveled to isolated regions in order to coordinate a hearing screening for school-age

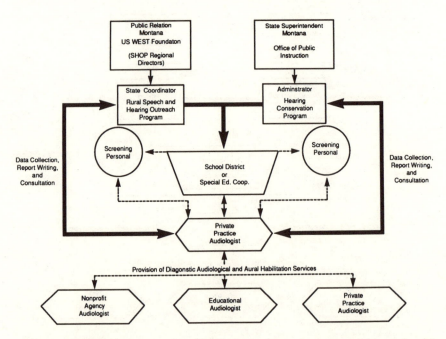

Figure 4. Nontraditional service delivery model using a school district or special education cooperative as the contract provider and a private practice audiologist as the service provider.

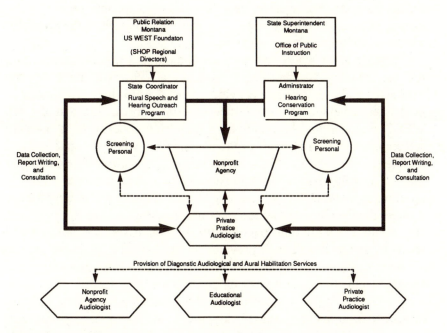

Figure 5. Nontraditional service delivery model using a nonprofit agency as the contract provider and a private practice audiologist as the service provider.

children. Since all children and adults identified as at risk for hearing loss were referred to all of the audiologists in the region for further evaluation, the private practice audiologist could contact clients to provide additional audiologic services, such as hearing aid follow-up or repair while visiting that region. In addition, the private practice audiologist had the option to contract with the University of Montana (already providing the audiologic services to the veterans in Montana) for hearing aid fittings and orientation for any veterans living in isolated regions who were not able to easily return to the university for these services. The integrity of these services was monitored by the two central administrators of the combined program. If an adult hearing aid user objected to the nature or costs of the services, the administrators would include the complaints in their annual evaluation of the contract provider's service. Thus, the administrators served as patient advocates and provided peer review of the quality of audiologic services delivered across the state. Fortunately, very few client complaints regarding the nature, extent, and quality of services were documented in the program, and these complaints were easily resolved.

In those areas where two or more audiologists were in competition for the delivery of audiologic services, all contacts made by the contracted audiology service provider were governed by the policies and guidelines developed by the Office of Public Instruction and the US WEST Foundation. Any individual requiring more than a hearing screening was referred to all of the audiologists within the state without preference or prejudice. Those children and adults identified as being at risk for hearing loss could freely choose any audiologist for the follow-up services. The children were eligible for funding for these services through the development of contracts between the contract provider and all audiologists within the region. Still, in most cases, the children and adults tended to choose their previous service provider, or in the case of a newly identified young child, the parents tended to choose to receive service from the audiologist of the contract provider. This open nonpreferential referral pattern allowed all audiologists within the state to benefit from the program. Finally, due to the nature of this program, a particular child could be followed by three audiologists, each responsible for a different component of the child's aural rehabilitation management program.

ADEPT MODEL

As a consequence of these various service delivery models, the continued funding of the program was highly dependent on the success of keeping all state, nonprofit, and private agencies as well as the consumers satisfied. That is, the program needed to ensure that all parties involved were profiting from the service delivery model in their region and that these benefits were easily recognized. Thus, the administrators of the program focused on providing an environment rich in autonomy for the audiologists funded by the programs, rich in referrals for those audiologists not directly funded by the programs, rich in audiologic services for the consumers, and rich in public relations to promote the public service image of the state and the US WEST Foundation. Furthermore, the leadership needed to be relatively transparent to the practicing audiologist while simultaneously being clearly visible to the legislature, the Office of Public Instruction, and the

US WEST Foundation. Borrowing from the philosophy of P.B. Crosby (1986), the programs adopted an ADEPT model of administration. This model of administration focused on the global preparation of the audiologists to run relatively autonomous programs rather than the development of a micro-management approach to the hearing conservation program. The ADEPT model of administration focuses on five characteristics of professionalism: Accountability, Discretion, Enthusiasm, Productivity, and Thrift.

ACCOUNTABILITY

The concept defined here revolves around two premises. The first premise states that individuals cannot be asked to do something "right the first time and every time thereafter" unless they know exactly what they are asked to do. Accountability in performance therefore depends upon the accuracy of the communication. Recognizing this premise, the administrators were concerned with system integrity from the initiation of the joint funding. The goals and objectives of the Educational Hearing Conservation Program needed to be integrated with the goals and objectives of the Rural Speech and Hearing Outreach Program. Once the final mission of the combined program was determined, the mission was communicated to all audiologists. To accomplish this mission, the program provided a minimum of two state meetings a year for all audiologists within the state of Montana and, in addition, scheduled a brief time to discuss issues at the state association's annual convention. Although the primary goal of each meeting was to provide continuing education, another important focus of these meetings was to promote group unity. In addition to the benefits of the continuing education activity, the audiologists received new information regarding the status of the hearing conservation program, provided feedback regarding the policies and procedures of the program, and discussed issues that directly and indirectly affected the practice of audiology in Montana. Participation in these meetings provided audiologists with an agenda addressing the future of their practice and with some direction regarding their professional goals. One basic premise of good business management is that individuals will never really put themselves into a project until they understand what their personal roles are in terms of making the project succeed. Thus, the administrative model in this program focused on providing an accurate assessment of the role and responsibilities of each participant and how these roles integrated into the overall project.

The second premise defining accuracy focuses on decision making. The administration of a large audiologic program rarely involves making simple decisions. Rather, the administration of a comprehensive hearing conservation program depends upon the accurate interpretation of the data and belief systems that are provided to the administrator. The validity and reliability of the data and belief systems can, and often do, influence the outcomes of decisions. As a consequence, every effort was made to test the accuracy of the data and belief systems provided to the administrators. In addition, every effort was made to ensure that each participant in the program strived to be accountable in data collection and reporting at all levels. The data, in turn, provided a guide that was used as a basis for future action and allocation of resources. In order to manage a program of this size properly, the administrators needed to know what was happening, when it was happening, where it was happening, and to whom it was happening. Once again, frequent and accurate communication across all participants was a key element to the success of this joint project.

DISCRETION

A project of any magnitude is rarely successful if discretion is not a key element of the administrative model. This premise was critical for the successful integration of the hearing conservation programs in Montana. Every audiologic community has its turf battles, and the audiology community in Montana is no exception. The key to the success of this program was the ability to effectively communicate and implement the goals and objectives of the program while simultaneously promoting each audiologic practice within a given region. The administrative model focused on selling all audiologic services and all audiologists. When turf issues arose, these issues were immediately resolved with discreet negotiations between the parties involved. In addition, the program strived to establish working relationships with other educational and health care professionals, their agencies, and their associations. Every effort was made to resolve discrepancies and conflict during their initial stages. The image of any program is directly dependent on the relationships the program has with its community. An image of success is therefore dependent on the harmonious relationships within and between agencies.

ENTHUSIASM

Crosby (1986) identified three phases in getting an organization or an individual to be productive in the very best manner possible: conviction, commitment, and conversion. *Conviction* is defined as the intellectual decision that something is desirable to do. *Commitment* is defined as the intellectual decision to seriously allocate resources to undertake the task. *Conversion* is defined as the passion that drives the intellectual decisions defined above. Little work was needed in this area because most audiologists had actively participated in the development and implementation of the hearing conservation program well before the public/private partnership was initiated. In fact, many private practice audiologists who were not directly involved with the project had made significant previous investments of their time and energy to providing a comprehensive audiologic program throughout the state, and provided strong support for this program. While in most instances, the leaders of a project generally set the tone, the administrators of this project simply needed to contribute to the existing esprit de corps of the audiologists.

PRODUCTIVITY

One of the key elements with this philosophy of administration is that the procedures and protocols should be prepared by those individuals who are doing the work. While the program had a set of state-mandated guidelines and requirements, the audiology program within each region was not micro-managed. In most regions, the existing hearing conservation programs were successful in providing comprehensive audiologic services to school-age children. The only change in the program that was needed in all but one region was the expansion of services to younger children and to adults. A change in service providers was deemed necessary in one area because the service provider claimed that there were no hearing-impaired children in the region and failed to achieve the 501(c)(3) tax status necessary to receive the US WEST Foundation funding. Bimonthly reports were collected describing the activities of the program. These reports were used to generate reports describing the breadth and extent of services to the state's Department of Education and to the US WEST Foundation. These reports were not intended to provide a means for evaluating the productivity of the audiologists (unless the data reports were simply incomplete or inaccurate representations of the service provided). Comparisons of the data across regions as a means of measuring productivity would have led to erroneous interpretations because the environmental, geographic, and climatic constraints changed dramatically as a function of each region.

THRIFT

To initiate a program, it is necessary to have a system to define goals and a means to measure progress toward those goals, but to get things done, it is necessary to have a budget. While the introduction of the US WEST Foundation's funding clearly saved the structural integrity of the Educational Hearing Conservation Program, this funding was tied to the expansion of audiologic services to populations that were not targeted in the development of the educational audiology program. In the business world, more companies fail due to the lack of proper control of the money than due to the lack of money itself. Audiologic programs are no different from other businesses. In fact, the lack of proper control of the state funding by the Educational Hearing Conservation Program led to the severe retrenchment of state funding prior to the initiation of the public/private partnership.

The first step in establishing a thrift philosophy with this program was to reduce the amount of indirect and administrative costs charged to the program. Convincing the service providers to reduce the overhead was fairly easy because the reduction in state funding placed many school districts and special education cooperatives at risk for failure to meet state and federal regulations for special education funding. Furthermore, the US WEST Foundation would not award any funding to any agency proposing indirect cost allocations of greater than 10% of the total direct costs. For the nonprofit agencies that subcontracted the audiologic services, even 10% of the total costs provided a relatively large contribution to the total operating costs of the agency, particularly in light of the relatively autonomous activities of the audiologists. In two regions, the service providers actually augmented the program by allocating their own funds to the program.

The second step in establishing the thrift philosophy was to identify the budget process as simply a financial agreement between the service provider, the Office of Public Instruction, and the US WEST

Foundation. The budget process throughout the project was intended to give as much autonomy to service providers as necessary to ensure that they had the appropriate resources to implement the program. That is, the budget process was not used to constrain the flexibility of the service providers. Instead, the budgets were used primarily to track overspending during the course of the year and underspending at the end of the budget period. Thus, the budget process helped the administrators and the service providers determine the need for any change within the system, the flexibility to execute that change, and the means to monitor the effects of the change. In essence, the budget process provided the basis for future action within the program.

The third and final element of the thrift philosophy of administration involved providing sufficient financial resources to promote the program, from within the program as well as external to the program. External promotion of the program was relatively straightforward because the US WEST Foundation encouraged the service providers to use company advertising. Consequently, preschool and adult hearing screenings were advertised in community newspapers. Additional public relation materials such as posters, promotional literature, and formal announcements were readily available for display. The internal promotion of the program was more difficult. Most audiologists who received funding from this program had long participated in the Educational Hearing Conservation Program. As a result, they were very familiar with the state's guidelines for audiologic services as well as their general role and function as educational audiologists within a specific geographic region. Adding a "corporate image" to this role was the challenge presented by the public/private partnership. The primary focus for the internal promotion was to provide opportunities for the audiologists to clearly recognize the contributions the US WEST Foundation was making to the program. In this case, "thrift" meant developing line item allocations for continuing education and development, salary increments, and equipment procurement. Even in times of fiscal contingency, this program strived to provide as many professional development opportunities as possible. Instead of eliminating the budget for personnel development, the program allocated additional funding to provide opportunities for professional growth.

RESPONSIBILITIES OF SERVICE PROVIDERS

While this ADEPT model of administration provides the basic foundation regarding the management of the program, it does not specify the roles and responsibilities of the key personnel within the program: the service providers. Any successful program must be constructed and managed by a definition of roles and responsibilities of those individuals who are truly implementing the program. By having a clearly defined scope of activities, the service providers can direct the appropriate resources to meet the program's needs and goals with minimal effort. In 1980 and in 1983, the Office of Public Instruction published a *Handbook of Hearing Conservation*, which defined the audiologist's role in the Educational Hearing Conservation Program. Due to the significant reduction in funding, the handbooks were modified to reduce the number of mandatory services in the program and to provide guidelines for the implementation of the combined programs. Appendix A presents the guidelines for the delivery of audiologic services offered to children (Montana Office of Public Instruction 1987). These guidelines are intended *not* to demonstrate a model program for the identification of hearing loss in children but to represent the compromise in services that were *minimally acceptable* for both audiologists and school administrators. In addition, while these guidelines delineate specific activities for the educational audiology program, they do not delineate any specific activities for the identification, evaluation, and management of hearing loss in adults. When working with adults, the audiologists were encouraged to develop their own screening protocols after consultation with the state coordinator of the Rural Speech and Hearing Outreach Program in Montana. In addition, Dr. Ronald Schow from Idaho State University (who served as a consultant for the Rural Speech and Hearing Program in Idaho) assisted the audiologists in the development and implementation of their adult hearing screening programs.

MARKETING

If any business is to survive, every individual associated with that business or project must contribute to a sales effort (Samony 1989). Private practice audiologists have recognized this basic business premise for years. Educational audiology is no different, particularly given the descriptions of educational audiology practices as described by English (1991) or Allard and Golden (1991). The simple fact is that all professional, technical, administrative, and clerical personnel are responsible for selling the program. If there is not an active sales effort promoting the agency or project made by any one or more persons directly involved, then they are not contributing to the survival and growth of the agency or project.

If there was any weakness in the combined hearing conservation program in Montana, it was the inability of most audiologists to recognize their responsibilities and opportunities for selling the program. Audiologists tend to be very competent in selling their professional services to the consumers of these services, whether they are engaged in private, nonprofit, or public sponsored activities. That is, audiologists recognize the need to present a professional image by being informed, attentive, and responsive to the hearing-impaired individual's communicative needs. That was the case in Montana. The program literally received thousands of written positive comments praising the professionalism and competency of the audiologists and the accessibility of the high quality audiologic services in rural areas. Still, the program was not as successful selling its own merits to two major clients: the Montana legislature and the US WEST Foundation. While this focus did not hurt the program, it did not significantly enhance the program in the long term.

The primary clients of the Educational Hearing Conservation Program and the Rural Speech and Hearing Outreach Program in Montana were the state legislature and the US WEST Foundation, respectively. As such, the marketing effort of the combined program attempted to focus on two central themes:

1. Convincing each legislator that the tax dollars allocated to the program are a needed and well-deserved investment, and
2. Communicating the "Good Corporate Citizen" image for the US WEST Foundation.

Due to the previous efforts of audiologists and speech-language pathologists, these clients recognized the value of investing resources into a statewide hearing conservation program. Consequently, the program itself had already been sold. What was needed in the marketing effort was an agenda to maintain the loyalty of these customers. Preserving client loyalty should be included in any strategic plan and budget, it should be monitored consistently by the administrators, and it should be practiced daily by all participants in the program.

In a sense, two marketing programs were developed and were at work within this partnership. On one side, the added visibility for the US WEST Foundation derived from the linkage between its corporate identity or logo and an important health care program was a very positive marketing plan. This partnership added value to the US WEST Foundation's corporate image in the form of "Good/Responsible Corporate Citizen." The synergy of this association has a "halo" effect on all forms of corporate advertising that carry the identifying signature of the program. Conversely, in the second marketing plan, the unique graphic elements of US WEST Foundation's corporate logo or trademark link the instant recognizability of the logo with an important health care program lending its credibility to selling the program.

Although the US WEST Foundation's Rural Speech and Hearing Outreach Program covered seven western states, the Montana program best demonstrated the win/win nature of the partnership from a marketing standpoint. Over and above the added value of tying the Foundation's sponsorship into traditional advertising vehicles such as newspaper advertisements and public relations programs, there also was the considerable value in a more nontraditional form of advertising—the interface with program participators. Montana's size and large rural population diminish the value of traditional advertising. The Foundation's sponsorship of the Rural Speech and Hearing Outreach Program in partnership with the state's Educational Hearing Conservation Program took on a very immediate meaning for the 75,000 people served annually by this program. Furthermore, because the combined program focused on children and young adults, the program also took on a very immediate meaning for their families. The goodwill ascribed to the program was transferred to the corporate sponsor. Testimonials captured by the program provided a record of this goodwill for possible future use.

The challenge of the second marketing plan was to get the word out to a largely rural public about the substantial benefits of early hearing screening for children and the importance of routine hearing screening for older adults. The Montana partnership developed the "Did You Know?" campaign, which was incorporated into the US WEST Foundation's advertising. The campaign posed a rhetorical question designed to educate the public about the availability of free hearing screenings and the quality of life implications related to the identification, evaluation, and remediation of hearing disorders. In this marketing program, the advertising monies from the US WEST Foundation's parent corporation contributed to getting the word out and added value to the program. This partnership was and remains truly a two-way street.

In the 1990s, public funding for health care programs is expected to be increasingly challenged for cost-effectiveness. The same holds true for corporate advertising budgets in a downsized and streamlined business environment. The Montana model could be utilized for a variety of health care screening programs and serves as an exemplary model where all partners derive substantial economies by working in tandem as well as enjoy significantly enhanced visibility in the community.

SUMMARY

The success of this public/private partnership in providing a comprehensive hearing screening program to the citizens in Montana is largely attributed to the effective development of functional policy adopted by all personnel associated with the project. Furthermore, all audiologists in the state of Montana had the opportunity to directly participate in the project, whether or not they directly received funding as contract providers. In his presentation at this International Symposium for Screening Children for Auditory Function, Dr. Alfred A. Baumeister (1991) stated that input on public policy by the professionals implementing that policy runs tandem with the ability of these professionals to influence decisions on whether the policy should exist. In other words, audiologists who believe in the need for a comprehensive hearing screening program should not limit their action to the simple expression of their belief systems. These audiologists are obligated to participate in the creation and implementation of a program that delivers a comprehensive hearing screening service to all individuals in the community.

Audiologists can have impact on public policy regarding the identification of hearing loss in children and adults. One only has to look as far as Dr. Marion Downs and the work she has achieved toward her goal of screening hearing in newborns (Downs 1990) to observe how one individual can influence public policy. One only has to look as far as the Educational Hearing Conservation Program and the Rural Speech and

Hearing Outreach Program in Montana to observe an exemplar of a multifunded, public/private partnership dedicated to identifying all individuals with significant hearing loss and then to providing the appropriate evaluation and intervention services necessary for these individuals. The integrated program described above provides an excellent model as to how each public policy can be successfully applied to provide comprehensive hearing screening services statewide.

First, this program demanded and obtained a specific and clear consensus about what must be done, who should do it, when it should be done, and where it should be done. In addition, the strategies used to implement the program changed as a function of the availability of resources to provide the audiologic services and the recognition by the community to take advantage of the resources.

Second, this program involved a few dedicated audiologists and service providers who contributed considerable time and energy to research and understand the political environment, the major players within this environment, and the obstacles to the implementation of a comprehensive hearing conservation program. From the very beginning stages of the program, this knowledge domain was continually and freely shared with all audiologists to ensure that each individual could contribute to the continued success of the program. Communication within and across all service providers was exceptional due to the established network of audiologists funded by the earlier hearing conservation program. This network was maintained and the linkages between the professionals were reinforced and expanded during frequent professional meetings including individuals not funded by the programs.

Third, the active involvement of the US WEST Foundation exemplifies the advantage to all participants when a large corporate foundation chose to act as one element in an advocacy group sharing a common cause.

Fourth, as audiologists recognized the role of a statewide hearing screening program and its benefit to their own practices, the public/private partnership served as the foundation for cooperative ventures rather than competitive activities. This cooperation delivered major benefits at all levels of activity, from the delivery of hearing screenings in schools to the discussions of policy formation and regulations in the political arena. By presenting a unified voice, the audiology community could begin to guide public policy rather than simply respond to it.

Finally, the ability for all individuals involved, from the funding agencies personnel to the screening personnel, to accept the need for high standards of performance while simultaneously compromising certain self-interests created an environment that facilitated program development and integration rather than permitted a continued deterioration in the availability and quality of hearing health care services. The end result was a public/private partnership that has established and maintained a comprehensive, active network of hearing health care professionals dedicated and able to serve all people in Montana.

ACKNOWLEDGMENTS

The authors wish to express their gratitude to Mark W. Grote, M.B.A., for his assistance in the preparation of this manuscript. In addition, the authors wish to acknowledge the significant contributions provided to this program by Ms. Barbara Ranf and Mr. Larry Nash of the US WEST Foundation, Dr. Peter Ramig at the University of Colorado, and Dr. Thomas Longhurst at Idaho State University. Finally, the authors wish to express their appreciation to, and admiration of, the audiologists in the state of Montana whose focus on unity in purpose and function serves as an exemplary model of effective teamwork.

REFERENCES

Allard, J.B., and Golden, D.C. 1991. Educational audiology: A comparison of service delivery systems utilized by Missouri schools. *Language, Speech, and Hearing Services in Schools* 22:5-11.

American Speech-Hearing-Language Association. 1984. Definitions of and competencies for aural rehabilitation: A report from the committee on rehabilitative audiology. *Asha* 26:37-41.

Baumeister, A.A. 1991. Influencing public policy. Paper read at the International Symposium on Screening Children for Auditory Function, June 1991, Nashville.

Board of Public Education, State of Montana. 1980. *Handbook of hearing conservation.* Available from the Office of Public Instruction, State Capital, Helena, Mont.

Board of Public Education, State of Montana. 1983. *Educational hearing conservation guidelines*. Available from the Office of Public Instruction, State Capital, Helena, Mont.

Crosby, P.B. 1986. *Running things: The art of making things happen*. New York: McGraw-Hill.

Downs, M.P. 1990. Twentieth century pediatric audiology: Prologue to the 21st. *Seminars in Hearing* 11:408-411.

English, K. 1991. Best practices in educational audiology. *Language, Speech, and Hearing Services in Schools* 22:283-286.

Johnson, S.J., Bain, B.A., Goldberg, D.M., and Wynne, M.K. 1986. Evaluation of contracted educational audiological services in Montana. Paper read at the 1986 Annual Convention of the American Speech-Language-Hearing Association, November 1990, Detroit.

Montana Office of Public Instruction. 1987. *Interim guidelines for an educational hearing conservation program*. Helena, Mont.:Office of Public Instruction.

Samony, J.M., Sr. 1989. Who, me sell? *Sound and Video Contractor* 7(1):46-49.

Appendix A
Guidelines for the delivery of educational audiology services in Montana

Purpose

The purpose of the program is to identify children with educationally significant hearing losses and to follow those children through the stages of evaluation, remediation, and placement.

I. Definition of Terms
    A. It is the policy of the Office of Public Instruction to interpret "those children allowed by Montana law" to mean that audiological services will be available to all children in Montana from birth through age 21, including those attending private and public schools or otherwise.
    B. It is the policy of the Office of Public Instruction to interpret "audiological services" to be comprehensive audiological services which may include the screening and identification of hearing loss, aural rehabilitation, consultation regarding hearing aids and assistive listening devices as appropriate, hearing aid orientation and monitoring, and other case management responsibilities including participating in the educational planning for hearing-impaired children.
    C. It is the policy of the Office of Public Instruction to interpret the "contracting for the delivery of audiological services" to require that service providers submit a complete and appropriate proposal, in accordance with these guidelines, to provide complete audiological advisement and consulting services to the schools which serve children in Montana.
    D. It is the policy of the Office of Public Instruction to interpret the term "hearing-impaired" to mean the deaf, deaf-blind, and hard of hearing as defined in 20-7-401 MCA.

II. Delivery of Services
    The integration of the Educational Hearing Conservation Program with the Rural Speech and Hearing Outreach Program sponsored by the US WEST Foundation should ensure a comprehensive school and preschool hearing screening program. The delivery of audiological services shall include the screening for and identification of hearing loss, the participation in case

management responsibilities for hearing-impaired children, and coordination of aural rehabilitation services.

A. Training of School Personnel

The audiologist in each area will have the responsibility for training the people responsible for hearing screening in his/her multi-county area. Repeat or updated training may be necessary throughout the school year.

B. Screening and Identification

1. Screening

Screening tests for the school-aged child are intended to identify those individuals in need of referral for further evaluation and identification. Services shall be conducted as prescribed in the descriptions below.

   a. The mandatory grades to be screened annually may be limited to grades K, 1, and 9 or 10. Other children who should be screened are teacher referrals, new children from out-of-state, and special education students whose three year re-evaluations are due.

   b. Pure tone screening for the school-aged child should be performed at 1000, 2000, and 4000 Hz with a calibrated audiometer. The screening levels should be 20 dB HL at 1000 and 2000 Hz, and 25 dB HL at 4000 Hz. The screening personnel should determine whether the ambient room noise levels in the screening environment will not confound the results. Every effort should be made to use the best room environment possible in each screening location.

   c. Whenever possible using the existing equipment and professional staff, impedance screening should be included in the screening process and conducted according to the guidelines described in the 1983 *Handbook of Hearing Conservation.*

2. Rescreening

   a. Follow-up rescreening should not be done until 4 to 6 weeks after the initial screening except where distance is a strong deterrent and then it may be done in a time frame consistent with the logistics of the screening program. Rescreening should be accomplished by personnel with a thorough knowledge of the screening process (audiologist, nurse, speech-language pathologist, etc).

   b. In appropriate environments or using specialized equipment such as insert earphones, the rescreening should attempt to approximate the pure tone thresholds to reduce the over-referral of stable mild hearing losses or stable mild to moderate, high frequency hearing losses. Preventing over-referral or under-referral is THE PRIORITY of a good screening program.

3. Preschool Hearing Screening
   a. Preschool screening should be accomplished by the audiologist with assistance from another person. Many methods have been used to screen hearing in preschool children and several of these methods have been described in the earlier handbooks.
   b. It is imperative that impedance audiometry be used in both the screening and rescreening of preschool children.
   c. There is agreement among all audiologists and special education professionals in the state of Montana that the screening and identification programs for preschool children should be as comprehensive as possible so that the follow-up services can be initiated prior to the child enrolling in public schools.

4. Audiological Referral and Assessment/Evaluation
   a. The purpose of assessment is to determine the specific auditory sensitivity or functioning of an individual referred due to failure on the initial hearing screening and/or rescreening. The audiological assessment shall be performed by a licensed audiologist or an audiologist with a provisional license.
   b. The need for referral for audiological evaluation will be determined by the audiologist in the child's geographical region. The audiological referral will be made to all audiological agencies within the area or within a reasonable distance. It may be assumed that a parent may choose the nearest agency, however, this may not always be the case.
   c. The expectation of a timely and comprehensive audiological evaluation report shall be made clear to each agency providing audiological services under this program.

5. Medical Referral and Assessment/Evaluation
   a. Medical evaluations are performed by physicians and are essential for the proper diagnosis of those children suspected of having hearing loss and for the treatment of those children with active ear diseases.
   b. The audiologist will serve to refer children needing medical attention and then monitoring the outcomes of these referrals.

C. Case Management
   1. The service provider shall assure that a licensed audiologist participates in the child study team process for those students known to have an educationally significant hearing impairment.

2. The scope of service provider's case management responsibilities shall include participation in services necessary to ensure a hearing-impaired child's optimum functioning within the school community, as specified in these guidelines. Provision of services may be indicated as a result of sensorineural, conductive, or central hearing loss, because of a condition that is a result of or interacts with a hearing loss, or for any combination of the above factors.

D. Aural Rehabilitation

1. Aural rehabilitation shall refer to services and procedures for facilitating adequate receptive and expressive communication in individuals with hearing impairment. Aural rehabilitation services and procedures shall include, but are not limited to, the following:
   a. Identification and evaluation of sensory capabilities.
   b. Interpretation of results, counseling, and referral.
   c. Intervention for communicative difficulties.
   d. Evaluation and modification of the intervention program.

2. Service providers shall participate in the provision of aural rehabilitation services, and in the coordination of effort with the school community for identified hearing-impaired children.
   a. Needs Assessment
      Service providers shall (when appropriate) provide a thorough needs assessment for each identified hearing-impaired child in the contract region. All of the following categories are to be considered to determine the need for counseling, referral, and/or the provision of intervention services, and reported to the child study team:
      1) Language
      2) Amplification
      3) Speech
      4) Auditory/Listening Skills
      5) Counseling
      6) Audiological Monitoring
      7) Academics
      8) Mainstreaming
      9) Classroom Acoustics
      10) Special Services (interpreters, note-takers)
      11) Related Evaluations/Services
      12) Consultation
      13) Curriculum
   b. Additional Service Provider Responsibilities
      Follow-up responsibilities shall include the following:

1) Mandated service to be delivered by service providers: audiological evaluation and monitoring and amplification evaluation and monitoring.

2) Services to be either provided by the service providers or referred to appropriately licensed and trained personnel: auditory training/listening skills, language, speech, counseling, academics, modification of classroom acoustics, consultation, and curriculum.

3. The Hearing Conservation Program area advisor should meet the minimal competencies and possess the special knowledge defined in the ASHA Committee on Rehabilitative Audiology Report (1984).

III. Administration of Service
   A. Administration of audiological services shall include the service provider's program management and program administration.
   B. Program Management
      1. Program management shall include, but not be limited to, the preparation, processing, and implementation of a service contract for the delivery of audiological services to all children in the contracted geographical region.
         Program management shall have two major components:
         a. The contract proposal which delineates the various components of the proposal submitted for the award of the service contract.
         b. The contract implementation which directs how the contract is executed as specified by the contract proposal and guidelines for services.
   C. Program Administration
      1. Program administration shall have two priorities:
         a. The service provider's internal administration to determine that the necessary staff, facilities, and equipment are available to undertake their charge.
         b. The service provider's interaction with the school communities in the contracted district to ensure that sufficient communication channels are present to meet the needs of the hearing-impaired children in the district.
   D. Records
      1. Service providers shall develop and maintain records as may be necessary or useful in assuring the quality performance of this contract.
      2. All program service, administrative, financial, client, or other records relating to the performance of this service shall be retained

by the service provider for the contract period. These will be placed in proper order by the provider on or before June 30 of each year and shall be made ready for transfer to the succeeding provider if service procedures change for any reason.

3. The State of Montana, the Montana Legislative Auditor, and Office of Public Instruction, the United States Department of Education, the Comptroller General or their duly authorized agents or representatives, shall have the right to access to any books, documents, papers and records of the service provider which are pertinent to the services provided. The State of Montana, the Montana Legislative Auditor, the United States Department of Education, the Comptroller General of the United States, or any of their duly authorized agents or representatives, shall, until the expiration of 18 years from the completion date, have the right to review those books, records, documents, papers and other supporting data which involve transactions or pricing data submitted, along with the computations and projections used therein.

E. Evaluation
1. The service provider shall guarantee that the Office of Public Instruction (OPI), and/or their representatives, may conduct periodic on-site assessments of provider's services and program management in order to ensure compliance with the terms of this contract. When an assessment is complete, the OPI will supply the service provider with a written summary of the assessment.

2. When the OPI specifies in the summary that the assessment reveals noncompliance of the terms of service provision, the service provider shall, within 30 days of receipt of the written summary, submit a detailed plan and time line for correcting the problems and coming into full compliance with the terms.

3. Failure to comply will be deemed a default by the service provider.

Chapter 24

The Selective Auditory Attention Test (SAAT): A Screening Test for Central Auditory Processing Disorders in Children

Rochelle Cherry

INTRODUCTION

In recent years, an increased amount of attention has focused on the need for early identification of children with central auditory processing disorders (CAPD) (Keith 1988; Musiek et al. 1990). CAPD has been linked to communication problems, school failure, and problems with social development. Children labeled as learning disabled may also have CAPD (Ferre and Wilber 1986).

Ideally, identification of CAPD should lead to a better understanding of a child's behavior and poor communicative and academic performance, which, in turn, can help generate more positive attitudes toward that child. Parents and teachers then will not "blame the victim" since disruptive behavior is not under his or her control. This better understanding of the problem should enable professionals to neutralize the antisocial behavior found in many of these children. Identification should also lead to remediation to minimize the educational deficits often found in these children. This remediation includes controlling the environment (room acoustics), using devices to improve listening (FM units), auditory training, developing compensatory strategies, and choosing appropriate educational placement (Sloan 1986; Lasky and Cox 1985; Cline 1988). Finally, medical referrals should be made for those children with neurologic problems, such as localized central nervous system (CNS) lesions.

Table 1

Criteria for Selecting Conditions for Screening and Application to Screening for CAPD in Children

1. Condition should be prevalent.	1. 6.5% of children 3 to 17 years old have LD (Zill and Schoenborn 1990). A high proportion of these have CAPD.
2. Condition is serious.	2. Academic achievement and social development can be adversely affected (Keith 1988).
3. Screening decreases time to diagnosis.	3. In the absence of screening, diagnosis of CAPD can be delayed until child begins to fail in school (Cherry 1980).
4. Diagnostic tests are available to confirm problem.	4. Comprehensive diagnosis is available.
5. Condition is treatable, and progress is improved with early identification.	5. Management is available and should begin as soon as possible—educational placement, auditory training, compensatory strategies, etc. (Sloan 1986).
6. Screening should not be harmful.	6. Screening procedure is noninvasive.
7. Cost of screening, diagnosis, and treatment is reasonable.	7. Cost of screening can be minimized by eliminating unnecessary follow-ups.

Adapted from Hayes and Pashley (1991).

Criteria used to determine the appropriateness of CAPD screening (table 1) indicate that screening is warranted. The screening process involves a series of decisions; among them, which populations should be screened, the test to be used, criteria used to determine follow-up, selection and training of personnel, and the method for monitoring screening program results (Musiek et al. 1990).

Several populations can be screened. The broadest approach involves mass screening of all young children in a particular educational placement in order to identify children at risk for auditory-based learning disabilities (LD) or CAPD before any problems emerge. A narrower approach is to screen all children who demonstrate behavior typical of

CAPD (Fisher 1976; Smoski 1990). These children are often referred for audiologic evaluations because they behave as though they have a peripheral hearing loss, especially when listening under adverse conditions. Audiologists typically rule out peripheral hearing loss as well as middle ear pathology. However, the typical audiologic evaluation does not adequately assess the more subtle problems found in children with CAPD. Parents and teachers are often told that there is no "hearing problem" (Musiek and Geurkink 1980). Many of these children should be screened to determine whether or not a potential CAPD exists.

The CAPD screening test should enable the clinician to identify which children require further and more specific testing, and which children do not. Screening procedures must be relatively quick and inexpensive since they are generally applied to a number of children (Lessler 1974). Therefore, before choosing a test, the following factors should be considered: length of time necessary for administration and scoring, equipment and personnel requirements, validity and reliability, and appropriateness for population (e.g., age and linguistic background).

DESCRIPTION OF SAAT

The Selective Auditory Attention Test (SAAT) was developed for both large-scale and individual screening of children with CAPD (Cherry 1980). The test is based on the assumption that poor selective auditory attention skills can interfere with learning (Hagen and Kail 1975; Ross 1976). The SAAT is quick to administer (approximately eight minutes) and can be administered by personnel other than audiologists, including speech-language pathologists and learning specialists. It can be administered using a portable cassette tape recorder either under headphones or in sound field. A 1000 Hz calibration tone is included, but the test can be administered at any comfortable loudness level in a quiet room. The SAAT is reliable and appropriate for young children (Cherry 1980; Chermack and Montgomery 1991). Currently, there is no gold standard by which we are able to measure sensitivity and specificity of any CAPD tests in LD children (Musiek et al. 1990). However, researchers have successfully differentiated normal achievers (NA) from LD children with CAPD tests (Ferre and Wilber 1986; Keith et al. 1989).

The SAAT has two subtests: (1) a list of 25 monosyllabic words prerecorded in quiet providing a speech recognition score, and (2) an equivalent list, prerecorded with a semantic distractor, which provides a selective listening score. The Word Intelligibility by Picture Identification (WIPI) Test (Ross and Lerman 1971) lists and test plates were chosen as stimuli because they (1) have stimulus words within the recognition vocabulary of young children; (2) involve a closed response task; (3) do not require the ability to read; (4) do not require a verbal response, eliminating the problem of misarticulations; (5) are an identification task rather than a same/different decision, minimizing short-term memory requirements; (6) utilize pictures that are clearly drawn in color; (7) contain four matched lists of 25 monosyllabic words; (8) use the same carrier phrase to introduce all words, eliminating context that may aid in the identification of target words; (9) minimize the influence of guessing on performance scores (with six pictures per test plate); (10) have at least four phonetically similar words among six words depicted on each plate; and (11) are demonstrated as valid and reliable measures of speech recognition for young children (Sanderson-Leepa and Rintelman 1976).

A great deal of variability in scores has been reported in the literature for speech-in-noise tasks (Mueller 1985; Musiek and Baron 1987). Factors that may contribute to the reported differences are type of noise used, mode of presentation, signal-to-noise ratio, and test material. Previously, we conducted a study to identify the most efficient

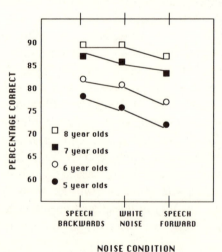

Figure 1. Group mean scores in percentage correct for each age group under each noise condition.

distractor (Cherry 1979; Cherry and Kruger 1983). Forty-four children (23 NA and 21 LD children), ranging in age from 7.0 to 8.9 years, were tested under three distractors using the WIPI as the stimulus. The distractors were (1) broadband noise (nonlinguistic), (2) speech backward (linguistic nonsemantic), and (3) speech forward (semantic).

For each age group, the performance scores of NA children were significantly higher than the performance scores of LD children, regardless of type of distractor chosen (figure 1). Mean scores of the NA were 8%, 10%, and 20% higher than LD children when the competing material was speech backward, broadband noise, and speech forward, respectively. However, there was no overlap in the individual performance scores between the two groups when the semantic distractor was used, once adjustment was made for age (table 2). This finding suggests that a semantic distractor is most efficient for identification of selective auditory attention difficulties associated with LD. A semantic distractor was, therefore, selected for the SAAT.

A diotic mode of presentation (same stimuli presented simultaneously to both ears) was chosen because it eliminates spatial location cues and is more difficult than a dichotic mode (Triesman 1964b). The stimulus words and the distractor (a story chosen for interest by a children's librarian) were both prerecorded by the same speaker, thus eliminating voice cues and, again, increasing the difficulty of the task (Triesman 1964a). To maximize difficulty, a 0 dB signal-to-noise (S/N) ratio was used (Hedrick and Kunze 1974).

Table 2
Range of Raw Scores in Percentage Correct for Each Subgroup on Each Noise Condition

Subjects	Speech Backward	White Noise	Speech Forward
7-Year-Old Children			
Normal Achieving	80-92	76-88	72-88
Learning Disabled	68-88	56-80	44-60
8-Year-Old Children			
Normal Achieving	80-96	84-92	80-92
Learning Disabled	72-88	72-88	56-72

SAAT FINDINGS

To establish the usefulness of the SAAT as a screening tool, it was administered to 325 children from preschool through second grade (4 to 9 years old). The children were divided into three groups: 201 NA, 36 LD, and 88 teacher concerned (TC). This information was not available to the tester until after all of the children were screened. All children in kindergarten through grade two who met the subject selection criteria were tested, as well as a random sample of children in prekindergarten who were preregistered for school. Students were designated as NA if they met the following academic criteria: (1) regular classroom placement; (2) no report of emotional or learning problems; (3) reading ability at or above grade level; (4) never failed a grade; and (5) not considered low achievers by their teachers.

Children were designated as LD if they met the following criteria: (1) classification as LD by a child study team; (2) attendance in special programs for the LD; (3) normal IQ (90-110) on at least one section of the Wechsler Intelligence Scale for Children (Wechsler 1974) and no less than 75 on the other section; (4) reading achievement at least one year below grade level for first and second graders; (5) no report of emotional problems; and (6) not taking drugs to control hyperactivity.

Children designated as TC met the following criteria: (1) regular classroom placement; and (2) teacher concerned about learning progress. Some of these children had been referred to the child study team for assessment and possible classification.

All children were required to pass a pure-tone hearing screening test at 20 dB HL for frequencies of 500, 1000, 2000, and 4000 Hz (ANSI S3.6-1969) in both ears since CAPD test results can be affected by a peripheral hearing loss (Katz 1978). Each child listened individually to the two WIPI lists on the same day. Each session took approximately eight minutes. The child first listened to a list in quiet (no distractor). The instructions, which were prerecorded, asked the child to listen to the man asking him or her to point to a picture, and then to point to that picture. Each child was required to obtain a score of 88% to 100% on the speech recognition subtest. This established the child's ability to perform the task and to point to the appropriate picture. The child received prerecorded instructions to ignore the other man telling a story and then listened to a list with the distractor.

Table 3
Mean Performance Scores in Percentage Correct by Age and by Subject Group
Under the Competing Message Condition

	Normal Achievers	Learning Disabled	Teacher Concerned	All Subjects
4-Year-Olds				
% correct	62.80	--------	50.00	60.67
(number)	(10)		(2)	(18)*
5-Year-Olds				
% correct	66.42	60.00	58.07	63.84
(number)	(38)	(1)	(27)	(77)*
6-Year-Olds				
% correct	70.61	56.00	67.28	69.25
(number)	(66)	(1)	(39)	(106)
7-Year-Olds				
% correct	74.57	57.17	69.87	72.63
(number)	(67)	(17)	(15)	(99)
8-Year-Olds				
% correct	79.40	66.79	76.00	76.52
(number)	(20)	(17)	(5)	(42)

* There were 6 4-year-olds and 11 5-year-olds who were unclassified and are only included in "All Subjects."

Statistical analysis of results with linear regression and analysis of variance techniques confirmed that selective listening skills improved with age for each of the three groups. While there was no significant difference between the three groups when tested in quiet, significant differences appeared under the distractor condition ($p < 0.01$). At each age level, LD children scored significantly lower than TC children who, in turn, scored significantly lower than NA children (table 3 and figure 2). These results are consistent with other studies (Cherry 1981; Katz and Wilde 1985; Rupp 1983; Keith et al. 1989).

CONCLUSIONS

The SAAT appears to be efficient at identifying those children who may be at risk for learning problems as measured by teacher concern. Table 4 is a distribution of percentile ranking based on age and

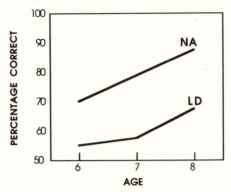

Figure 2. Group mean scores in percentage correct for normal achieving (NA) and learning disabled (LD) children. The younger age groups (4- and 5-year-olds) were omitted due to small numbers in the LD group.

performance score. Only 13% of NA children but 40% of TC children and over 90% of LD children scored at risk (their scores falling into the lower 25th percentile of all children tested). Using the Pearson product movement correlation, a test-retest coefficient 0.94 for list 1 (no distractor) and 0.89 for list 2 (with distractor) was obtained. Chermack

Table 4
Distribution of Percentile Ranking by Age and by Classification

Age (years)	Normal Achieving		Teacher Concerned		Learning Disabled	
	Pass	At Risk*	Pass	At Risk*	Pass	At Risk*
4	9	1	0	2	--	--
5	33	5	14	13	1**	0
6	56	10	26	13	0	1
7	57	10	9	6	1**	16
8	20	0	4	1	1**	16

* All children whose percentile ranking was 25% or less.
** Of these three, one 5-year-old was classified solely on the basis of visual and motor problems, and the 7- and 8-year-olds were in the process of being unclassified and mainstreamed by their respective schools.

and Montgomery (1991) found high intertest equivalence for the matched forms of the SAAT.

These findings have clinical implications. Specifically, it appears that the SAAT is an efficient screening device for identification of children with learning difficulties due to CAPD. Thus, this test can be used as a screening tool for deciding when to administer a lengthy battery of central auditory processing tests. This is important because the earlier these children are correctly identified, the better their prognosis for remediation (Pinheiro and Musiek 1985).

SUMMARY

This chapter includes a discussion of some of the issues that must be considered if screening for CAPD can be accomplished feasibly. The need for such a screening appears to be present. One such screening test is the SAAT, which is quick, easy to administer, and requires no special equipment or personnel. Following an at-risk score on the SAAT, children should be evaluated using more costly and time-consuming procedures. This two-step process should lead to earlier diagnosis and treatment for many children with CAPD.

REFERENCES

American National Standards Institute. 1970. *Specification for audiometers*. ANSI S3.6-1969. New York: American National Standards Institute.

Chermack, G.D., and Montgomery, M.J. 1991. Interlist equivalence of the selective auditory attention test. Paper presented at the American Academy of Audiology Conference, Denver, Colorado.

Cherry, R. 1979. Effects of competing message content on selective auditory attention abilities of normal achieving and learning disabled children. Unpublished Ed.D. dissertation, Columbia University.

Cherry, R. 1980. *Selective auditory attention test-manual*. St. Louis: Auditec of St. Louis.

Cherry, R. 1981. Development of selective auditory attention skills in children. *Perceptual and Motor Skills* 52:379-385.

Cherry, R., and Kruger, B. 1983. Selective auditory attention abilities of learning disabled and normal achieving children. *Journal of Learning Disabilities* 16:202-205.

Cline, J. 1988. Auditory processing deficits: Assessment and remediation by the elementary school speech language pathologist. *Seminars in Speech and Language* 9:367-382.

Ferre, J., and Wilber, L. 1986. Normal and learning disabled children's central auditory processing skills: An experimental test battery. *Ear and Hearing* 7:336-343.

Fisher, L.I. 1976. *Fisher auditory problems checklist.* Cedar Rapids, Iowa: Grant Wood Area Educational Agency.

Hagen, T., and Kail, R. 1975. The role of attention in perceptual and cognitive development. In W. Crickshank and D. Hallahan (eds.), *Perceptual and learning disabilities in children*, vol. 2 (pp. 165-194). Syracuse N.Y.: Syracuse University Press.

Hayes, D., and Pashley, N. 1991. Assessment of infants for hearing impairment. In J. Jacobson and J. Northern (eds.), *Diagnostic audiology* (pp. 251-266). Houston, Tex.: Pro-ed.

Hedrick, D.L., and Kunze, L.H. 1974. Diotic listening in young children. *Perceptual and Motor Skills* 38:591-598.

Katz, J. 1978. The effects of conductive hearing loss on auditory function. *Asha* 20:879-886.

Katz, J., and Wilde, L. 1985. Auditory perceptual disorders in children. In J. Katz (ed.), *Handbook of clinical audiology* (pp. 664-688). Baltimore: Williams and Wilkins.

Keith, R. 1988. Central auditory tests. In N. Lass, J. McReynolds, and D. Yoder (eds.), *Handbook of speech-language pathology and audiology* (pp. 1215-1236). Toronto: B.C. Decker.

Keith, R.W., Ruby, J., Donahue, P.A., and Katbamna, B. 1989. Comparison of SCAN results with other auditory and language measures in a clinical population. *Ear and Hearing* 10(6):382-386.

Lasky, E., and Cox, L. 1983. Auditory processing and language interaction: Evaluation and interaction strategies. In E. Lasky and J. Katz (eds.), *Central auditory processing disorders* (pp. 243-268). Baltimore: University Park Press.

Lessler, K. 1974. Screening, screening programs, and the pediatrician. *Pediatrics* 54:608-611.

Musiek, F., and Geurkink, N. 1980. Auditory perceptual problems in children: Considerations for otolaryngologists and audiologists. *Laryngoscope* 90:962-971.

Musiek, F., and Baron, J. 1987. Central auditory assessment: 30 years of challenge and change. *Ear and Hearing* 8:22S-35S.

Musiek, F., Gollogly, K., Lamb, L., and Lamb, P. 1990. Selected issues in screening for central auditory processing dysfunction. *Seminars in Hearing* 4:372-384.

Mueller, G. 1985. Monosyllabic procedures. In J. Katz (ed.), *Handbook of clinical audiology* (pp. 355-382). Baltimore: Williams and Wilkins.

Pinheiro, M., and Musiek, F. 1985. Special considerations in central auditory evaluation. In M. Pinheiro and F. Musiek (eds.), *Assessments of central auditory dysfunction* (pp. 257-266). Baltimore: Williams and Wilkins.

Ross, A.O. 1976. *Psychological aspects of learning disabilities and reading disorders*. New York: McGraw-Hill.

Ross, M., and Lerman, J. 1971. *Word intelligibility by picture identification*. Pittsburgh: Stanwix House, Inc.

Rupp, R. 1983. Establishing norms for speech-in-noise skills in children. *The Hearing Journal* 36:16-19.

Sanderson-Leepa, M.E., and Rintelman, W.F. 1976. Articulation functions and test retest performance of normal-hearing children on three speech discrimination tests: WIPI, PBK-50, and NU Auditory Test no. 6. *Journal of Speech and Hearing Disorders* 41:503-519.

Sloan, C. 1986. *Treating auditory processing difficulties in children*. San Diego: College Hill Press.

Smoski, W. 1990. Use of CHAPPS in a children's audiology clinic. *Ear and Hearing* 11:53S-56S.

Triesman, A.M. 1964a. Verbal cues, language and meaning in selective attention. *American Journal of Psychology* 77:206-219.

Triesman, A.M. 1964b. The effect of irrelevant material on the efficiency of selective listening. *American Journal of Psychology* 77:533-546.

Wechsler, D. 1974. *Wechsler intelligence scale for children* (revised test manual). New York: Psychological Corp.

Zill, N., and Schoenborn, C. 1990. *Health of our nation's children, United States, 1988*. Baltimore, Md.: National Center for Health Statistics.

Chapter 25

Screening for Auditory Disorders in Psychiatric Hospitals

Judith A. Marlowe, Tamara Lewis Engels, and
Robert W. Keith

INTRODUCTION

Throughout the past decade, an increasing body of research and greater clinical attention have focused upon those children who exhibit delays or dysfunction in the development of perceptual mechanisms involved in the organization and integration of sensory input (ASHA 1988). Included in this group are those children who, despite normal audiograms, behave as though they have a hearing disorder. Various labels are applied to this phenomenon, including central auditory deficit, auditory language learning disorder, auditory perceptual disorder, nonsensory auditory deficit and, more recently, auditory processing disorder (Cohen 1980; Keith 1981). Additionally, there is considerable debate over the relationship of such auditory disorders to language-learning disabilities, dyslexia, attention deficit disorder, and attention deficit hyperactivity disorder, or ADHD (Bashir, Wiig, and Abrams 1987; Johnson 1987; Keith 1981; Zinkus 1986).

Not surprisingly, this debate has generated confusion and some controversy about the relative role of various professionals in the identification and remediation of auditory processing disorders (Keith 1981). Today, a host of individuals and facilities including psychologists, reading specialists, tutoring clinics, developmental education centers, hospitals, speech-language pathologists, and audiologists present themselves as resources for families seeking relief from the educational and behavioral consequences of these listening difficulties. Each professional employs a variety of assessment techniques aimed at delineating the nature and extent of the underlying cause for the problem. In addition, many interact with other professionals for a multidisciplinary evaluation approach.

An important recent development in the provision of these services is the increasing number of psychiatric hospitals with a primary marketing effort directed toward diagnosis and treatment of children's learning and socialization problems. Managed by a number of nationwide corporations, there are now at least 250 such facilities operating in the United States. Each facility admits approximately 300 children and adolescents annually for inpatient treatment.

FEATURES OF AUDITORY PROCESSING DISORDERS

Auditory and verbal communication is our primary means of sharing feelings, attitudes, and beliefs, informing others, learning new information, and controlling or structuring our environment in order to manage it. Thus, disruptions of auditory reception and verbal expression can render the communication process ineffective and frustrating (Bashir, Wiig, and Abrams 1987). The presence of chronic communication disorders during the preschool years, in particular, exerts an impact upon later academic achievement and social adaptation (Zinkus 1986). Specifically, children with auditory disorders are typically described as inattentive, and inconsistent and inappropriate in responding to auditory signals. They are easily fatigued, easily distracted, and are unable to localize sound or differentiate soft versus loud sounds. They require frequent repetition of information, are unable to remember information presented verbally, offer delayed responses to questions, and have difficulty appreciating puns, jokes, or idiomatic expressions (Bashir, Wiig, and Abrams 1987; Cohen 1980; Keith 1981). Children with auditory disorders often exhibit disorganized verbal communication efforts and may rely upon nonverbal "acting out" behaviors for self-expression (Bashir, Wiig, and Abrams 1987; Johnson 1987). Keith (1986) depicts the complexity of the clinical picture in a model that illustrates the cumulative and interactive factors contributing to the diagnostic puzzle (figure 1).

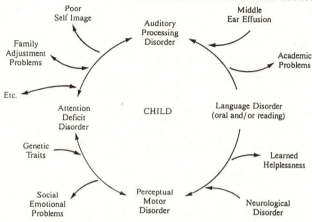

Figure 1. A model of possible factors contributing to a child's performance problems. From Keith 1986, reproduced by permission The Psychological Corporation.

EVALUATION OF AUDITORY PROCESSING DISORDERS

Even though there is great interest in formal assessment of auditory complaints, a survey of available test instruments reveals that recording techniques, material selection, length of administration time, and adequacy of normative data vary widely (Keith et al. 1989). Moreover, some tasks combine auditory/visual modalities or depend upon higher level language skills. With such tests, it may be difficult to confidently identify what role auditory processing plays in the child's problem and to plan effective remediation approaches (Keith 1981).

A Screening Test for Auditory Processing Disorders (SCAN) was designed as an easily and rapidly administered normed tool for clinicians (Keith 1986). The battery is composed of three subtests. The Filtered Word Subtest is an auditory closure task in which two lists of twenty monosyllabic words low pass filtered at 1000 Hz with a filter roll-off of 32 dB per octave are presented monaurally to assess the child's ability to recognize words when a portion of the acoustic spectrum is reduced. The Auditory Figure Ground Subtest examines word identification skills in the presence of competing multitalker speech babble at a +8 dB signal-to-noise ratio. The unrecognizable babble was selected for its uniform intensity and had been compressed to further reduce any acoustic peaks. Both test items and background babble are monaurally presented to the ear under test. The Competing Word Subtest is a dichotic task in which two different monosyllabic words matched for duration within five milliseconds are presented to each ear simultaneously. Both words are reported. However, during the first half of the test, the subject repeats the right ear stimuli first. During the second half of the test, subjects respond with the left ear item first. An ear advantage score is computed, as well as the standard score for this portion of the SCAN. A standard score profile, an auditory age equivalent, and an analysis of subset differences allow the examiner to derive useful information using age-related norms that extend from 3 to 12 years of age.

SCREENING WITH SCAN

A survey of children admitted to a psychiatric hospital who were evaluated audiologically and screened with SCAN was undertaken by one of the authors (T.E.) to determine if auditory processing disorders contribute to the behavioral disorders under treatment. A similar review was completed by the first author (J.M.) who serves as an allied medical staff consultant to two psychiatric hospitals in another state. All three institutions, while unrelated, are affiliated with corporations whose marketing thrust is aimed at families whose children are experiencing academic and behavioral difficulties. The descriptive data accumulated from an analysis of nonselected sample of referrals are presented below.

RESULTS

The records of 92 children were reviewed for this report. Sixty-eight (74%) of these were males, consistent with estimates that males comprise 75% of those children with learning disorders (Cohen 1980; Keith 1981). Twenty-four (26%) of the sample were female. Eighteen (19.5%) of the original total sample were excluded from further review since they were older than 12 years, the limit of currently published norms available for SCAN. Seventy-four children under 12 years remained appropriate subjects for this report (80% of the total referred for evaluation). Children as young as age 3 were admitted for evaluation and treatment at the three facilities.

Acoustic impedance measures and pure-tone audiometry were administered in an initial stage of the evaluation of the 92 children. Surprisingly, 21 children (23%) demonstrated a peripheral hearing loss. These percentages are constant for both facilities. Since SCAN is intended for use only with children whose peripheral hearing is within

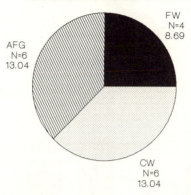

Figure 2. Distribution of significantly decreased (≥ 2 standard deviations) SCAN scores by subtest. Number of subjects = 7. AFG=Auditory Figure Ground Subtest, CW=Competing Word Subtest, FW=Filtered Word Subtest.

normal limits, these children with a peripheral loss were excluded from SCAN analysis. Forty-six children met age and peripheral hearing criteria for SCAN and completed the test. Of the 46, 7 children (15%) earned standard scores two standard deviations below their respective age norms indicating auditory processing disorders of significance. Inspection of the individual subtests revealed that the lowest scores were obtained for the Auditory Figure Ground Subtest and the Competing Word Subtest. In 2 youngsters, only the Auditory Figure Ground score was depressed, whereas in 5 subjects, more than one test result was depressed (figure 2).

For 33 of the 92 cases under review, one of the authors (J.M.) had access to additional diagnostic information. This subset of children was further examined to gain information regarding admitting diagnosis and outcome of language evaluation. Fourteen of these children were admitted for treatment of depression, 10 for ADHD, 7 for conduct/oppositional disorder, and 1 each for treatment of schizophrenia and drug dependency (figure 3). Fourteen of this group (42%) were referred to a speech pathologist instead of an audiologist. Eleven children were found to exhibit language disorders, most commonly in the areas of auditory comprehension and memory that led to recommendations for further auditory assessment (figure 4). Five children (15%) were discharged without completing any hearing or language evaluations.

Although the original focus of this case review was screening for auditory processing disorders, the finding of peripheral hearing loss in

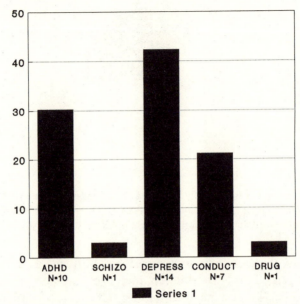

Figure 3. Distribution of admission diagnoses in select sample of 33 subjects. ADHD=attention deficit hyperactivity disorder, SCHIZO=schizophrenia, DEPRESS=depression, CONDUCT=conduct/oppositional disorder, DRUG=drug dependency.

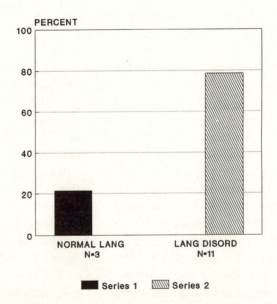

Figure 4. Results of language evaluation in a select sample of 14 subjects.

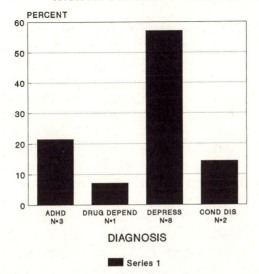

Figure 5. Distribution of presence of peripheral hearing loss by diagnostic category within select sample of 14 subjects. ADHD=attention deficit hyperactivity disorder, DRUG DEPEND=drug dependence, DEPRESS=depression, COND DIS=conduct disorder.

23% of the original 92 subjects is interesting. These children did not have a homogeneous admitting diagnosis. Eight were undergoing treatment for depression, 3 were labeled ADHD, 2 were identified as having conduct disorders, and 1 was drug dependent (figure 5).

IMPLICATIONS

Our review of the case information from these 92 children suggests that the number of children admitted to psychiatric hospitals with auditory disorders, both peripheral and central, is sufficient to warrant routine inclusion of auditory screening measures. A surprising finding was the incidence of undetected peripheral hearing loss, especially in older children who, presumably, had been previously screened in physicians' offices or at school. Of concern was the realization that multiple evaluations of language, cognitive, and affective dimensions of behavior had already been performed and interpreted without the benefit of information about hearing. Treatment plans that were under way did not take into account the influence of auditory disorders on the child's clinical picture. Further study is needed to determine how information on auditory factors might affect diagnostic and treatment strategies.

Several issues emerged that pose a dilemma if routine auditory screening is to be offered to children admitted to psychiatric hospitals. Cost and timing concerns arise. In particular, the question is whether these hospitals need their own audiology facilities, equipment, and personnel for auditory screening as opposed to contractual arrangements to transport inpatients to established community facilities for evaluation. While referral for testing might appear to be a logical solution, liability concerns and scheduling difficulties cannot be overlooked. These youngsters exhibit behavior that is difficult to manage under ordinary circumstances. Offices that do not routinely serve psychiatric patients may not be equipped to deal with contingencies that may arise. Scheduling is a major problem because these children undergo multiple assessments within a relatively brief period prior to discharge. An alternative, that is, screening by case history to select those patients who require further evaluation, also may be less effective. Access to pertinent information regarding history of ear disease and academic performance may vary according to the admitting diagnosis and the subsequent focus of examination. In view of the percentage of children reported here who have peripheral or central auditory disorders, we would argue that on-site audiologic procedures, including at least impedance and pure-tone thresholds, and a screening test for central auditory disorders, should be administered to all children in this population.

Perhaps the most daunting issue to be confronted is the inability to provide appropriate follow-up for children identified with auditory disorders. Reasons for poor follow-up include brief hospitalization, due to limits of insurance coverage, failure of many insurance providers to underwrite outpatient services, and difficulties in obtaining family cooperation. The latter can be worsened by the lack of direct contact between families of hospitalized children and audiologists or speech pathologists. Information is customarily relayed to the family via the admitting physician and/or case workers who may be unfamiliar with audiologic information. Parents may feel frustrated and overwhelmed by the magnitude of behavioral problems they face with their child and, therefore, may elect to focus upon other issues that seem more directly related to solving their problems. Or parents may assume that the public schools will address any auditory difficulties. The need for appropriate communication of audiologic findings, and interacting with educational and medical systems that serve the child, is essential because lack of follow-up will negate the benefit of screening.

Summary

Today, more than ever before, audiologists are challenged to provide a variety of screening services in diverse settings. One population that appears to merit our concern is the growing number of youths with emotional and behavioral problems of sufficient magnitude that families, schools, and the traditional structures for managing these difficulties must be supplanted by specialized care facilities. Valuable hearing health services, which can be provided in that venue, offer an important opportunity for audiologists. Audiologists can ensure that effective screening to detect auditory disorders becomes a regular component of the diagnostic and management programs for those youths for whom communication, learning, and socialization are in jeopardy.

References

American Speech-Language-Hearing Association. 1988. *Audiological assessment of central auditory processing: An annotated bibliography.* Rockville, Md.: American Speech-Language-Hearing Association.

Bashir, A.S., Wiig, E.H., and Abrams, J.C. 1987. Language disorders in childhood and adolescence: Implications for learning and socialization. *Pediatric Annals* 16(2):145-156.

Cohen, R.L. 1980. Auditory skills and the communicative process. In R.W. Keith (ed.), *Seminars in speech, language and hearing.* New York: Thieme-Stratton.

Johnson, D.J. 1987. Nonverbal learning disabilities. *Pediatric Annals* 16(2):133-141.

Keith, R.W. 1981. Tests of central auditory function. In R. Roeser and M.P. Downs (eds.), *Auditory disorders in school children.* New York: Thieme-Stratton.

Keith, R.W. 1986. *SCAN: A screening test for auditory processing disorders.* San Antonio, Tex.: The Psychological Corporation.

Keith, R.W., Rudy, J., Donahue, P.A., and Katbamna, B. 1989. Comparison of SCAN results with other auditory and language measures in a clinical population. *Ear and Hearing* 10(6):382-386.

Zinkus, P. 1986. Perceptual and academic deficits related to early chronic otitis media. In J. Kavanagh (ed.), *Otitis media and child development*. Parkton, Md.: York Press.

PART V.

Intervention

Chapter 26

Current Issues in Early Intervention

Donald B. Bailey, Jr.

INTRODUCTION

Early intervention may be defined as the provision of educational, therapeutic, preventive, and supportive services for young children with disabilities and their families. From an historical perspective, early intervention grew out of the basic assumption that providing services at the earliest possible time would maximize the benefits that might accrue to the child, the family, and society. For example, it is assumed that early intervention will facilitate children's development, help support families in coping with the tasks associated with care of children with a disability, and reduce the need for costly specialized services in later years.

Formal early intervention efforts at the federal level first focused on children living in poverty. A number of special programs were established in the 1960s in an effort to remediate the devastating influences of poverty on children and families. Perhaps the most relevant of these efforts for early intervention was the establishment of Head Start programs in an attempt to provide enhanced early experiences for preschoolers living in poverty, a program that is still growing and expanding today.

Services for children with disabilities have emerged more slowly. In 1968 Congress established the Handicapped Children's Education Program in order to develop and demonstrate models for serving young children. Although nearly 600 such projects have been funded since that time, services for young children with disabilities have, until recently, remained scattered and often inaccessible. In 1972, the first national mandate to serve young children with disabilities was built into the Economic Opportunity Act by requiring that at least 10% of the children served by Head Start programs have disability.

It was not until 1986, however, with the passage of Public Law 99-457, that legislative provisions were established that set the stage for widespread services for all young children with disabilities. The legislation required public schools to provide free and appropriate educational services to all children ages 3 to 5 years with disabilities. In addition, incentives are provided for states to provide services for infants and toddlers under 36 months of age, although these services are not required. While for 3- and 4-year-olds the law represents a downward extension of previous legislation for school-age children, the infant and toddler component reflects a substantial change in the nature and focus of services, with the role of family support emerging as significant.

An analysis of current services for young children with disabilities reveals a diverse system serving a heterogeneous group of children and families. Diversity in children is reflected in changing demographics related to both age and etiology of disability. Programs are increasingly serving the very youngest children, often providing services in the hospital. Complications related to low birth weight, prematurity, maternal drug and alcohol use, HIV infection, and adolescent pregnancy have expanded the traditional categories (e.g., hearing impaired, mental retardation) to an inclusion of children who are at risk for a variety of developmental or behavioral outcomes. The families served often represent a group that is diverse with respect to culture, socioeconomic status, parental age, views of service providers, and goals for treatment.

Just as there is variability in children and families, so too is there variability in programs and services that constitute early intervention. Included in this diversity are various settings (e.g., homes, child-care centers, hospitals, clinics, evaluation centers), treatments (e.g., education, therapy, counseling, family support, medication, surgery, specialized equipment), and philosophical perspectives.

Given this ecological context, what are some of the major issues currently facing professionals who work in early intervention programs? Historically, the field has been preoccupied with a single primary issue: Is early intervention effective? A large number of studies have investigated this question with children living in low socioeconomic conditions. The general conclusion from this research is that early intervention can produce significant gains in children's intellectual functioning and socioemotional development, although the gains generally decline within a few years. There is also evidence that early intervention programs for low-income children reduce grade retention and the need for special education services (Haskins 1989). Research on children with disabilities, however, has been less conclusive. Reviews of this research (e.g., Casto and Mastropieri 1986; Ottenbacher 1989; Shonkoff and Hauser-Cram 1987) suggest that early intervention may be effective, but strong proof is still forthcoming.

Most researchers today acknowledge that the question of whether early intervention is effective is deceptively simple. How early is the intervention provided? Who are the targets of intervention? What is the treatment? What outcomes are important? The complexity of the question, combined with the legal mandate for early intervention services, has led most researchers and clinicians away from asking whether early intervention is effective to asking a more complex question: What interventions are best for which children/families in order to achieve a particular type of outcome? Although the effectiveness of early intervention remains an important conceptual and practical issue, the issue has come to be viewed in the context of a set of complex services that are already in place or are being planned.

Many issues could be identified as current in early intervention. Some are at a general policy level (e.g., what criteria should states use to determine whether a child is developmentally delayed?), whereas others are very specific (e.g., does approach A work better than approach B in facilitating communication skills?). This chapter addresses four that are likely to be important across disciplines, etiologies, and service delivery settings. The first is an examination of the goals of early intervention. The second and third issues reflect a more detailed examination of two goals of early intervention: family-centered services and normalization. The final issue addresses the need for strategies that will enhance the change process and improve current practices.

THE GOALS OF EARLY INTERVENTION

From an historical perspective, the primary goal of early intervention has been to foster children's development. Usually the extent to which this goal has been achieved has been assessed through the measurement of changes in children's IQ scores. In recent years, however, parents, professionals, and policy makers have questioned both child development as the only goal of early intervention and the reliance on a relatively meaningless measure of competence for providing the worth of early intervention. This state of affairs has forced an introspective examination of the reasons why early intervention is provided. The result of that process has been the identification of a wide array of purposes of early intervention and many thoughtful discussions and arguments about the relative worth of each. Bailey and Wolery (in press) have synthesized this literature and suggest that seven goals have emerged as relevant for early intervention:

SUPPORTING FAMILIES IN ACHIEVING THEIR OWN GOALS

Public Law 99-457 emphasizes the importance of family support as a primary goal of early intervention, especially for infants and toddlers, with the requirement for an Individualized Family Service Plan (IFSP) for each child and family served. In addition to child goals and services, the plan must include a statement of family needs and describe family support services, including case management. This reflects a growing philosophical shift in early intervention to a more family-centered approach (Bailey 1987; Dunst 1985; Shelton, Jeppson, and Johnson 1987). For example, Dunst (1985) argues that "enabling and empowering" families ought to be the primary goal of early intervention.

PROMOTING CHILD ENGAGEMENT, INDEPENDENCE, AND MASTERY

This goal emphasizes the importance of focusing on immediate rather than long-term goals of early intervention. Research on children with disabilities often demonstrates delays or disabilities related to interactions with the environment and independent behavior. Thus, a major goal of early intervention is to promote children's engagement with the mastery of environments in which they spend time, such as homes, child-care centers, and community sites (e.g., parks, churches, grocery store).

PROMOTING DEVELOPMENT IN IMPORTANT DOMAINS

This has been the historical goal of early intervention and remains an essential purpose. The term *development*, however, is increasingly recognized as a broad construct covering many aspects of children's growth and functioning. These include basic areas of cognition, communication, social, self-help, and adaptive skills, as well as constructs such as self-esteem and self-control.

BUILDING AND SUPPORTING SOCIAL COMPETENCE

The ability to interact with other persons is probably the most important skill one learns. Many studies over the years have documented that young children with disabilities often have poor social skills. The parallel finding of social skills deficits in older persons with disabilities (including adults) suggests that this is a critical aspect of early intervention, although often it is relegated to a secondary position because of focus on other areas.

FACILITATING THE GENERALIZED USE OF SKILLS

Another finding that permeates the research literature is that children with disabilities often do not use the skills they have learned in a variety of contexts or when presented new problems. Thus, a fifth goal of early intervention is to facilitate the widespread or generalized use of learned skills.

PROVIDING AND PREPARING FOR NORMALIZED LIFE EXPERIENCES

How can children with disabilities best be integrated into the mainstream of society? This question reflects an important value base of all services for children with disabilities, and is especially important in the context of early intervention. One major goal of early intervention is to provide normal life experiences and help children acquire the skills needed to succeed in "normalized" settings.

PREVENTING THE EMERGENCE OF FUTURE PROBLEMS OR DISABILITIES

A final goal of early intervention is related to prevention. Many children served in early intervention programs demonstrate minimal delays in development, yet because of a diagnosed disability (e.g., Down syndrome, hearing impairment, cerebral palsy), health history (e.g., prematurity, low birth weight, maternal drug or alcohol use), or environmental circumstances (e.g., poverty) are considered high risks for delay or disabilities. Thus, a final goal of early intervention is to prevent the emergence of delays of problems whenever possible. A related goal is to prevent the need for specialized services or equipment.

These seven goals represent an extraordinarily broad mandate for early intervention and constitute perhaps the most important issue facing early intervention professionals today: Why are we here, and what do we want to achieve as a result of these services? The answer to this question is likely to be individualized according to each child and family served. The question, however, bears important implications for another important issue: Is early intervention effective? This question can be answered only after determination is made of the goals for early intervention.

PROMOTING FAMILY-CENTERED SERVICES

Promotion of family-centered services has emerged as one of the most significant issues facing professionals working directly in early intervention programs as well as professionals working in clinics, schools, evaluation centers, and other programs whose clients include young children. A family-centered approach to service delivery means that professionals (1) consider the child's family to be the client seeking services; (2) include families as partners in identifying needs and resources most likely to meet child and family needs; (3) respect family values and priorities in the ultimate determination of goals and approaches to service delivery; and (4) provide services and conduct all professional activities in a way that helps families feel competent and respected (Bailey 1987; Dunst 1985; Zigler and Black 1989).

A family-centered approach is one in which family concerns are integrated into every aspect of service delivery rather than isolated as a service provided by one team member such as the social worker or psychologist. Although specialized expertise in working with families is a necessary part of any treatment team, effective implementation of a family-centered philosophy can occur only if every team member implements it as a part of his or her work.

Why provide family-centered services? This question is asked by many professionals whose primary concern is with the well-being of the child with a disability. At least three reasons for family-centered services can be identified (Meyer and Bailey in press). First, many families have expressed, either directly or through personal stories, their frustration with a service system that has not met their needs. Second, many programs have found that activities they assumed to be important to families (e.g., parent meetings, parent-implemented curriculum or therapeutic activities) are not well attended or utilized, often because programs have failed to listen to clients, involve them in the decision-making process, or provide services that are feasible and consistent with client expectations (Cadman, Shurvell, Davies, and Bradfield 1984). Finally, it has been suggested that well-intentioned services sometimes have negative consequences for families. This was evident in the research of Affleck, Tennen, Rowe, Roscher, and Walker (1989), who studied the effects of a hospital-to-home support program for mothers of high-risk infants in the neonatal intensive care unit. They found numerous positive outcomes of the program, but only for mothers who, at the onset, felt a need for the program. Those who did not feel a need for it, but got it anyway, reported less competency, had a lower sense of control, and were less responsive to their infants after the program than before. The authors suggested that the program may have had a negative effect on the self-confidence of these mothers by suggesting that they really did need help.

Bailey, McWilliam, Winton, and Simeonsson (1991) have suggested that programs serving young children and their families ought to address at least seven questions regarding family-centered services: (1) What is our philosophy about working with families? (2) How will we involve families in child assessment? (3) How will we assess family needs and resources? (4) How will we involve families in team meetings and decision making? (5) How will we incorporate family goals into the individualized plan? (6) How will we implement the plan and provide case management services? and (7) How will we involve families in the transition process? These questions emphasize the need for professionals to examine all aspects of service delivery to determine the extent to which services are family-centered.

The remainder of this section draws on one of these questions—How will we involve families in child assessment?—to illustrate selected issues and considerations regarding family-centered practices. The traditional model of child assessment usually involves parents whose child is suspected of having some form of disability. The professional is the expert who is expected to provide information and answers regarding the presence of a disability, its etiology, prognosis for the future, and suggestions for treatment. Professionals rely on sophisticated equipment and measurement tools to assess children, usually in isolated contexts away from normal activities and routines. The child is tested alone, without peers and often without parents. The primary purpose of the assessment is to identify deficits for purposes of remediation.

This model of child assessment evolved as professional expertise grew and standardized measures evolved. Although the model has many necessary and important components, it also has numerous possibilities for negative outcomes (Bailey and Wolery 1992). For example, by building on the professional-as-expert model, the approach reinforces the notion that parents know very little about their children when, in fact, they often have much information that is essential to a full understanding of the child's functional abilities and limitations. Parents often do not feel that they are part of the assessment process and consequently may not agree with the conclusions or recommendations that emerge, especially if they are not perceived as functional recommendations or consistent with family priorities or values. As a result, follow-through on recommendations may be minimal. Furthermore, the very nature of the assessment process often means that it focuses primarily on identifying children's deficits rather than strengths and coping styles.

How might a family-centered approach change the child assessment process? The following suggestions are offered in this regard:

1. Realize that assessment is also an intervention activity. The way assessments are conducted inevitably influences families by shaping the ways they view themselves and affecting the extent to which they initiate or follow up on treatment recommendations. Assessment should be viewed as an activity designed not just to identify children's problems but also to determine family priorities for their children, understand how they perceive their child's strengths and needs, build and reinforce parents' sense of competence and worth, and develop a shared perspective on the child as well as a shared commitment to intervention goals and activities.

2. Determine parent goals for child assessment. What do parents want from the assessment process? The answer to this question ought to drive much of the assessment activity. Although professionals often will want to ask and answer other questions, the concerns of parents should drive the assessment activities and the informing process.

3. Determine parent preferences for roles in child assessment. Families can engage in a variety of roles in the assessment process: receiving information, determining the types of information to gather or where assessments are conducted, observing assessments, providing information, and collecting data. Families will vary in their preferences for roles. Some will only want information from professionals, whereas others will want to be involved in decision making about assessment as well as data collection. A family-centered approach would provide families with an array of alternatives and respect family desires for involvement. An especially important consideration, however, is making sure that families perceive the array of roles as meaningful and not a waste of their time.

4. *Make every effort to ensure that assessment information is conveyed in a sensitive and jargon-free fashion.* Increasing specialization and knowledge development often result in a new vocabulary that is known only by experts within a given field. Assessment reports invariably are characterized by families as confusing due to use of jargon and scores that are not easily understood. Also reports have been described as technical and insensitive, ignoring the human qualities that make each child unique and special. Reports should be written in ways that clearly communicate findings in a positive fashion.

5. *Involve families in the decision-making process.* The natural extension of family involvement in child assessment is family involvement in decisions that are based on assessment activities. This implies that rather than the traditional meeting in which professionals inform parents of the results of their assessment, a meeting is held in which parental and professional perspectives are merged into a coherent view of the child and his or her needs.

PROMOTING AND PROVIDING NORMALIZED EXPERIENCES

The next issue to be discussed in this chapter is the goal of promoting and providing normalized experiences for young children with disabilities and their families. Public Laws 94-142 and 99-457 require that children with disabilities be served in the *least restrictive environment* and, to the extent possible, be educated with children who do not have disabilities. These requirements are based on a philosophical value base related to normalization, or the notion that children and adults with disabilities ought to be able to experience life as normally as possible (Nirje 1985; Wolfensberger 1972). The normalization principle bears implications for early intervention professionals in at least three areas: opportunities for interacting with normally developing children, normalized intervention strategies, and normalized family involvement

(Bailey and McWilliam 1990). Since family involvement has already been discussed, this section addresses the first two of these concerns.

Should children with disabilities be served in "mainstreamed" programs with normally developing children? Very few professionals or parents would disagree with the philosophical goal of mainstreaming, but many are concerned about whether its implementation is feasible and most effective for children with disabilities. A large number of studies have examined mainstreaming in the context of early intervention, and several conclusions now appear warranted. Many observational studies have documented that children with disabilities do, in fact, interact with normally developing children when placed in mainstreamed programs, although interactions have repeatedly been shown to be facilitated by active teacher involvement in play. A recent review of studies comparing mainstreamed and specialized placements for children with disabilities (Buysse and Bailey in press) found strong support for the beneficial effects of mainstreaming on children's social behavior. Although mainstreaming has not been shown to be superior to specialized programs in enhancing children's development, the fact that they generally result in progress that is no different from that observed in specialized programs raises serious concerns about the value of segregated services.

Although mainstreaming is an essential part of normalization, the use of normalized intervention strategies also is an important consideration. In essence the question is as follows: To what extent should children with disabilities be taught or treated in ways that differ from those used with normally developing children? The fact that a child has a disability almost inevitably means that some form of special education or treatment is needed. But often the question of normalization has not been asked of treatments, only the question of effectiveness. If the normalization principle were implemented, however, professionals (and parents) would evaluate treatment goals and alternative procedures in part on the extent to which they are typically used with other children as well as on the extent to which they would ultimately facilitate integration into society at large. An example of this debate, of course, is whether children with hearing impairments should rely exclusively on sign language as a mode of communication. Also, in early intervention, a current issue is the extent to which guidelines for developmentally appropriate practice, such as recommended by the National Association for the Education for Young Children (Bredekamp 1986), are appropriate for young children with disabilities (Carta, Schwartz, Atwater, and McConnell 1991; Wolery, Strain, and Bailey in press).

FACILITATING CHANGE AND INNOVATION

The identification of issues in early intervention directly implies that some changes are needed in the field. This brief paper suggests that early intervention programs need to rethink the goals of early intervention, with a special focus on family-centered practices and normalization. The final issue to be discussed here is the manner by which these changes are likely to occur. Because of the research in this area, implementation of family-centered practices is used to illustrate some of the challenges.

Despite legislative guidelines and numerous professional publications, it is likely that a shift from child-focus to family-centered services will be challenging for many professionals. Research has shown that most professionals have received little training in working with families (Bailey, Simeonsson, Yoder, and Huntington 1990), and those who work in early intervention feel their skills are stronger in work with children (Bailey, Palsha, and Simeonsson 1991). Professionals in many states report a significant discrepancy between current and desired practices in working with families (Bailey, Buysse, Edmondson, and Smith 1992; Mahoney and O'Sullivan 1990). Although most value family roles, they have many concerns about how a family-centered philosophy could be implemented and what effects it would have on them and the children and families they serve (Bailey, Palsha, and Simeonsson 1991).

These findings suggest that changing to family-centered services, just as other significant changes in practices, will not be a quick or an easy process. Winton (1990), drawing on the literature of organizational processes, suggests that the likelihood of change occurring will be increased if training and the change process (a) are based on the perceived needs, values, and goals of the professionals involved; (b) are supported by administrators and policy makers; (c) include a goal-setting phase; and (d) involve follow-up and support for change to occur. These issues are not unique to early intervention. Because of the significant and rapidly occurring changes in the field, however, research on enhancing the change process in this context is essential.

SUMMARY

This chapter has presented a brief overview of four major issues confronting professionals who serve young children with disabilities and their families: determining the goals of intervention, providing family-centered services, promoting normalization, and facilitating systems change. The issues are interrelated and point to the complex ecology in which early intervention programs and services are operating. These and other issues will continue to be discussed as we seek to operationalize "best practice." It is likely that these issues will only be resolved when sufficient research has been conducted allowing for meaningful evaluation of alternatives, and when parents, professionals, and other key decision makers agree on the goals of an important societal activity.

REFERENCES

Affleck, G., Tennen, H., Rowe, J., Roscher, B., and Walker, L. 1989. Effects of formal support on mothers' adaption to the hospital-to-home transition of high-risk infants: The benefits and costs of helping. *Child Development* 60:488-501.

Bailey, D.B. 1987. Collaborative goal-setting with families: Resolving differences in values and priorities for services. *Topics in Early Childhood Special Education* 7(2):57-71.

Bailey, D.B., and McWilliam, R.A. 1990. Normalizing early intervention. *Topics in Early Childhood Special Education* 10(2):33-47.

Bailey, D.B., Simeonsson, R.J., Yoder, D.E., and Huntington, G.S. 1990. Preparing professionals to serve infants and toddlers with handicaps and their families: An integrative analysis across eight disciplines. *Exceptional Children* 57:26-35.

Bailey, D.B., McWilliam, P.J., Winton, P.J., and Simeonsson, R.J. 1991. *Promoting family-centered practices in early intervention: A team-based model for change.* Chapel Hill, N.C.: Frank Porter Graham Child Development Center, University of North Carolina.

Bailey, D.B., Buysse, V., Edmondson, R., and Smith, T.M. 1992. Creating family-centered services in early intervention: Perceptions of professionals in four states. *Exceptional Children* 58:298-309.

Bailey, D.B., Palsha, S.A., and Simeonsson, R.J. 1991. Professional concerns, skills, and perceived importance of work with families in early intervention. *Exceptional Children* 58:156-165

Bailey, D.B., and Wolery, M. 1992. *Teaching infants and preschoolers with disabilities.* 2d ed. Columbus, Ohio: Macmillan.

Bredekamp, S. (ed.). 1986. *Developmentally appropriate practice in early childhood programs serving children from birth through age 8.* Washington, D.C.: National Association for the Education of Young Children.

Buysse, V., and Bailey, D.B. In press. Behavioral and developmental outcomes for young children with disabilities in integrated and segregated settings: A comparative review. *Journal of Special Education.*

Cadman, D., Shurvell, B., Davies, P., and Bradfield, S. 1984. Compliance in the community with consultant's recommendations for developmentally handicapped children. *Developmental Medicine and Child Neurology* 26:40-46.

Carta, J.J., Schwartz, I.S., Atwater, J.B., and McConnell, S.R. 1991. Developmentally appropriate practice: Appraising its usefulness for young children with disabilities. *Topics in Early Childhood Special Education* 11(1):1-20.

Casto, G., and Mastropieri, M.A. 1986. The efficacy of early intervention programs: A meta-analysis. *Exceptional Children* 52:417-424.

Dunst, C.J. 1985. Rethinking early intervention. *Analysis and Intervention in Developmental Disabilities* 5:165-201.

Haskins, R. 1989. Beyond metaphor: The efficacy of early childhood education. *American Psychologist* 44:274-282.

Mahoney, G., and O'Sullivan, P. 1990. Early intervention practices with families of children with handicaps. *Mental Retardation* 28:169-176.

Meyer, E.C., and Bailey, D.B. In press. Family-centered care in early intervention: Community and hospital settings. In J. Paul and R. Simeonsson (eds.), *Working with families and children with special needs.* 2d ed. New York: Holt, Rinehart, Winston.

Nirje, B. 1985. The basis and logic of the normalization principle. *Australia and New Zealand Journal of Developmental Disabilities* 11(2):65-68.

Ottenbacher, K.J. 1989. Statistical conclusion validity of early intervention research with handicapped children. *Exceptional Children* 55:534-540.

Shelton, T.L., Jeppson, E.S., and Johnson, B.H. 1987. *Family-centered care for children with special health care needs.* Washington, D.C.: Association for the Care of Children's Health.

Shonkoff, P.J., and Hauser-Cram, P. 1987. Early intervention for disabled infants and their families: A quantitative analysis. *Pediatrics* 80:650-658.

Winton, P.J. 1990. A systemic approach for planning inservice training related to Public Law 99-457. *Infants and Young Children* 3(1):51-60.

Wolery, M., Strain, P., and Bailey, D.B. In press. Applying the framework of developmentally appropriate practice to children with special needs. In S. Bredekamp (ed.), *Appropriate curriculum and assessment.* Washington, D.C.: National Association for the Education of Young Children.

Wolfensberger, W. 1972. *The principle of normalization in human services.* Toronto: National Institute on Mental Retardation.

Zigler, E., and Black, K.B. 1989. America's family support movement: Strengths and limitations. *American Journal of Orthopsychiatry* 59(1):6-19.

Chapter 27

Birth to Five: The Important Early Years

Marie Thompson

INTRODUCTION

The early years, from birth to 5, are very important years for all children. They learn about language and how to use it. They learn to speak, and they learn about themselves and their environment. These early years help young children establish positive and firm foundations for language, reading, learning, self-esteem, and family relationships, or they can be filled with negative messages that contribute to the child not reaching his or her potential as a well-educated, well-adjusted, independent young adult. The early years are especially important for the very young hearing-impaired child who receives imperfect messages, often a product of body language and facial expressions rather than true oral language. If these early years are critical to the hearing-impaired child's future, as they are, then what can professionals and families do to develop a rich and positive environment in which this special child can begin to grow toward his or her potential? To identify the characteristics associated with a positive learning environment, we identified 6- to 7-year-old successful hearing-impaired children and their families with whom we have worked for the past 17 years in early childhood. Then, we examined the program elements that, in our opinion and the families' opinion, contributed to the excellent achievements these children have made. These "successful" young children are ones who are functioning as productive members of their families, have excellent functional language, and are achieving in school like their age-related *hearing* peers.

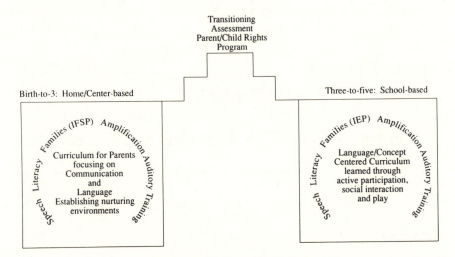

Figure 1. Critical elements for programs serving hearing-impaired children, birth to 5 years of age. Notice that the basic elements of speech, auditory training, and literacy are all approached through social interaction and language. Families play a key role in all early education of hearing-impaired children.

The critical elements of programs that contribute to the growth of young hearing-impaired children are found in figure 1. Many of these critical elements are the same as those that contribute to the success of hearing children, such as family involvement and a focus on language, literacy, and play. There are obvious differences in programs for hearing-impaired children. We must use amplification and *teach* listening skills, speech production, and language. All of the elements identified in figure 1 are equally important in programs for children from birth to 3 and from 3 to 5 year of age. The following elements were addressed in this paper because they often receive little or no attention and often raise questions from both parents and professionals: family systems; communication, language, and speech; early literacy; play; transitioning; and curriculum for 3- to 5-year-olds.

FAMILY SYSTEMS

Families are children's first teachers. No matter how large or small a family is, or what its constellation, children learn from their families. Language is learned through interactions between the child and caregivers at home (mother, dad, grandparent, older sibling). For example, adults interpret infant behaviors as communicative long before children have language and respond accordingly. In the very early stages of infancy, most caregivers use language as one means of communicating socially. Although adults are aware that infants do not yet understand language, they use language as if the child is understanding what is said and is an integral part of the communication process. For example, Snow (1977) provides us with such a "conversation" that includes the "teaching" of language as well as the "teaching" of social interaction and turn taking:

Mother	*Ann*
	(smiles)
Oh what a nice little smile.	
Yes, isn't that nice?	
There.	
There's a nice smile.	(burps)
What a nice wind as well!	
Yes, that's better isn't it?	
Yes.	
Yes.	
Yes!	(vocalizes)
There's a nice noise.	

Moses (1985) points out that families also impact emotional development:

> *Do you want to know the single, strongest element that impacts development? The attitude of the parent toward the child, which is affected by the impact on the parent of having an impaired child.*

Families are, of course, important to children at all times, but perhaps most especially during the early years of birth through 5 when children are literally learning everything from scratch. Professionals have a tremendous influence on families during these early years as well. Parents often describe a long-lasting impact from intense negative interactions with professionals, especially if they feel that they are viewed as "abnormal" and/or their knowledge about their child is not valued (Halpern and Parker-Crawford 1982).

Families of hearing-impaired children play a significant part in the success of the children, especially during the early years. During this period, so much depends upon the parent's acceptance of the child and the ability to provide a stimulating and nurturing environment at home, and then support for beginning school programs. As professionals, we must recognize that each hearing-impaired child is an integral part of the family and what affects the family affects the child, and vice versa. If, as professionals, we understand that the child is indeed an integral part of the total family system, then working with the child will always include and, in fact, will begin with the parent(s) and other family members involved in the child's life. It is therefore critical that, whether we work with a hearing-impaired infant or a 4- or 5-year-old, we do so from a family systems perspective.

Viewing a family from a systems perspective does not mean that professionals are to pass judgment and identify the family as good or bad. It can, however, help them step back and gain perspective on the child they are working with if they can visualize the child as one part of the total system. Figure 2 is a representation of one family system. Within this system are often many subsystems, such as mother and hearing-impaired child, which may create problems between the mother and father. The child may recognize that there is not a strong coalition between the mother and father, and may use this information to play one against the other or may start developing behavior problems. Or the father may feel left out and drift farther away from developing a close relationship with the child. Subsystems may shift and change at different times, but they contribute to the way in which the family and special child behave.

Some family systems are very open and make changes with every suggestion made. Others are closed and will not allow external influences to enter the system. Either one of these types of systems can affect the success of intervention. A more closed family will make a strong attempt to maintain homeostasis or to make sure that the way the family functions remain the same. In terms of intervention, this might mean the family would agree with what you suggest but would not implement the suggested activities. In a totally open system, a family may flit from one professional to another and attempt to respond to every suggestion that

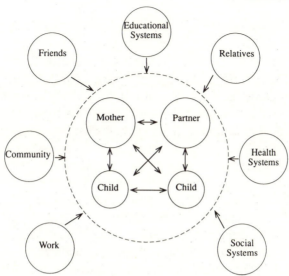

Figure 2. The family as a system. The hearing-impaired child is part of the total family system. Each family system will differ. In order to provide the most appropriate education for each child, it is essential to understand how the entire system and subsystems interact with each other and with the child—and that systems and subsystems can change.

is made. In a *relatively* open system, a family will maintain a balance of stability and make appropriate changes as needed.

Family systems are influenced by the immediate family and by relationships, myths, and rules that have been handed down through one or more generations. These intergenerational influences might affect how the family views education or whether the child wears a hearing aid. Looking beyond the immediate family to the extended family may provide insights and make sense of current problems.

As seen in figure 2, multiple systems may also influence the family and child. These influences range from the parent's type of job to hours that adults work to change in jobs (Brofenbrenner 1986). While the impact of all these systems on the family may appear to be overwhelming at first, the framework can provide a useful perspective to consider when working with families. That is, you are not the only one interacting with them and attempting to influence their lives. Awareness of the multiple factors that impact the family does not mandate that professionals act on each one. Rather, awareness can perhaps help shape intervention strategies that take into account the often complex reality of the family's situation.

Stress. Learning that a child is hearing impaired causes stress and affects the entire family system. Often many other systems, external to the family, become involved. This also impacts the family and may cause additional stress. It is helpful for professionals to recognize that, although proposed intervention strategies may help the hearing-impaired child, the family may not be able to implement these strategies. Family implementation depends on how this system is able to cope with either acute (diagnosis, telling friends and family, finding resources, etc.) or chronic (general, ongoing management) stress, or the *ongoing* process of grieving (denial, anxiety, guilt, depression, anger), which recurs throughout the hearing-impaired child's life (Moses 1985).

Being aware of, and at least attempting to understand, the child and family as a holistic system is a key to influencing a hearing-impaired child's potential for achievement and success as a well-adjusted human being. Legislators and professionals who were responsible for writing Public Law 99-457 recognized the importance of families and mandated that an Individual Family Service Plan (IFSP) be written whenever a child age birth to 3 entered a program. What is intended is that families be included as part of the team that decides what is desirable for all members of the family, including the special child.

Service delivery for families of children age birth to 3 years. Centers offer exciting opportunities for parent support groups and interaction among young children. Homes offer a natural, familiar, and consistent environment. A combination of center- and home-based intervention is optimal for families and hearing-impaired children from birth to 3 years. The children belong to a very low incidence population. Consequently, there are often not enough children in a given geographic area to justify developing a well-coordinated center-based program specifically designed to meet the special needs of hearing-impaired children. This is especially true in rural areas and small towns. Family needs may also make center programs impractical. Families with only one car that is used by one parent for business have no private transportation to travel to a center, or there may be insufficient funds for gas. Public transportation may be totally inconvenient, and school buses are not available for children from birth to 3 years. It is possible that there are siblings who have their own needs, such as transportation to or from school, or a nap. Meeting center-based schedules is not possible under those circumstances.

Home visits can be arranged at times convenient to the entire family so that dad or other adults and siblings can be involved in the learning process. Further, as stated earlier, it is critical to address the needs of the entire family because, following the identification of the hearing impairment, the parents' own needs may be neglected and the needs of the other children in the household may be overlooked. If left unaddressed, these instances of neglect can produce dysfunction within the family and have negative impact on the hearing-impaired child. Conducting at least the major portion of the program in the home and involving the whole family can help avoid these problems.

Some suggest that home-based programs require parents to be the primary teachers and, further, that many parents do not have the skills to teach or would prefer not to teach (Bailey and Simeonsson 1988). However, parents, other adult caregivers, and older siblings of hearing-impaired children, by their very interactions with the children, do provide ongoing teaching just as families of young normal hearing children do. It is much better for all of them to be well informed about how to use the home environment, utensils, and toys to provide the most enriching experiences, experiences that will help the hearing-impaired child to make continued progress, especially in such important and new areas as auditory training and language. Tharp and Wetzel (1969) assert that parents may be more effective than professionals. Parents have greater opportunities to influence behavior during more frequent interactions with the child in a wider range of settings than do "therapists" or teachers. The home is the natural environment for the young child, a place where he or she spends most of the time with important others, such as parents and other family members. Professionals can show parents how to use available materials and how to use them naturally every day at home while preparing food, eating, getting up, and going to bed. The optimal approach is when home visits are combined with a well-planned center-based program.

The importance of a curriculum written for parents. Most hearing parents of children whose hearing loss is newly identified need information—all kinds of information. A curriculum, written in nontechnical language, can provide information about the auditory system and hearing loss and also guidelines for working naturally with the child

Table 1
Birth to Three Years of Age Curriculum: Suggested Table of Contents

Introduction ....
Rationale for Home Visits ....
Parents and Trainers Working Together ....
Some General Suggestions About the Home Visits ....
Efficacy of Early Childhood Intervention ....
P.L. 99-457 and P.L. 101-476 ....
Assessment ....
IFSP ....
Family Systems ....
Communication and Language-Speech ....
Early Literacy ....
Play ....
Social Development ....
Total Communication (including various sign systems) ....
Early Environments that Encourage Communication, and Language
Development ....
      Part I: Communication Lessons ....
      Part II: Language Lessons ....
Auditory System (audiograms) ....
Amplification ....
Auditory Development ....
Auditory Training Lessons ....
Speech Development ....
      Speech Production Lessons ....
Transitioning ....
      Final Report ....
      Assessment ....
      Laws ....
      Rights ....
      Programs for 3 years to 5 years ....
Appendices ....
    A. Resources
    B. Charts of Normal Development

in such areas as language, auditory training, and speech. The curriculum should include basic information, be easy to follow, and provide a beginning for developing a partnership between the parents and whoever is working with them. Parents should have a copy of their own that they can read as they have time. This provides them with easily accessible and valuable information. A suggested table of contents (table 1) illustrates the many areas of content and activities that need to be provided in a comprehensive curriculum that will assist parents.

COMMUNICATION AND LANGUAGE—SPEECH

COMMUNICATION

Communication is the act of receiving and transmitting messages so that they are understood. Communication is the "umbrella" under which messages are communicated through facial expressions, body movements, music, and painting as well as *language* and *speech* (see figure 3). Communication is the primary function of language; it is the giving and/or receiving of information, signals, or messages in any form such as a glance, smile, nod, frown, pat on the shoulder, and more. Communication includes "reading" the nonverbal messages of others as well as listening to what they are communicating via speech and language. A child learns to see herself through her parents' eyes; her feelings of self-worth depend upon the messages her parents send. Children, according to Bruner (1978), communicate before they have language, and the development of language, a subset of communication, depends upon the prior development of communication (Kaye 1979).

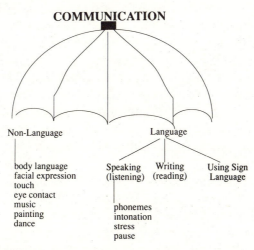

Figure 3. The umbrella of communication. Communication is essential to all human beings. It is important to recognize that young children, including hearing-impaired children, communicate first through looks and gestures. Later, children learn to use language to communicate and express their language through sign and speech.

Infants, early on, become communication partners because parents treat them as if they can make meaningful conversational contributions such as gazing, smiling, and cooing (Snow 1977). Very young children communicate intentionally by pointing, gesturing, or indicating in some nonverbal way what they want or need (e.g., Halliday 1975; Bates 1976).

It is very important to help parents identify the communicative intentions of their young hearing-impaired children. Many parents, even though they have other children, may fail to respond to their hearing-impaired child's attempts such as pointing to or picking up and giving a toy. Perhaps that is because these gestures are not always accompanied by vocalizations or because the parents are concentrating too hard on eliciting language or speech. Whatever the reason, we must assist parents in recognizing and rewarding the communicative attempts of their children, accompanying this recognition with appropriate language such as, "Oh, you want your bottle. Here it is." Reinforcing these early attempts encourages the continuation of communicative interaction and assists in building self-esteem.

LANGUAGE AND SPEECH

Language is composed of arbitrary symbols (words) that are agreed upon by a given society (or social group, such as teenagers). These words represent concepts and are combined using rules established and agreed upon by the same society or group. English is a language, whereas speech is one way to express language. Language, however, can also be expressed through writing or the use of sign. By using some form of signed English, one can maintain English word order and use English endings, or one can use American Sign Language (ASL or Ameslan), which is a separate language with its own rules. The main point is that speech is *not* synonymous with language and is not essential to expressing language.

"Language is a very complex system of symbols and rules for using those symbols" (Owens 1988). Hearing children apparently have little trouble learning the symbols of our language and the rules that direct use of these symbols. They receive language directly and indirectly for approximately 12 months before they begin to use it, and by 3 to 4 years are quite proficient in its use. As adults we have learned enough about our language and its rules to be able to identify language errors even though we cannot state the rules.

The socially agreed upon "code" of language allows people from that particular social group to communicate with each other. The code allows each person "to represent an object, event, or relationship without reproducing it" (Bloom and Lahey 1978). For example, if someone were to request that you help him find his red nylon jacket, you would be able to form a mental picture of the jacket and begin the search. You could also describe an airplane trip to friends. The friends could easily follow your story without being physically there because they have referents for and understand the language "code" you and they are using.

Language and hearing-impaired children. The focus on helping young hearing-impaired children get a good start in developing language is critical. Because we do not know how much distortion is present within the auditory system in these young children, we cannot be sure how much oral language is being received or understood. Therefore, while working on training the auditory system, it is essential to ensure that each child is also receiving consistent language input. One way to accomplish this is to help parents learn to use TC or total communication (Thompson and Swisher 1985). TC, when used as originally intended, stresses auditory input and oral production and, at the same time, recognizes the importance of ensuring *language* input. Therefore, TC would include use of amplification, lip reading, auditory training, training speech production, playing with and imitating sounds with infants and toddlers, encouraging vocalizations, providing good, consistent speech models, reinforcing the use of consistent sound patterns to represent an object or action, use of verbal language, and use of sign language (English). Although some parents and professionals believe that learning sign will be detrimental to learning speech, no *data* support this belief (Lowenbraun and Thompson 1988).

Speech production. Speech production, by producing language orally, is one way of expressing our language and communicating with others. We can also express our language by writing, or signing and fingerspelling. Speech production is complex because it involves very precise coordination between the neurologic, muscular, and motor systems to produce the sounds as well as an intact auditory system so that we can monitor and revise our speech errors. We have rules that tell us what speech sounds are in our language and how to put them together to form words (phonology). When we combine speech sounds according to the rules and articulate them in an acceptable fashion, we have produced speech.

Summary. Communication is the act of receiving and sending messages in many different ways whereas language is a complex system of symbols and rules. Language can be expressed by both speech and sign. The importance for young hearing-impaired children and their families is that they communicate in ways that are clear and supportive.

EARLY LITERACY

One might wonder how literacy is relevant to a discussion of very young children, especially those who are hearing impaired. It can, and does, but is not utilized as a "tool" for teaching as often as it could be. First of all, what is meant by early literacy? There is no dictionary definition, but early literacy includes the use of language, scribbling, and an interest in books. All of these activities appear to lead to increased use of language, reading, and writing later, in school. According to Morrow (1989), "the success of the school literacy program frequently depends on the literacy environment in the home." Since the ability to read becomes more critical to success the longer a child is in school, and since language is involved in the reading process, it is essential that we incorporate what is known about early literacy into programs for hearing-impaired children from birth to 3 and from 3 to 5 years of age.

FACTORS THAT AFFECT EARLY LITERACY

Many researchers have provided us with information about factors that appear to influence early literacy (e.g., Teale 1978; Morrow 1983), such as interpersonal interaction between the child, parents, siblings, and other adults, and the availability of materials such as books, paper, crayons, and pencils. Parents read newspapers, magazines, and books and spend time reading to their children. When children scribble and look at books, the behavior is rewarded by the parents. Parents also take their children to bookstores and libraries. These activities are not forced or *focused* on literacy but evolve through social interaction during each day through routines such as writing a grocery list, going to the store and reading the list, paying bills, recognizing fast-food stores, identifying license plates, writing and receiving "thank you" notes.

ACTIVITIES AT HOME

Morrow (1989) offers suggestions that will encourage literacy for young children. She recommends having both adult and children's books throughout the home and, in addition to crayons, paints, and pencils, providing felt boards and story tapes. Reading books and talking about the stories daily appear to provide an excellent beginning for literacy. It also can be a warm, social, pleasurable time for parents and children, and a time to use language in a meaningful way.

Parents can provide a model by reading and writing and by calling attention to all the things they do "read," from recipes to cereal boxes to constructing an item using written instructions. They can "read" to their children from the very beginning by looking at picture books and identifying people, objects, and actions. Although initially infants may mouth books, Lamme and Packer (1986) have an excellent description of how babies respond to "book reading" from birth to 15 months. They point out that babies who have been read to since birth will have definite "favorite" books at 6 months, and by 9 months will predict actions and make appropriate noises and gestures for the stories they favor. By 1 year, children are still listening but are almost taking the lead, especially if it is a familiar story. Initially, parents are pointing and labeling, then adding language about action. Eventually they ask questions about what will happen next. As children mature and can concentrate more on the story, parents can read the text rather than simply talk about the story, and children will begin to sense the relationship between the language of "telling" and the language of "writing."

The interactive language used during reading time also demonstrates a relationship between the real world and the world of books. For example, a parent might point to the shoes on the little girl in the book and then point to the child's shoes, labeling them and talking about them being the "same," an important concept for hearing-impaired children. Children gradually begin to use language themselves to label, tell parts of the story, and "make up" new endings. Ninio and Bruner (1978) call this type of parent-child reading routine "scaffolding dialogue" because the parent leads the child into labeling and "telling about," and provides assistance as necessary until the child can take over. As children's language skills increase, they can "scribble" representations of both pictures and the written word, thus completing the circle of oral/signed, written, and read language.

Table 2
Early Literacy at School

Student-centered curriculum
Teacher reads to students each day
    (later as children read, teacher reads to herself)
Teacher tells/writes stories each day
    make-believe
    events from home
    events at school
Children tell/"write"/draw stories each day
    (teacher actually writes stories at first)
    make-believe
    events from home
    events at school
    rhymes
Children "read" each day
Everyone talks about/dramatizes/draws stories
All components of language are simultaneously present
Positive classroom atmosphere (risk-free environment)
Learning is an active, constructive process

As children move into school at age 3, the same approach can be continued by using a student-centered curriculum or a whole language approach that involves principles of natural language learning (Norris and Damico 1990). Using such an approach, the teacher tells and reads stories every day. Children retell stories. The teacher writes these stories, which can then be "read" by the teacher and children and taken home to share and "read" with parents. The children can role-play or "act out" the stories and paint pictures depicting parts of the stories. Music for singing or dancing that relates to the stories can be employed (table 2 summarizes early literacy classroom characteristics). Such a classroom environment fosters relevant language, and the children are active participants. It is especially important for hearing-impaired children because it makes language useful, helps develop concepts, establishes an atmosphere of collaboration, provides auditory training experiences that are meaningful, and continues progress toward reading.

PLAY

Play is an activity to which young children devote a significant amount of time (Rubin, Fein, and Vandenberg 1983). The importance of play in children's lives has been recognized by including the right to play in the United Nation's Declaration of the Rights of the Child, along with adequate nutrition, housing, health care, and education (Almy 1984).

Since the late nineteenth century, theorists and researchers have acknowledged the influence of play on the child's cognitive, social, and emotional development, and have suggested a number of ways in which play facilitates various aspects of development. Piaget (1951) viewed play as an assimilatory activity in which the child could exert control over self and the environment and consolidate recently acquired skills, free from externally imposed rules and constraints. Vygotsky (1986) attributed a major role to pretend play in the acquisition of language and problem solving, maintaining that the symbolic nature of play serves as an essential link between early practical activity and later abstract thinking.

One line of current research has empirically investigated the role of pretend and sociodramatic, make-believe play in facilitating the cognitive and social development of young children. These studies have shown play as related to problem-solving abilities (e.g., Vandenberg 1981), measures of divergent thinking (e.g., Dansky 1980; Pepler and Ross 1981), social knowledge (e.g., Rubin 1980), and language (e.g., Rubin 1980). Findings from recent studies provide evidence that pretend play positively impacts various aspects of cognitive, social, and language development (e.g., Clark et al. 1989; Dansky 1985).

One possible explanation for the relationship found between pretend play and cognitive abilities, in particular, is that play enhances creative thought and active problem solving by allowing children to act and think in a flexible manner, to freely transform objects and situations, and to explore and generate novel ideas (Bruner 1972; Rubin et al. 1983; Trostle and Yawkey 1988).

Play is as universal to children as the stages of development, and that is certainly no coincidence. In fact, play and development are so linked that there is some confusion about which impacts the other. Does a child's developmental stage determine the kind of play the child will engage in, or does play allow learning that furthers the developmental progression? Actually, both statements can probably be made about the relationship between play and development. Play and development are mutually reinforcing (Athey 1984), and together they equip the child for managing her or his environment. Quinn and Rubin (1984) put it this way: "While play behavior reflects a child's development and thus follows a regular developmental sequence, play also serves as a way for children to focus and strengthen newly developed skills."

Since play is linked so closely to development, it is an appropriate subject for further investigation. In fact, there is a great deal about the subject that might not be apparent to the casual observer. This may come as a surprise to those who thought play was a frivolous, unimportant part of childhood that actually interfered with learning. Play is connected with every aspect of development, including cognitive, social, emotional, and physical development. However, the interaction of play and development is most plainly seen in the areas of cognitive and social development (Quinn and Rubin 1984).

DEFINING PLAY

Play is a category of human activity that is so common that the average person doesn't spend much time thinking about what play actually "is." If asked to define play, people are likely to first respond with familiar examples but then experience difficulty when they try to express just what it is about those examples that makes them "play." In fact, there are several kinds of play. The definition of play is subject to change depending on what type of play is being addressed. Piaget spoke of three stages of play—practice, pretend play, and games-with-rules—that apply from infancy through adolescence (Fein 1986). These kinds of play share three characteristics. First, they are motivated from within the child. Second, they are pleasurable and enjoyable to the child. Finally, attention is given to the performance of play behavior rather than the outcome of the behavior. This latter mind-set, however, changes as the child moves into the games-with-rules stage (Smith, Takhvar, Gore, and Vollstedt 1985). While these things are held in common, the various stages of play, have there are distinguishing characteristics.

PRACTICE PLAY

Practice play is not the first kind of play that usually leaps to mind when one thinks of playing. Practice play, or exploratory play, does not involve the pretending or game playing found in later stages of play. Exploratory play is performed by infants as they repeat newly acquired skills in response to objects around them or in response to a caregiver (Athey 1984). The very act of manipulating objects serves an important function in furthering motor development. Play contributes to the development of a child's mind. As infants play with objects, they learn about the properties of those objects. For example, they become familiar with hard and soft, bright and dim, smooth and rough, pliable and firm, mobile and stationary. In addition, the infant learns to define his or her self as separate from the surrounding objects, as an individual who acts on those objects (Athey 1984), another important aspect of cognitive development.

Infant exploratory play takes on an interactive flavor as caregivers participate in the child's playing. This kind of playful "exploration" is more social than the play discussed thus far and involves different kinds of learning. Children learn the basics of social behavior through caregiver-infant games, learning the social significance of gestures (such as smiling and waving) and eventually words (McHale and Olley 1982; Ninio and Bruner 1978). Infant play becomes increasingly sophisticated as the child learns turn taking during interactive games like peek-a-boo (Power and Parke 1982). Turn taking also becomes a part of language play between adults and infants, a type of exploratory play important to the discussion of language-delayed children.

An infant's first attempts at language are called "babbling," a behavior that is repetitive, pleasurable, instigated by the child, and not goal directed. Babbling can therefore be considered play (Athey 1984). Infant language play becomes interactive as caregivers respond to their child's sounds by actions like smiling and repeating sounds. The positive response of parents to infantile attempts at language rewards the behavior. The repetition of the baby's sounds can influence the selection of sounds made by the child (Athey 1984). Language learning takes place through the playful interactions naturally occurring between children and their parents.

PRETEND PLAY

Pretending is a magical kind of play. According to Piaget, pretend play is the act of changing the world into whatever a child desires, allowing the child to experience mastery and power (Bailey and Wolery 1989). In pretend play, the child has the freedom to try out new strategies for dealing with the world and to soar with the imagination into fantastic and impossible situations. These are fairly advanced levels of pretend play. However, as we will see, pretend play has much more down-to-earth beginnings.

Pretend play begins around 12 months of age. The first instances of solitary pretend play involve a child using a practical object to enact a familiar activity, with him- or herself as the reference point. An example is when a child pretends to feed him- or herself (Fein 1986). In the next level of solitary pretend play the child uses another object as the reference point of the play activity. An example is when a child pretends to feed a doll. This level of play takes place from about 15 to 21 months (Fein 1986). A more advanced level of solitary play is when the child steps out of the pretend situation and manipulates an object as if it were performing the actions. As an example, the child pretends that one doll is feeding another (Fein 1986).

In the beginning of solitary play, children play completely separate from one another. Eventually, though, children engage in parallel play, a kind of solitary play in which children proceed with their own individual activities with other children nearby (Athey 1984). That is, they play "next to" others without playing "with" them. At around 3 years of age, the child begins moving from solitary play to social play (Athey 1984). At first this is merely associative, but it turns into cooperative play as children mature (Mann 1981). In the social stage of pretend play, children enact miniature versions of adult activities as they learn to master motor skills (Athey 1984). Abstract thought begins to make its appearance in play as children apply problem solving and creativity to play situations (Athey 1984).

A number of studies have found relationships between pretend play in young children and various measures of divergent or creative thinking, such as ideational or associative fluency, and alternative or novel uses of objects. Dansky and Silverman (1973) found that preschoolers exposed to free play conditions generated more nonstandardized responses to objects than control subjects and subjects exposed to imitative play. Li (1978) found that kindergarten children assigned to a pretend play treatment group outperformed free play and control subjects on tests of alternative uses of unfamiliar objects. Clark et al. (1989) reported a longitudinal study indicating a relationship between children's symbolic play at preschool and aspects of creative behavior measured three years later. Pelligrini (1980) demonstrated the relationship between the skills needed for dramatic play demonstrated by kindergarten children and those required later for reading and writing.

Play is a medium through which children can learn new cognitive and language skills. For example, the first time a child pulls a string that makes the music, play may be considered work and an adaptive process by which the child learns a new skill and new thought process. Afterward, the child does it for pleasure, and it becomes "play." Play, then, promotes the consolidation of newly learned principles and actions through repetition. Although there is no *causal* relationship between language and play, there is certainly a correspondence between play and the *use* of language on the child's part. (See Appendix A.) Obviously, the adult-child interactions through play provide the perfect opportunity for language input. As children mature, play provides highly motivating opportunities for them to *use* language in meaningful ways, such as making pretend cookies for daddy or "writing" and "mailing" letters in the pretend post office. Finally, because play is relaxed and tension-free, it provides a risk-free environment in which children can explore materials, social interactions, and language that might be inhibited under more controlled formal conditions.

The inability to hear does not necessarily inhibit exploratory play. Young hearing-impaired children can, and do, explore the environment through vision, touch, taste, and smell. However, studies have found that hearing-impaired children are delayed in the onset of pretend play (Casby and McCormick 1985; Esposito and Koorland 1989; Higgenbotham and Baker 1981; Schirmer 1989).

Play is a child's work. Play is an activity that is highly motivational. Children, without any kind of prodding, willingly engage in all types of play, which leads to developmental progress and learning in *all* domains. It is a "naturally occurring" behavior that can be utilized by parents, teachers, and other caregivers to ensure that children continue to learn and to love learning. It needs to be included in every curriculum for the early years (birth through 5) of the hearing-impaired child.

TRANSITIONING

Transitioning is the bridge between programs for children from birth to 3 and from 3 to 5 years old. If the transition process is well planned and orchestrated, it can prove to be an exciting time for the family and the hearing-impaired child. Most hearing-impaired children, by age 3, are ready to join peers on a daily basis and enjoy new, more mature activities. Parents are delighted to see their hearing-impaired child progress. However, unless the transition is well planned and work with families is begun early, it can be a time of great stress for parents of hearing-impaired children because invited family participation is often reduced; therefore, problems may arise. In order to assist families during the transition period, it is critical to begin serious discussions about the *transition* process with the parents *at least one year* before the child enters school. There is a tremendous amount of information for them to digest. It usually takes a year for them to really begin to understand it all and to ask the questions they need to ask. Parents need to be informed about the initial intake process, which includes assessment and an IEP (Individual Education Plan), as well as similarities and differences between the programs and their rights as defined in P.L. 94-142.

Assessment. Most birth-to-3 programs use one or more developmental scales to determine the functional level of each child in the various domains (cognition, motor, social, language, etc.) and to monitor progress over time. For example, in our program (ECHI), we use a battery of scales and checklists to determine functional levels, including the Rockford Infant Developmental Scales (Project RHISE 1979), the Communicative Intention Inventory (Coggins and Carpenter 1981), the SKI*HI Language Development Scale (Tonelson and Watkins 1979), a cognitive checklist based upon Piagetian tasks, an auditory checklist based upon normal auditory development, and a speech checklist adapted from Ling (1976; 1988). Using these scales and checklists over time assists us in determining whether or not a child is progressing appropriately and provides us with a long-term overview of the child's behaviors. No test-taking skills are required.

When children enter school programs at 3 years of age, the assessment process is usually quite different. Children are expected to perform on standardized tests administered in a strange room by professionals they have never seen before. Often these professionals are not trained to work with hearing-impaired children. Nevertheless, the children are expected to respond by pointing or performing as instructed in a given period of time. They may even be removed from their parents. The separation can intensify the strangeness of the situation and reduce the ability of the child to communicate and to perform as required. All of these factors can result in poor test performance and lead to inaccurate conclusions about the child's ability. Poor results derived from such a "test" situation can be devastating to parents who have watched their child progress over time and know how well their child performs in a comfortable environment with familiar people. If the parents know their rights or have an advocate with them, they may refuse to accept the results. In addition, they may have their child entered into the program for the hearing impaired and observed for a period of time prior to making a final decision about placement. In the worst scenario, the child is misdiagnosed and placed in a program designed for severely delayed children with no other hearing-impaired children; a program that is not designed for hearing-impaired children will not focus on language, auditory training, and speech. There is a distinct difference between formal testing and the use of developmental scales and checklists. Parents also need to be advised that they can (1) take with them to the assessment process a professional who knows their child, (2) request further testing, (3) request placement and observation before further testing, and (4) not sign the IEP until they are totally satisfied with test results, placement, and program.

IEP VERSUS IFSP

Parents also need to be informed about the distinction between the IEP and the IFSP. During their involvement in the birth-to-3 programs, the entire family as well as the child with the hearing impairment are the focus of concern. The parents are encouraged to identify information they want and any needs they may have as well as what they want for their child. Parents are integral to developing the Individual Family Service Plan (IFSP). There is usually intensive involvement with the program and the professionals working in the program. When the child transitions to school, the IEP is usually developed by the multidisciplinary team and is focused on the child. Family needs are no longer addressed. Although by law (P.L. 94-142), parents are supposed to participate in developing the IEP, they often are only invited to a final meeting where already developed plans for the child are presented and they are asked to sign in order to indicate that they agree with the goals and objectives as written. Unless parents are informed ahead of time, they do not know that it is their right to participate in the entire process and to assist in identifying educationally appropriate goals and objectives for their child.

In addition to assessment, the IEP, and placement, parents need to discuss busing. Recognition that their small child has to ride a bus, often for an extended period of time, is an additional stress to the family. It often helps if parents understand that they will be able to follow the bus for a few days and determine for themselves that most children rather enjoy the ride. Parents will not be included as extensively in the school program as they were previously in the birth-to-3 program. In order to prevent feelings of being "left out" or "no longer needed," parents need to learn as much about school programs as possible and the school rules for visiting and participating. It is important for them to understand that, because their child is older and entering school, their involvement will change but will not be any less important.

WHAT CAN HELP

As mentioned earlier, it helps to start discussing the transitioning process with parents at least one year before the child enters school. At that time, parents should be provided with a packet that includes information about P.L. 94-142, assessment, the IEP, and their rights. Rules and regulations from the state where their child will attend school are also helpful and should be included in the packet. Such information should specify steps parents can take if they are not satisfied with the assessment process, IEP, and/or placement. It is important and helpful to have a sample IEP in the packet for the parents to review. A checklist of what to look for in a program for 3- to 5-year-olds should also be included so that parents know what to look for when they visit. If possible, parents should visit several programs so they can observe similarities and differences and decide what is appropriate for their child's education. Parents whose child is entering the program will benefit from talking to parents whose child entered school one or two years previously. We have found that writing a very complete final report that provides all information about the child and family from entry to exit from the birth-to-3 program is also very helpful to parents and school districts. When districts have a complete report with accompanying documentation, they are less likely to rely as heavily on the results of their brief assessment. If the birth-to-3 program is monitoring all domains, it also facilitates the transition process if birth-to-3 personnel transfer their results to the specific forms of the receiving school district.

It is very beneficial to parents, school personnel, and child if personnel from the birth-to-3 program are personally acquainted and work closely with personnel from the programs for 3- to 5-year-olds, sharing information and taking parents and child to visit before starting the program. During the visit, the parents can meet the principal, teacher, and others who will provide services to their child, such as the audiologist and speech-language pathologist. Parents can observe the curriculum being implemented, ask questions about it and other facets of the program, while the child participates with the other children. Visits, if handled appropriately, help everyone become acquainted, reduce tensions, and generally facilitate a smoother, friendlier transition for child, family, and school personnel.

CURRICULUM: 3 TO 5 YEARS

A curriculum can be viewed as a road map—a means of helping us get from one place to another. It can be very structured and specify step-by-step how to help a child accomplish a new objective. Or a curriculum might, instead, be a set of goals and objectives. No matter what the type of curriculum, one of the major determinants of *quality* is the degree to which the program is developmentally appropriate (Bredekamp 1987). Young children need both active and quiet times. They learn best through play and through doing, not through the use of inappropriate formal teaching techniques where they must always sit quietly and listen while adults talk to them. It is important to resist the demand for formal teaching techniques that overemphasize narrowly defined academic skills and that use strictly supervised pencil and paper activities that are developmentally inappropriate (Bredekamp 1987). According to Elkind (1986), the stress on early academic skills is a result of a misconception about how children learn. Developmental learning will make content more relevant to the young child (such as learning to button a sweater and count the buttons at the same time) and integrate learning from two content areas such as learning to print your name so you can "sign" your dictated story or your artwork. From experts such as Piaget (1951), Bruner (1978), Cazden (1988), and Kamii (1985), we know that learning is a very complex process and that children learn best by being active participants in the learning process: exploring, experimenting, questioning, and learning to use increasingly more complex language to facilitate the entire process.

Although all of the above information relates to normal hearing children, it is of the utmost importance that we, as professionals, remember that hearing-impaired children are children first and that most follow the same developmental patterns and have the same developmental needs as hearing children. Therefore, the same approach to learning that benefits normal hearing children will also benefit normally developing children who have a hearing impairment.

Appropriate curriculum goals will therefore

1. Encourage learning in all domains: physical, social, emotional, cognitive, language/literacy, speech, and audition.
2. Encourage learning through play.
3. Encourage active participation in the learning process.
4. Ensure that each child is appreciated for his or her uniqueness in ability, development, interests, and style of learning.
5. Help develop a sense of curiosity about the world.
6. Help instill a love of learning by providing a risk-free environment in which to learn.
7. Encourage children to develop positive feelings about themselves and others.

PARENTS

During the early stages of birth to 3 years, curriculum for the hearing impaired focuses on parents, providing them with information and suggesting ways for them to interact with their child in warm, creative ways and in natural environments. As the hearing-impaired child reaches 3 years of age and enters school and the curriculum focus shifts more toward the child, it is important to remember that the child is still one part of a total family system. Parental involvement and participation still need to be considered in curriculum development so that the relationship between home and school is strengthened and the hearing-impaired child benefits from continuity of learning. This can be accomplished in several ways, such as parents participating in the classroom when they can, visiting periodically, having evening preschool parent group meetings, sending a notebook back and forth on a daily basis to describe special events and activities, or scheduling one day each week when teachers make home visits. A positive partnership will increase the potential learning for each child. The emphasis is on developing *positive* interactions from the beginning, not waiting until something "bad" happens to make the first contact with parents.

LANGUAGE

Language is central to learning and communication for all humans. It is essential that young hearing-impaired children learn all aspects of language and how to use language appropriately in different environments. The curriculum for 3- to 5-year-old hearing-impaired children is language centered (see figure 1). It is also concept based because "language maps onto or encodes a child's existing knowledge" (Mclean and Snyder-Mclean 1978). Although they may first learn a concept from an intuitive perspective and use a label for it before they have fully realized the adult concept, children begin by talking about things they know and grafting language onto their existing knowledge about their world (Owens 1988). They must be actively involved in the learning process because their experiences are the basis for early language development.

ENVIRONMENT

The arrangement of the environment, or the classroom, reflects the philosophy of the curriculum and of the adults responsible for implementing it. Children learn best by being active participants in the learning process and, therefore, need enough space for active learning. This is particularly important for hearing-impaired children who need an experiential approach to learning concepts. Seeing, tasting, feeling, and smelling are very effective channels of sensory input for all children, especially for the hearing impaired.

To facilitate this particular style of learning, it is helpful to establish "learning" or "interest" areas within a large room. Children then can move from one area to another and can be provided with new information in each area. Each area provides special materials and different learning opportunities. The various areas would include (1) a messy area for painting, water and sand play, and cooking; (2) a building area with different size blocks, boxes, boards for ramps and roads, wood scraps, barns, doll houses, cars, and trucks; (3) a quiet area with pillows, crayons, paper, and picture books; (4) a home center with child-size sink, stove, refrigerator, beds, dolls, dress-up clothes, dishes, and play foods; (5) a science area, which might change with the seasons as well as house the class pet; (6) a snack area; and (7) a large area for group activities such as language and auditory training including marching or dancing. Every curriculum should include large muscle activities. Therefore, a gym and playground with equipment would also be a part of the necessary environment. Equipment within the interest areas should be kept on shelves or in cabinets that are readily accessible to young children. Such an arrangement assists in learning self-help skills and responsibility, which contribute to social development and positive self-esteem. Field trips to parks, stores, classrooms with older hearing-impaired children, homes of classmates, and so forth should also be included in the curriculum. The environment, therefore, is established to encourage children to learn through active participation (play) with materials, adults, and peers. A daily schedule within the curriculum would include group and individual times, physical (fine and gross motor) development, social interaction, and cognitive development all with the central focus on language development. Every daily schedule must be *flexible* to take advantage of *spontaneous learning events*.

A sample schedule might include the following:

Arrival. Adults greet the children. Depending upon language level, they ask about how they are and what they did last night, and receive notebooks from home. This interaction builds upon the *social* use of language. Each child has a special place for clothing and personal items for sharing time, and then puts his or her things away (with or without assistance as necessary). Activities such as these contribute toward the development of independence and identification of "me" as a person who has a special place to keep things. With the assistance of the teacher, audiologist, or speech-language pathologist, each child checks his or her hearing aids and batteries or replaces the personal hearing aid with an FM instrument. This activity ensures that hearing aids are in good working condition and also helps children learn that *they* are responsible for the maintenance of their hearing aids.

Free choice. Children select the interest (learning) center they are interested in and play (work) there until everyone has arrived. Adults who are not involved in greeting or checking hearing aids monitor the learning centers and provide appropriate assistance and language input.

Group time. This may include calendar time and may be divided into different levels depending upon concept-language development. It might also include a time for sharing something special, either something concrete such as a baseball cap or a new stuffed animal, or telling about a special treat such as going to a party or to the ice-cream store with the family. It is also the time to talk about what will happen during the school day and who the helpers are for the various tasks.

Group auditory training and speech. Five to ten minutes are spent on something active such as marching to music or playing musical instruments to accompany a recording or dancing. This is active and involves whole body movement, which is essential for young children. Marching and dancing also provide a nice transition from one activity to another. During the second part of group time, the children are divided according to language-concept level into two or three groups. The auditory training might be combined with language-math concepts, for example, and involve feeding the cookie monster one, two, three, or more cookies. Depending upon the language level of the child, the interaction might be between the adult and child or one child telling another child "how many" cookies to feed cookie monster and checking to see if the amount was correct. The children are "working" on many skills through play. They are interested because the subject (cookie monster) is known to them and is a fun character they like, and they are actively involved. In a public school program, the speech-language pathologist who works in the classroom might be responsible for one group or move from group to group.

Gym or outdoor play. Large muscle development is important and would include running and skipping, climbing, riding trikes, swinging, and so forth. This is an excellent time for providing language input and, as children are able, having them *use* language themselves.

Washing and snack time. As children return to the classroom, some facility is available for toileting and washing hands. The "helpers" distribute napkins, placemats with each child's name, and whatever else is appropriate. While the "helpers" are busy, the other children are involved in a story, fingerplay, poem, or song. When snacks are ready, each child is assisted in finding her place by "reading" her name. Snack time is an excellent time to learn to try new foods, learn good manners, learn about reading labels and, of course, receive and use language.

Cleanup time. Each child is responsible for disposing of "throw away" products or putting dishes in the sink. "Helpers" collect placemats and wash tables. The other children are given different color tags and directed to their color group. As helpers finish, they also receive a color and find the appropriate group.

Group time. This is a time for a variety of activities that relate to social interaction through sharing, telling, dramatizing, concept development, and language. One day might be making and baking cookies for Father's Day. The baking of cookies could be followed by creating a card (painting, cutting and pasting, crayoning, etc.) for Dad and writing something special inside. Another day might involve the teacher reading a story, the children telling their version of the story to the teacher who writes it down and helps read it back. The story might be dramatized, or an art project might be planned where the children paint or draw pictures about the story. Children who need it can spend time on individual work and still be able to participate in the group activities.

Cleanup and dismissal. If props or art materials have been used, it is important to help children understand that they are responsible for assisting in cleanup. After cleanup is a good time to read a short story, poem, or rhyme, or sing a song. Children collect their wraps, art projects, notebooks, etc., and say good-bye to teachers and each other—important for good manners and appropriate social use of language.

Although arrangement of time and variety of activities will vary from place to place, the above schedule is used to demonstrate how much content a curriculum can offer to children in an environment that fosters active participation and learning through play. Work on speech production and auditory training can occur within a meaningful context so that young hearing-impaired children will learn how important and useful these skills are and also learn how to use them in "real-life" situations. While they are learning language, they are expanding their cognitive knowledge, social skills, responsibility, and self-esteem.

SUMMARY

The early years from birth to 5 are important years for all children, especially those who are hearing impaired. Professionals and families need to ensure that those years are rich and positive so that the children's potential to learn can be enhanced. Although there are some differences between programs for hearing-impaired children from birth to 3 years and from 3 to 5 year, such as greater involvement of parents in the earlier years, there are many similarities. These include an emphasis on an experiential approach, often referred to by adults as "play";

reinforcement of the child's *communication* attempts; consistent auditory training; and language as the central focus.

Enjoyable and exploratory early years will assist young children in developing positive self-concept, language, and social skills that will help them the rest of their lives.

REFERENCES

Almy, M. 1984. A child's right to play. *Young Children* 39(4):80.

Athey, I. 1984. Contributions to play of development. In T.D. Yawkey and A.D. Pellegrini (eds.), *Child's play: Developmental and applied* (pp. 11-27). Hillsdale, N.J.: Lawrence Erlbaum Associates.

Bailey, D.B., and Simeonsson, R.J. 1988. Home-based early intervention. In S. Odom and M. Karnes (eds.), *Early intervention for infants and children with handicaps* (pp. 199-215). Baltimore, Md.: Paul H. Brookes Publishing Co.

Bailey, D.B., and Wolery, M. 1989. *Assessing infants and preschoolers with handicaps*. Columbus, Ohio: Merrill.

Bates, E. 1976. Language and context. In *The acquisition of pragmatics*. New York: Academic Press.

Bloom, L., and Lahey, M. 1978. *Language development and language disorders*. New York: John Wiley and Sons.

Bredekamp, S. (ed.). 1987. Developmentally appropriate practice in early childhood programs serving children from birth through age 8: Expanded ed. Washington, D.C.: NAEYC.

Bronfenbrenner, U. 1986. Ecology of the family as a context for human development: Research perspectives. *Developmental Psychology* 22:723-742.

Bruner, J. 1972. The nature and uses of immaturity. *American Psychologist* 27:687-708.

Bruner, J. 1978. Learning how to do things with words. In J. Bruner and A. Burton (eds.), *Wolfson College lectures 1976: Human growth and development*. Oxford: Oxford University Press.

Casby, M.W., and McCormick, S.M. 1985. Symbolic play and early communication development in hearing impaired children. *Journal of Communication Disorders* 18:67-78.

Cazden, C. 1988. *Classroom discourse: The language of teaching and learning*. Portsmouth, N.H.: Heinsmann.

Clark, P.M., Griffing, P.S., and Johnson, L.G. 1989. Symbolic play and vocational fluency as aspects of the evolving divergent cognitive style in young children. *Early Child Development and Care* 51:77-88.

Coggins, T., and Carpenter, R. 1989. The communicative intention inventory: A system for observing and coding children's early intentional communication. *Applied Psycolinguistics* 2:235-252.

Dansky, J.F. 1980. Cognitive consequences of sociodramatic play and exploration training for economically disadvantaged preschoolers. *Journal of Child Psychology and Psychiatry* 20:47-58.

Dansky, J.F. 1985. Questioning "A paradigm questioned": A commentary on Simon and Smith. *Merrill-Palmer Quarterly* 31(3):279-284.

Dansky, J.F., and Silverman, I.W. 1973. Effects of play on associative fluency in preschool-aged children. *Developmental Psychology* 9:38-43.

Elkind, D. 1986. Formal education and early childhood development: An essential difference. *Phi Delta Kappan* 631-636.

Esposito, B.G., and Koorland, M.A. 1989. Play behavior of hearing impaired children: Integrated and segregated settings. *Exceptional Children* 55:1095-1118.

Fein, G. 1986. The affective psychology of play. In A. Gottfried and C. Brown (eds.), *Play interactions: The contribution of play materials and parental involvement to children's development.* Lexington, Mass.: Lexington Books.

Halliday, M. 1975. *Learning how to mean: Explorations in the development of language.* London: Edward Arnold.

Halpern, R., and Parker-Crawford, F. 1982. Young handicapped children and their families: Patterns of interaction with human service institutions. *Infant Mental Health Journal* 3:51-63.

Higgenbotham, D.J., and Baker, B.M. 1981. Social participation and cognitive play differences in hearing-impaired and normally hearing preschoolers. *Volta Review*, April, 135-149.

Kamii, C. 1985. Leading primary education toward excellence: Beyond worksheets and drill. *Young Children* 40(6):3-9.

Kaye, K. 1979. Thickening thin data: The material role in developing communication and language. In M. Bullowa (ed.), *Before speech.* New York: Cambridge University Press.

Lamme, L.L., and Packer, A.B. 1986. Bookreading behaviors of infants. *The Teaching Teacher*, February, 504-509.

Li, A.K. 1978. Effects of play on novel responses in kindergarten children. *Alberta Journal of Educational Research* 24:31-36.

Ling, D. 1976. *Speech and the hearing-impaired child.* Washington, D.C.: A.G. Bell Association.

Ling, D. 1988. *Foundations of spoken language for hearing impaired children.* Washington, D.C.: A.G. Bell Association.

Lowenbraun, S., and Thompson, M.D. 1988. Environments and strategies for learning and teaching. In *Handbook of special education: Research and practice.* Vol. 3: *Low incidence conditions.* New York: Pergamon Press.

McHale, S.M., and Olley, J.G. 1982. Using play to facilitate the social development of handicapped children. *Topics in Early Childhood Education* 2:76-86.

Mclean, J., and Snyder-Mclean, L. 1978. *A transactional approach to early language training.* Columbus, Ohio: Merrill.

Mann, L. 1981. *Play and the non-verbal child.* Paper presented at the Annual Meeting of the National Association for the Education of Young Children.

Morrow, L.M. 1983. Home and school correlates of early interest in literature. *Journal of Educational Research* 76:221-230.

Morrow, L. 1989. The home as a vehicle for literacy development. In *Literacy development in the early years: Helping children read and write* (pp. 22-37). Englewood Cliffs, N.J.: Prentice Hall.

Moses, K.L. 1985. Dynamic intervention with families. In E. Cherow, N. Matkin, and R. Trybus (eds.), *Hearing impaired children and youth with developmental disabilities* (pp. 82-98). Washington, D.C.: Gallaudet College Press.

Ninio, A., and Bruner, J. 1978. The achievement and antecedents of labeling. *Journal of Child Language* 5:5-15.

Norris, J., and Damico, J. 1990. Whole language in theory and practice: Implications for language intervention. *Language, Speech, and Hearing Services in the Schools* 21:212-220.

Owens, R. 1988. *Language development: An introduction.* 2d ed. Columbus, Ohio: Merrill.

Pelligrini, A. 1980. The relationship between kindergartner's play achievement in prereading, language, and writing. *Psychology in the Schools* 17:530-535.

Pepler, D.J., and Ross, H.S. 1981. The effects of play on convergent and divergent problem-solving. *Child Development* 52:1202-1210.

Piaget, J. 1951. *Play, dreams, and imitation in childhood.* New York: Norton.

Power, T.G., and Parke, R.D. 1982. Play as a context for early learning. In Laosa and Sigel (eds.), *Families as learning environments for children.* New York: Plenum Press.

Project RHISE. 1979. *Manual for administration of the Rockford infant developmental evaluation scales (RIDES).* Bensenville, Ill.: Scholastic Testing Service.

Quinn, J., and Rubin, K. 1984. The play of handicapped children. In T. Yawkey and K. Rubin (eds.), *Child's play: Developmental and applied.* Hillsdale, N.J.: Lawrence Erlbaum Associates.

Rubin, K. 1980. Fantasy play: Its role in the development of social skills and social cognition. *New Directions for Child Development* 9:69-84.

Rubin, K., Fein, G., and Vandenberg, B. 1983. Play. In E.M. Hetherington (ed.), *Handbook of child psychology: Socialization, personality, and social development*, vol. 4 (pp. 693-774). New York: Wiley.

Schirmir, B.R. 1989. Relationship between imaginative play and language development in hearing-impaired children. *American Annals of the Deaf* July, 219-222.

Smith, P.K., Takhvar, M., Gore, N., and Vollstedt, R. 1985. Play in young children: Problems of definition, categorization, and measurement. *Early Child Development and Care* 19:25-41.

Snow, C. 1977. The development of conversation between mothers and babies. *Journal of Child Language* 4:1-22.

Swisher, M.V., and Thompson, M.D. 1985. Mothers learning simultaneous communication: The dimensions of the task. *American Annals of the Deaf*, July, 212-217.

Teale, W.H. 1978. Positive environments for learning to read: What studies of early readers tell us. *Language Arts* 55:922-932.

Tharp, R., and Wetzel, R. 1969. *Behavior modification in the natural environment*. London: Academic Press.

Thompson, M.D., and Swisher, M.V. 1985. Acquiring language through total communication. *Ear and Hearing* 6:29-32.

Tonelson, S., and Watkins, S. 1979. *The instruction manual for the ski*hi language development scale*. Logan, Utah: Project SKI*HI.

Trostle, S., and Yawkey, T. 1988. Facilitating creative thought through object play in young children. *The Journal of Creative Behavior* 17(3):181-189.

Vandenberg, B. 1981. The role of play in the development of insightful tool-using strategies. *Merrill-Palmer Quarterly* 27:97-109.

Vygotsky, L. 1986. *Thought and language*. 3d ed. Cambridge, Mass.: MIT Press.

Appendix A
Approximate Age, Play, and Corresponding Language

Play	Language

Six to Seven Months:

Play	Language
Holds toy and plays actively with rattle.	Makes an increased variety of sounds.
Looks at self in a mirror, smiles, vocalizes, and pats the mirror.	Listens to own voice.
Watches things and movement about her.	
Can amuse self and keep busy for at least 15 minutes at a time.	

Nine Months:

Play	Language
Bangs one toy against another.	Combines syllables.
Imitates arm movements such as splashing in the tub, crumpling paper, shaking a rattle.	Copies sounds when she hears them, such as voice sounds or other sounds with tongue or mouth.
Manipulates all objects within reach.	
Pleasure of motor activities dominates.	Pays attention to own name and to "no-no."

Twelve Months:

Play	Language
Responds to music.	Can imitate some familiar words.
Examines toys and objects with eyes and hands, feeling them, poking them, and turning them around.	Meaningfully uses some other words in addition to "ma-ma" and "da-da."
Likes to put objects in and out of container.	Will hand you a block or a toy or familiar object upon request.
Instrumental activity, e.g., hits one toy with another.	
May use just one toy in an activity.	
Activities change quickly.	
Strategies used in grouping objects not clear.	
No make-believe.	
Activities may involve own body, e.g., items on head, items in mouth.	
More complex activities begin with some activities adapted to conventional use of objects.	
Activity more restrained and localized on fewer objects.	
Uses brush to brush, for example, but activity deteriorates quickly.	

Play	Language

Eighteen Months:

Purposefully moves toys and other objects from one place to another. Often carries a doll or stuffed animal about with her.

Likes to play with sand, letting it run between fingers and pouring it in and out of containers.

Hugs a doll or stuffed animal, showing affection or other personal reaction to it.

Likes picture books of familiar objects.

Scribbles spontaneously with a pencil or crayon.

Plays with blocks in a simple manner—carrying them around, fingering, and handling them gathering them together—but does not build purposefully with them. It takes many trials before she can make three to four stand in a tower.

Imitates simple things she sees others do, such as "reading" a book.

Activities more dispersed.

Toys may be adequately chosen but not always used appropriately, e.g., child may brush hair and socks.

Items are grouped by spatial, functional criteria used in grouping not always clear.

Vocabulary consists of from 5 to 20 single words, usually names of people, familiar objects, or activities. Chatter in nonverbal sounds or jargon, which often takes on adult inflections of voice and sounds as if she were "talking" in another language.

Understands some language, often responding to such directions as: "Come here," "Give me a hug," "Do you want some milk?"

Can point to familiar objects in pictures, to objects in the room, and to parts of the body such as eyes, ears, and nose.

Listens to rhymes and songs, and interesting repetitions of sounds for short periods.

By Nineteen to Twenty Months:

Begins to use toys only for designated purpose, i.e., use brush only to brush hair.

Twenty-four Months:

Likes to investigate and play with small objects such as toy cars, blocks, pebbles, sand, and water.

Has a vocabulary of from 18 to several hundred words.

Play	Language

Twenty-four Months: (continued)

Likes to play with large objects such as buggies and wagons, which she can push, and in which she can carry things.

Likes to play with messy materials such as clay, patting and pinching and fingering it.

Can snip with scissors but is awkward.

Imitates everyday household activities such as cooking, hanging up clothes. These are usually activities with which she is closely associated and things she sees rather than remembers.

Plays with blocks, lining them up or using them to fill wagons or other toys. Can, with urging, build a tower of six or seven blocks.

Knows function of objects and uses appropriately.

Symbolic play; box used as bed, pretends to drink.

"Make-believe" play emerges; teddy bear becomes a playmate.

Uses less nonverbal jargon.

Tries to use words in telling physical needs or answering simple questions, but does not carry on conversations.

Is beginning to use pronouns, especially "me" and "mine."

Combines two and three words to express an idea, such as "Daddy gone," or "Want a drink."

Understands simple directions and simple requests.

Carries on a "conversation" with self or with dolls.

Talks about what she is doing, though much of the "conversation" may still be jargon.

Asks the names of things, "What's that?" "What's this?"

Listens to simple stories, especially liking those she has heard before.

Three Years:

Pushes trains, cars, fire engines in make-believe activities.

Cuts with scissors, not necessarily in a constructive manner.

Makes well-controlled marks with crayon or pencil and sometimes attempts to draw simple figures.

Gives rhythmic physical response to music, clapping or swaying, or marching.

Initiates own play activities when supplied with interesting materials.

Likes to imitate activities of others, especially real-life activities.

Uses language easily to tell a story or relay an idea to someone else.

Expresses feelings, desires, and problems verbally.

Uses longer sentences, often with complex structure.

Uses plurals, past tense, personal pronouns, and prepositions such as "on," "behind," "under," "in front of."

Listens and can be reasoned with verbally.

Refers to self as "I."

Play	Language

Three Years: (continued)

Makes playhouses for dolls in corners or under tables.

Plays going to the store or going traveling; imitates activities she has closely observed.

Is beginning to make simple forms with clay, such as little round balls or long "snakes."

Uses blocks with more imagination, making trains and fences and streets and piling them into trucks for coal. Plays with them in combination with other toys.

"Make-believe" with dominant interest in animated toys such as dolls, teddy bears.

Play partner (doll) becomes more active, e.g., doll is fed, washed, put to bed, read to.

Absent objects or people introduced in play and symbolic substitutions are made.

Knows many such items as last name, sex, the name of the street she lives on (but not the number), and a few rhymes.

Listens to longer and more varied stories.

Speech may be infantile, but is usually understood, even by those outside the family.

Chapter 28

An Ecological and Developmental/Contextual Approach to Intervention with Children with Chronic Otitis Media

Lynne V. Feagans, Kristi Hannan, and Elizabeth Manlove

INTRODUCTION

Educators and developmental psychologists have only recently been involved in studying the relationship between health and development in normally developing young children. Although there has been a recognition that serious chronic and acute illnesses affect developmental processes (e.g., childhood cancer, diabetes, and other disabilities), the realization that mild illnesses may affect development has come more slowly. Interventions designed to promote children's development in the face of chronic illness have taken even longer.

The case of otitis media is an especially important one to consider for three reasons. First, it is the second most frequent reason parents take their children to the doctor (Teele, Klein, and Rosner 1984). Second, up to one-third of infants and toddlers have chronic middle ear disease (more than three reported episodes a year in the first three years of life). The third reason relates to the developmental consequences of the disease that may result in a host of delays or problems as the child grows older. Because many of the episodes of otitis media are silent, with no overt symptoms, it is often difficult to diagnose every episode. This is especially true in the crucial early years of life when the child cannot tell anyone that he or she has otitis media. Additionally, while antibiotics can be effective in treating a bacterial infection, they are not effective in reducing the fluid that builds up in the middle ear. This fluid usually causes a mild-to-moderate hearing loss that has been shown to be related to short- and long-term effects on language development, mother-child interaction, attention in the classroom, and standardized test performance (Lim in press).

Because otitis media is so frequent and may cause developmental delays, it is important to understand the nature of these problems in order to develop effective interventions. At the recent Fifth International Symposium on Otitis Media, researchers reported findings from a number of different recent studies. Friel-Patti and Finitzo (1990) reported from a cross-sectional study that children's early experience with otitis media related to hearing over time and emerging receptive and expressive language skills. Better language was associated with better hearing levels, suggesting that the relationship between otitis media and language is mediated by hearing. In a study of 106 children followed prospectively, Wendler-Shaw, Menyuk, and Teele (1991) found a negative correlation for male subjects between the amount of otitis media in the first 2 years of life and scores on the Peabody Picture Vocabulary Test (PPVT), a measure of receptive vocabulary. Friel-Patti and Finitzo (1990) found similar results in a study of 483 children followed prospectively from enrollment in day care at 6 months. Hearing levels between 6 and 12 months were significantly related to PPVT scores at 36 months of age. Several other studies indicated that children with chronic otitis media had poorer phonological skills and were less intelligible at 1 and 2 years of age (Luloff, Menyuk, and Teele 1991; Feagans and Blood 1991).

Feagans and Blood (1991) reported that children between 12 and 18 months of age with many bouts of otitis media attended less well to language during book reading in comparison to children who had few bouts of otitis media, suggesting that attention may also be affected by otitis media. They also found that these children with chronic otitis media were rated by their parents as more distractible.

Finally, several papers (Wallace, Gravel, and Ganon 1991; Chase, Teele, Klein, and Rosner 1991) suggested that otitis media may actually affect the way parents interact with their children, with parents of high otitis children using less optimal strategies. These authors speculate that otitis-prone children display behavior that can adversely affect the way parents interact with them.

In summary, there is now good evidence that at least some children experience hearing loss and other developmental delays linked to experience with otitis media early in life. But who are the children most at risk? And how can interventions be designed to prevent problems?

RISK GROUPS TO BE TARGETED FOR INTERVENTION

Some children are more likely than others to get this disease and thus to suffer effects on development. There are a number of risk factors for otitis media. Nine of them will be discussed below.

First, otitis media is most prevalent in the first 2 years of life, then decreases over the later preschool years (Paradise 1980). Thus, children are most at risk for having chronic problems with otitis media in the first few years of life when many skills are being developed (Giebink 1988).

Second, children who suffer their first episode in the first year of life are those who will most likely continue to get frequent episodes (Lundgren, Ingvarrson, and Olofsson 1984; Klein in press). Clearly, the earlier the onset, the more likely that the child will have chronic problems with this disease early in life.

Third, day-care attendance, especially in the early years of life, has also been linked to higher rates of otitis media. This is probably due to the fact that the children are exposed to large groups of peers, and that otitis media is often a secondary infection from contagious upper respiratory infections (Fiellau-Nikolajsen 1979; Lundgren et al. 1984). A recent study from the Centers for Disease Control (Hurwitz, Gunn, Pinsky, and Schonberger 1991) indicated a complicated picture of the increased risk of upper respiratory infection in day care: Infants and toddlers were at increased risk of illness, as were children in day care who had no siblings. The study also concluded that among children aged 36 to 59 months, those who had been in day care for 27 or more months had a lower risk of illness than those unexposed to day care, suggesting that long periods in day care can lead to lower rates of illness. A recent study of 1,335 children from birth to 60 months (Froom and Culpepper 1991) found that histories of recurrent acute otitis media, poor hearing, and tonsillectomy or adenoidectomy were all more frequent in day-care-attending children, ages 25 to 60 months. On the other hand, they found that day-care children were brought to the doctor more promptly after the onset of symptoms than non-day-care-attending children.

Fourth, children from lower socioeconomic status homes have been reported to have more episodes of otitis media than children from middle-income homes. This has been shown in the U.S. and other countries (Cambon, Galbraith, and Kong 1965; Pukander, Sipila, and Karma 1984). One factor that might account for the higher incidence in poor families is crowding, since urban children have more otitis media than rural children. In addition, poor families often have more people living in a small space. It is estimated that children in these families have five or six times the incidence of otitis media (Paradise 1980).

The fifth risk factor is season of the year. Upper respiratory infections are more frequent in the winter than the summer months. Since otitis media is often associated with an upper respiratory infection, its incidence, too, is much higher in the winter. Figure 1 shows the incidence of otitis media by month in 80 infants and young children from the Pennsylvania State University Health and Daycare Project (Feagans and Blood 1991). The frequency of otitis media varies systematically by season, with otitis media higher in the winter months and lower in the summer months. The overall frequency of otitis media and other upper respiratory infections in these young children is very high, with the average child experiencing middle ear effusion about 25% of the time.

Sixth, children with various health or genetic problems have also been shown to be at increased risk for otitis media. Children who are premature tend to have more otitis media (Berman, Balkany, and Simmons 1978). In addition, children with Down syndrome and those with cleft palate also have more otitis media (Paradise 1980).

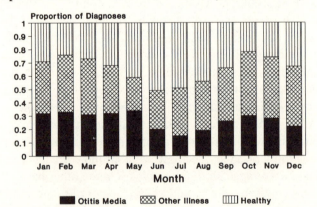

Figure 1. Incidence of otitis media and other illness from the Pennsylvania State University Health and Daycare Project.

Seventh, there does seem to be a genetic component in this disease. Although the mechanism is not clear, many studies have reported that certain families have more otitis media than others (Paradise 1980). This may be due to the inheritance of certain structural features of the ear as well as susceptibility to upper respiratory infections, which often lead to otitis media.

Eighth, certain ethnic groups seem to be more predisposed to otitis media. American Indian and Eskimo populations have much more otitis media than whites and especially than African-Americans (Giebink 1988). Again, this may be due to differences in structural features of the ear and susceptibility to illness.

Finally, recent evidence suggests that there may not be differences in the rates of otitis media for boys and girls. The effects on development, however, may be more pronounced for boys than girls (Wendler-Shaw et al. 1991).

An implication of the data on risk factors is that interventions should be targeted at those most at risk for otitis media and at the adverse effects associated with otitis media. This chapter will focus on interventions to prevent the negative effects of otitis media. Two models will be presented as a framework for examining these issues.

THE ECOLOGICAL AND DEVELOPMENTAL/CONTEXTUAL MODELS

Two overlapping theoretical models may be helpful in framing the way in which otitis media affects development. More important for this chapter, the models will highlight how developmentally and contextually appropriate interventions can be structured. Each perspective will be briefly reviewed to argue for its centrality in designing interventions. They will then be integrated for the purpose of proposing specific intervention strategies.

THE ECOLOGICAL PERSPECTIVE

Bronfenbrenner (1979) proposed a model in which the developing child is viewed within the context of multiple settings and layers of environmental influence. The child's development is seen as influenced by these multiple settings as well as the interrelations among people, objects, and activities in these settings. Development is also influenced by settings that the child does not participate in but that can indirectly have a large effect on the child.

The most immediate settings in which the child participates, and that presumably affect the child the most, are referred to as microsystems. They include the child's home, neighborhood, church, and school or day-care setting. These are the major settings in which the child actively participates. Microsystems affect development directly through reciprocal interactions between the developing child and significant people and events in these settings. The settings are seen as presenting the child with certain demand characteristics, some of which are similar across settings and others that are particular to one setting. The day-care/school microsystem may set limits on children's activity in the classroom that may not apply in the home setting. Children are asked to adapt their behavior to fit the demands of the various settings or microsystems. Thus, the ecological perspective sees the child's behavior as influenced greatly by the demands of the microsystems.

The links between these microsystems are called mesosystems and are important for the child's smooth transition from one microsystem to the next. For example, the communication between the child's parents and teachers is important for continuity between home and school. If the parent and the teacher understand the expectations for behavior in both settings and communicate about possible or current problems, it is likely that the child will adjust well in both settings. On the other hand, if communication is poor, as it often is between home and school, it will

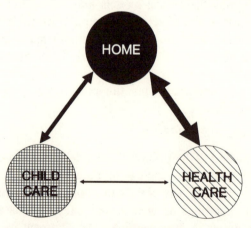

Figure 2. Major microsystems and mesosystem links for the young child with chronic otitis media.

be more difficult for the child to make the transition. Thus, mesosystems are critical links in this model. Figure 2 shows graphically the major microsystem and mesosystem links for the preschool child that will be discussed in this chapter. The thicker the mesosystem lines, the stronger the link between the microsystems as conceptualized in this chapter.

The next level of influence involves the exosystems, or settings in which the child does not participate directly but that influence the child indirectly because these larger contexts affect family attitudes and resources. For instance, a parent's workplace influences not only the child's financial resources and the child's access to the parent but also the child's beliefs about the workplace.

The child is also influenced indirectly by the even more remote macrosystems. Macrosystems include institutions such as the economic, sociocultural, and political systems. These larger institutions affect the philosophy as well as the resources in each microsystem. Figure 3 depicts the full Bronfenbrenner model as it will be used in this chapter.

THE DEVELOPMENTAL/CONTEXTUAL PERSPECTIVE

The developmental/contextual perspective complements Bronfenbrenner's model by adding more dynamic developmental processes that address the mechanisms of development while focusing on individual differences among children and environments. Lerner (Lerner and Lerner 1987; Lerner 1989) typifies this approach. He argues that there are two key propositions in this perspective: *embeddedness* and *dynamic interaction*. These concepts are described as follows:

> The idea of *embeddedness* is that the key phenomena of human life exist at multiple levels of being (e.g., the inner-biological, individual-psychological, dyadic, social network, community, societal, cultural, outer physical-ecological, and historical); at any one point in time variables from any and all of these levels may contribute to human functioning. However, it is important to have a perspective about human development that is sensitive to the influences of these multiple levels because the levels do not function in parallel; they are not independent domains. Rather, the variables at one level influence and are influenced by the variables at the other levels. There is a *dynamic interaction* among levels of analysis: As such, each level may be a product

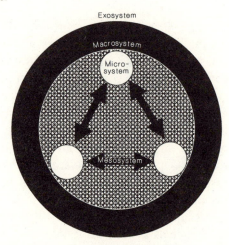

Figure 3. Bronfenbrenner's ecological model (1979).

and a producer of the functioning and changes at all other levels. (Lerner and Lerner 1987, p. 378)

This perspective adds to the model by providing the concept of the changing nature of the individual child over time as well as the changing demands of the environment. The perspective also emphasizes that there are different levels of functioning within the child that interact with each other to produce the characteristics displayed by the child. For instance, at the biologic level of functioning, a child may have otitis media, and at the behavioral level, he or she may be somewhat impulsive. The interaction between these two levels may produce dysfunctional behavior in particular settings.

There are a number of implications from this view of development. Three are particularly relevant to this chapter. First, the individual child is seen as having great plasticity in development according to Lerner and Lerner (1987). Since changes at one level of functioning affect other levels and then interact with setting or microsystem characteristics, there is always possibility for altering the status of the individual for better or worse (plasticity in development). Second, this perspective offers great potential for intervention because when development is plastic, change is always possible. Third, it endows the individual child with the ability to change the course of development (under the right circumstances), empowering the individual to be the producer of his or her own development.

The concept of "goodness-of-fit" espoused by Lerner and others (Lerner and Lerner 1987; Thomas and Chess 1977) helps to merge the ecological and developmental/contextual perspectives. In this view, the child's characteristics interact with the demands and characteristics of the setting to produce what might be called a "goodness-of-fit." In other words, goodness-of-fit indicates how well the individual fits with the characteristics of particular microsystems. Individuals receive feedback from the microsystem in the form of feedback loops that continually alter the person or setting to form a better or worse fit. The impulsive child may fit well in the home environment where the child gets feedback that the behavior is acceptable, while the school environment may not tolerate the behavior and give the child negative feedback that can lead to a host of poor developmental outcomes. The kind of feedback the child gets, as well as the child's ability to adapt his or her behavior to the setting, determines the goodness-of-fit.

INTERVENTION AND THE TWO MODELS

The purpose of this chapter is to suggest ways to prevent and minimize negative outcomes for young children with otitis media by planning interventions that (1) take into account microsystem, mesosystem, exosystem, and macrosystem influences on the child's development and (2) acknowledge the nature of the child in different settings and at different levels of functioning. This rather complex model may seem a bit unwieldy for the development of interventions; however, only a complex view can address all of the issues involved in truly effective interventions.

MICROSYSTEM AND MESOSYSTEM LEVEL INTERVENTION STRATEGIES

THE HEALTH CARE SETTING

Identification and assessment of otitis media. In general, the health care system has rather rigid demands for behavior on the part of the child and health care providers. It is the most formal setting that the child must operate within. Although the expertise that health care professionals possess is critical for successful identification and correct remediation of the problem, the demands within the setting and the mesosystem connections to other important microsystems of the child are often weak, making the health care setting less effective than it could be.

The identification of otitis media is routinely done in the health care system, but the intervention models proposed here suggest that the way in which identification is done can have enormous implications for the child's view of the health care system. An example of how this intervention model could change some health care practices may help.

Many children in our research projects have had negative experiences in health care settings, and the feedback over time has exacerbated the problem, producing a poor goodness-of-fit in the health care setting that hinders identification and remediation of otitis media. This can happen not because the physician or nurse is poorly trained but because health care professionals may not understand the implications of a poor fit with the health care setting. In addition, they are often not trained about the need for developmentally appropriate practice. Although otoscopy is not generally a painful procedure and can be done with almost all children in a gentle and nonthreatening way, many physicians merely operate at a technical level, making sure the child cannot move during the examination and failing to take the time to make sure the child feels comfortable about the procedure. When the child experiences pain and has arms restrained, an extremely aversive procedure for children, a negative feedback loop is set up within this setting. If reinforced on subsequent visits, this can cause children to fear and avoid any connections with this setting.

In the Penn State Project, we spent almost two years gaining the trust of some of our children who screamed at the sight of a nurse or physician, and especially the otoscope. Parents were often reluctant to have their children in our study, even though their children were otitis prone, because of the negative reactions their children had to the health care system.

Thus, a health care system that tries to be sensitive and responsive to the characteristics of young children creates positive feedback loops. This may initially cost time and money, but over time the positive feedback loops will make the fit between the child and the health care setting positive. As a result, examinations of the child will take less time, and parents will trust the system to be sensitive to their individual children.

Mesosystem connections: Remediation and referral. Once a diagnosis of otitis media has been made by the health care system, a program of medical treatment begins. Along with this treatment, continual monitoring of the child's hearing and development is done. This is especially important in cases where otitis is chronic, lasting months during the early years of life. The health care setting usually refers families for further evaluation of hearing and development. The mesosystem connections to the expertise needed for hearing and developmental evaluation are critical. Most physicians have these formal connections, but the best health care settings make the transition to these other professional settings easier for the family. This means stressing the importance of these other health-related professionals as well as giving families information about procedures and people in the settings. It is critically important, for instance, that children with chronic otitis media be seen quickly for a hearing evaluation to assess the degree of hearing loss. Making sure that this happens is not always easy, so the health care system must spend time to build in the mesosystem connections that assure a quick and easy transition for families.

Other types of developmental assessments are also important in cases of chronic otitis media where language and other cognitive processes might be affected. Again, referral may be made to other health care settings. The actual assessment and intervention may not be the responsibility of the health care system itself, but monitoring is critical for the long-term development of the child.

Although the health care system is set up to have formal connections with other formal health-related settings, it is not as well connected to either the home or day-care/preschool settings in which the child spends most of his or her day. Information from the microsystem may be critical to the physician in the kind of referral and follow-up recommended. The physician needs to understand these settings by asking questions of the family. In this way, the physician will be aware of how the otitis-prone child functions in the home and day-care settings as well as how a hearing loss may affect functioning in those settings. For instance, a child with many siblings in a home with the TV on most of the time may be at higher risk for poor developmental outcomes related to a temporary hearing loss compared to an only child in a family that rarely has the TV on. Likewise, a child in day care may be at higher risk because of the high level of ambient noise in the day-care environment. The health care system that has good connections to the home and the preschool setting can maximize the possibility of good outcomes for the child. Unfortunately, while most health care systems have some connections to the home, they have almost none to day care programs and schools, settings in which young children spend a major portion of the day.

In summary, the health care setting is critical for correct diagnosis, and if structured well, it can set up positive feedback loops that have a positive influence on the attitudes of parents and young children. Although a good formal mesosystem exists between the health care system and other professional settings like audiology, there needs to be more personal involvement by the health care system in making sure there is a good transition to these other professionals. The mesosystems to the home and school setting are much less developed and need to be strengthened if the health care setting is to have a positive impact on the child's total development.

THE HOME SETTING

Clearly, the most important microsystem for the preschool child is the home. This is the setting where there is the most investment in the child's well-being and that will probably have the most influence over early development. Thus, it is very important that the people in this setting are closely tied through strong mesosystems to the other microsystems of the child, namely, the health care system and the preschool/day-care setting. Overall, the people in the home have modest mesosystem connections to the health care system and to the school. These mesosystems can be critical in the child's adjustment to each setting and in providing information to other settings about the individual nature of the child in response to the setting. The parents, in particular, can be helpful in making sure the child has the best goodness-of-fit with the setting demands. For instance, if parents are enlisted to hold and entertain the child during an ear examination, the exam can be much less aversive. Health care settings that enlist and promote the participation of parents can strengthen the child's mesosytem connections and the ultimate adjustment of the child to the setting. The connection between home and the child-care setting is also crucial. Most children attend some form of preschool, and over half the married women with preschool children are working full time (Feagans and Manlove in press). Thus, the relationship between the home and the school is important for the child's adjustment in that setting also. The following section will focus on what can be done in the home as well as the relationship among the home, the school, and the health care settings.

Identification of the problem. The initial challenge in the home setting is to identify when a child has otitis media and then subsequently whether the child has a hearing loss associated with otitis media. Most parents can identify when a child has an acute episode of otitis because the child is irritable and in pain. Silent episodes can occur in over half the cases of otitis media (Feagans, Blood, and Tubman 1988). These episodes are difficult to identify, but they are important to detect if there is hearing loss associated with the episode.

If a child is otitis prone, parents should be alert to changes in the child's behavior when he or she has an upper respiratory infection that could eventually lead to otitis media. McConkey and Price (1986) offer a number of suggestions parents can use to informally assess a child's hearing when the child has otitis media as well as when the parents think the child is at risk for a silent episode of otitis media. First, they suggest speaking softly since a child with a mild hearing loss will easily hear if one speaks at a normal volume. Second, adults should check both ears, since unless the child has bilateral otitis media, the hearing loss will affect only one ear. Third, different types of sounds should be used. Low frequency sounds such as "oo" may be heard while higher sounds such as "sss" may be inaudible. Fourth, parents should be sure that the child is responding only to sound. Particularly with infants, other sense modalities, such as smell, gesture, and vibration (such as from a person walking across a springy floor), can lead to responses that seem to be to verbalizations. Finally, when attempting to assess a child's hearing, the adult should be sure that the child is in a context in which he or she will want to respond. A child very involved in play may be so engrossed that he or she does not want to be disturbed. In such a situation the lack of response may be due not to hearing loss but to the child's concentrating deeply on something else.

Fostering language development. Parents can be the critical element in preventing the poor outcomes in children with chronic otitis media. This means careful monitoring of the disease but also careful documentation of development that can help identify any developmental problems. In the home setting, parents can keep lists of gestures and words an infant or young toddler uses along with the corresponding meaning. Parents, by virtue of the fact that they spend more total and one-on-one time with their children, are in the best position to interpret the meaning of their children's communications. This is even true of parents who work full time. A recent study (Feagans and Manlove in press) found that working parents with an infant in day care were with the child two-thirds of the child's waking hours. Parents can share their knowledge with caregivers, thus improving the mesosystem links between home and school, and thereby improving the caregivers' abilities to understand the child.

Parents can also try to alleviate ambient noise in the environment to make sure the child has the best chance to differentiate sounds. In addition, parents may want to set aside time to talk to their child on a one-to-one basis about topics of interest to the child. Parents who spend time reading books to their children can also have a positive influence. A parent who spends time not just reading to the child, but also interacting over the pictures in the books and elaborating on sections of the book the child likes, can help the child develop a larger vocabulary and enjoy this time with the child. This activity has been called joint book reading and has been linked to better vocabulary in children and better reading skills when children enter elementary school (Ninio 1980; Teale 1984; Wells 1985).

Fostering social development. Since parents are children's "first teachers," they play an important role in facilitating the social development of young children with chronic otitis media. For example, the use of a disciplinary style that relies on reasoning and is based on a warm, nurturing relationship with the children is expected to be more effective in promoting prosocial behavior in young children than permissive or authoritarian methods (Zahn-Waxler, Radke-Yarrow, and King 1979; Baumrind 1977).

Second, parents can encourage group play by giving the child opportunities to interact around common activities with siblings. Siblings of different ages and skill levels will learn social behavior from one another when given opportunities to interact with limited adult intervention (Rogers and Ross 1986).

Finally, parents are powerful models for their children and can check their own behavior to make sure they are modeling verbal, problem-solving behaviors with their young children (Yarrow, Scott, and Waxler 1973). Combined with the efforts of adults in day-care and preschool settings, these techniques can help prevent social and behavior problems in children with otitis media.

Mesosystem connections. The parents are critical members of the home microsystem and are the most motivated to set up good mesosystem connections for the child. Although the intention to do so may be there, barriers to successful connections among the settings are common. As we have already discussed, the health care microsystem may not be initially responsive to parental initiations. Parents who insist that physicians take time and patience to allow their child to adjust to the diagnostic procedure help the health care system and their child. This can often be difficult for everyone when parents and the physicians have little time and when the health care setting can be intimidating.

The connections to the school may be critical not only in the identification of otitis media but in the way staff handle a child who has otitis media. Communicating to the school about the child's hearing loss or change in behavior will help staff at the school or day care deal with the child more effectively. Finding the time to talk to the day-care staff or school personnel can be frustrating. For instance, Zigler and Turner (1982) reported that parents spent less than eight minutes per day in a child-care setting that emphasized parental involvement. Such brief stays mean that communication with caregivers is apt to be limited. Parents and teachers need to find time to communicate regularly about the child's development since good mesosystem connections can be critical for the continuity of intervention and monitoring of the child's development.

THE DAY-CARE/SCHOOL SETTING

The day-care/school setting is the other important setting for the child. This setting provides the child with activities and skills that help develop cognitive and social skills. Teachers in these settings deal with many different children and usually are not trained to deal with children with otitis media. This section will try to illustrate a number of ways teachers may intervene to help the otitis-prone child as well as ways teachers can build better mesosystems to the home and the health care system.

Identification of the problem. When a child has otitis media, caregivers may know because they will be administering medication. Yet as noted earlier, over half of the episodes are silent episodes of otitis and will probably go undetected. Even when teachers know a child has otitis media, many are unaware that a child can suffer a significant concomitant hearing loss. Caregivers should be alerted that all children, but especially otitis-prone children, can have otitis media as a result of an upper respiratory infection. Children at risk for chronic otitis (see previous section) should be monitored carefully for hearing loss. Caregivers will need to use different methods to detect hearing loss from those suggested for the home. The ideas presented in the home setting section of this chapter can work quite well in the relatively quiet setting of the home; in a busy and noisy day-care center using those ideas may be more difficult. One solution is for caregivers to have some one-on-one time with children away from the larger group (Feagans 1986). In this quieter setting the caregiver could try some of the suggestions of McConkey and Price (1986), for example, checking both ears and using different kinds of sounds. If this is not possible, the caregiver may have to rely on even more informal assessments. For example, the caregiver should note whether the child seems to ignore adult verbalizations, particularly in situations where the adult and child are not face-to-face. Such "ignoring" may, in fact, be due to hearing loss.

Assessing and fostering language development. Once it can be established that a child has otitis media and there is likely to be some hearing loss, it is important that the child has every opportunity to get good language input in all the settings in which he or she functions. Children with chronic otitis media may articulate words less clearly and use more nonverbal gestures for communication (Feagans and Blood 1991). They also may be delayed in language and not attend or listen to language as well as others. Teachers can use a number of strategies to identify problems and promote good language.

While home assessments and language activities are apt to be relatively informal, the child-care setting offers the possibility of more formal assessments. Caregivers or support staff of a child-care program can do annual or semiannual developmental assessments of children to evaluate whether language is developing as expected. As with any assessment, multiple measures should be used. Currently, there are a number of screening instruments on the market, including the Early Language Milestone Scale (Copland 1987) and the Clinical Linguistic and Auditory Milestone Scale, or CLAMS (Capute, Shapiro, Wachtel, Gunther, and Palmer 1986). Although these instruments are useful in detecting a significant language delay, they are not, in our experience, sensitive to the subtle delays evidenced by otitis-prone children. A more subtle approach to assessment is needed to identify these delays.

Teachers should be aware of poor articulation and less attention during book reading and other oral language tasks, as well as problems with behavior and social interactions. Of course, the occurrence of these problems in an otitis-prone child may have other causes; but the interventions suggested should help all children. Two particular approaches seem particularly appropriate for the otitis-prone child. We will discuss them in more detail.

Both Tough (1977; 1982) and Blank (Blank, Rose, and Berlin 1978; Blank 1982) have proposed programs for young children that emphasize helping the child extend language in discourse or dialogue with an adult. Emphasis is placed on trying to engage the child in a sustained dialogue on a topic of the child's interest. In this way the adult can help the child reflect on the past, relate this topic to others, and in general explore more abstract and complicated concepts. These skills have been shown to be critical for school success and reading (Feagans 1982) and are not as well developed in otitis-prone children (Feagans et al. 1987).

Blank proposes four levels of abstraction of language and outlines a program for teachers to follow so that their strategies fit the language level of the child. Achieving this goodness-of-fit is important in helping the child develop further. She suggests activities to foster language and gives numerous examples. Tough emphasizes creating what she calls enabling environments that foster extended dialogues between adult and child. She also sees this as important in the preschool years and especially important for children who are at risk for language delay, like the otitis-prone child.

These intervention/prevention strategies are not always easy to employ in a busy and noisy child-care setting. McConkey and Price (1986) make a number of suggestions for ways to make communication easier. First, when communicating with the child, the adult should be in close proximity and face-to-face. This provides the child with visual as well as auditory cues and helps to focus his or her attention. Second, adults should speak clearly, and background noise such as radios should be minimized. Child-care programs can help reduce noise by installing acoustic ceiling tiles and by using carpeting and upholstered furniture (a sofa, for example), which will help to absorb sound. Thus, reducing the ambient noise is important for otitis-prone children (Feagans 1986). In addition, teachers can make sure that otitis-prone children are seated close to them when talking and exposed as little as possible to large, noisy groups where speech discrimination may be especially difficult.

Fostering social development. The social development of children with chronic otitis media has been largely unexplored. However, three areas of research suggest that children with otitis media who attend group programs may benefit from efforts to facilitate social skills.

First, several studies have found relationships between otitis media and potentially problematic social behaviors, including hyperactivity, short attention span, restlessness, and off-task and destructive behavior (Feagans 1986). Second, research has demonstrated links between otitis media in children and deficits in using and attending to language (Feagans et al. 1987). Third, research on the effects of day care on children's development has found that some children in day care may demonstrate more aggressive behavior than children not attending day care (Finkelstein 1974; Belsky 1988).

Given language deficits and the frustration stemming from difficulty in communicating, it seems likely that children with chronic otitis media may resort to physical means to get their needs met in the day-care setting. For these reasons, day-care children with chronic otitis media may need help from early childhood professionals in developing verbal and prosocial skills.

A number of authors have studied effective methods of promoting prosocial development in young children. Prosocial behavior includes helping, cooperating, empathizing, sharing, and comforting (Marantz 1988; Finkelstein 1982; Rogers and Ross 1986).

Several studies have found that inductive disciplinary techniques (i.e., labeling the inappropriate behavior, giving reasons for rules and consequences) combined with a warm, nurturing relationship with the child are effective in increasing prosocial behavior in young children (Zahn-Waxler et al. 1979; Baumrind 1977). In addition, such "authoritative" adults who were less controlling of children's behavior have been found to be more effective than those who exerted more control (Sparks, Thornburg, Ispa, and Gray 1984). Another technique that was found to be effective was modeling of specific prosocial acts by adults (Yarrow et al. 1973). For example, teachers can demonstrate appropriate ways of resolving conflicts over toys.

Rogers and Ross (1986) suggest additional ways that teachers and caregivers can foster prosocial development of young children. First, encouraging group play provides children with opportunities to practice and learn positive ways of interacting. Adults can promote group play by helping children see connections between their activities and engaging children in one another's play (Smilansky 1971; Christie 1982). In addition, grouping less socially skilled children with those who are more skilled encourages less skilled children to model the behavior of their more competent peers (Hartup and Coates 1967; Moore 1981; Vaughn and Waters 1980).

Another method of promoting prosocial development is to help children develop communication skills. Children who are able to talk about their own feelings and needs, as well as recognize the feelings and needs of others, are better equipped to interact in positive ways (Hughes, Tingle, and Sawin 1981; Hill 1983; Asher, Oden, and Gottman 1977). Caregivers can help children develop these abilities by labeling the child's feelings and identifying the effects of the child's behavior on others (e.g., "When you hit Derek, it makes him sad"). In addition, adults should encourage children to talk about their feelings, needs, and wishes (Schacter, Kirshner, Klips, Friedricks, and Sanders 1974).

Other techniques include role-playing and discussing problem situations and solutions (Krogh 1982), and helping children learn negotiation with others using verbal reasoning (Asher, Oden, and Gottman 1977). Finally, Rogers and Ross (1986) suggest providing activities that require limited adult intervention to give children opportunities to interact and work on resolving conflicts on their own.

When combined with efforts to identify and treat otitis media and its associated problems, methods to teach children prosocial skills in the day-care or preschool setting are expected to help prevent potential language, social, and behavioral problems as the children develop.

Mesosystem links. The links among day-care, home, and health care settings are not strong, but there is an especially poor link between the child-care setting (day care or preschool) and the health care system. This link is weak in at least two ways. First, the vast majority of child-care programs have no regular contact with health care providers. Second, in 1986 only 36 states had some form of health training requirement for caregivers in centers. Of these, only 16 states required health training for all staff (Morgan 1987). The ability of child-care staff to recognize illness, including otitis media, in a child depends largely on what teachers have learned on their own. Strengthening links between child-care settings and health care providers can include regular training for staff as well as having a health care professional available to the program on a regular basis to be used much in the way the school nurse is used in elementary school.

The Pennsylvania Chapter of the American Academy of Pediatrics is currently involved in developing a statewide network linking health care providers with early childhood programs. The ECELS program (Early Childhood Education Linkage System) offers a context in which health professionals can offer training and technical assistance to early childhood programs (American Academy of Pediatrics 1990). Presumably, forging links between health care and child-care providers will have the added benefit of strengthening links between child care and parents. This is expected to occur as child-care providers pass on the information they have acquired from health care providers to parents.

In addition, it is important for day-care staff to form specific mesosystem links to the pediatric care units in their community. For instance, this may be done by contacting various pediatric offices or public health offices (i.e., visiting nurses, etc.) and developing information links that can help their child-care setting function with respect to young children's health. Alerting the health care system to interest on the part of child-care settings about children's health can promote good relations and flow of information. Many communities have a Child Development Council that represents child-care needs in the community. This intermediate link may aid in specific child-care settings in making connections with the health care settings in the community.

EXOSYSTEM LEVEL INTERVENTIONS

WORKPLACE POLICIES

The lack of flexible work policies in many parents' workplaces may prevent parents from obtaining immediate health care for their sick children, keeping their sick children at home, and taking time for conferences with day-care providers and teachers about their children's language and social development. Offering flextime work options and cafeteria benefits are two ways employers can be more responsive to parents. Cafeteria benefits can offer parents the opportunity to select additional "sick child days" as part of their benefits package. Flextime options can allow them to leave work for parent-teacher conferences, making up the time at another point in the workday.

SCHOOL POLICIES AND PRACTICES

School system policies and practices related to health education have the potential to help children learn to manage their health and recognize difficulties they may be having related to illness and hearing loss. Requiring teachers to have knowledge or skill in identifying otitis media and its possible consequences could be an important step in helping these otitis-prone children.

MACROSYSTEM LEVEL INTERACTIONS

Broader, macrosystem influences also must be considered when planning interventions for young children with otitis media. The lack of a national health care policy at the macrosystem level also affects the child. In 1987, one in eight preschoolers had no health insurance. In addition, one in ten had not seen a doctor in the previous 12 months (Edelman 1987). National beliefs about the care of children in general affect children as well by influencing levels of government assistance. Access to health care influences the timing and quality of care parents obtain for their sick children. Since early treatment is important for preventing serious outcomes of otitis media, availability of health care can be a factor in the outcomes associated with otitis media for some children. A second, related macrosystem influence is socioeconomic status (SES). A number of studies have found links between SES and otitis media, possibly mediated by microsystem factors, such as crowding in the home, number of siblings, and urban versus rural residence (Feagans 1986). Families at lower socioeconomic levels are also less likely to be able to afford health insurance.

There have been recent macrosystem level responses to the need for expanded health care for children. Recently, legislation was passed that requires states to phase in Medicaid for children older than 6 as well as younger children. As a result, all children under age 18 are expected to receive coverage by 2002. In addition, a number of states have passed their own health insurance plans for children who are not covered by Medicaid or private plans (Children's Defense Fund 1991). The debate about the merits of a national health plan indicates that politicians and policy makers recognize this as an important issue to many Americans, children as well as adults.

The special vulnerability of children and the long-term cost-effectiveness of early health care interventions are well known. For example, neonatal intensive care for a low-birth-weight infant costs over $1,000 per day; yet comprehensive prenatal care costs only about $600. Similarly, it costs approximately $600 per day to hospitalize a child for a preventable illness but only $40 a year for preventive checkups through Medicaid (Edelman 1987). Despite this knowledge, not enough is being done to prevent health problems in young children.

Conclusions

The model of intervention presented in this chapter uses a conceptual framework that includes the importance of prevention and intervention in all the settings in which the child operates. The microsystems and the mesosystem connections between them are important for all children, but especially for children, like the otitis-prone children, who are at risk for developmental delays and problems. According to this framework, we need more integrated programs for these children that focus on all the microsystems. An understanding of these settings and their connections is critical for a successful intervention strategy. Further, the outside forces that often influence the microsystems and their connections may have a powerful influence on how effective the microsystems can be in adapting to the needs of children. Even if individual professionals cannot immediately change many of these exosystem or macrosystem forces, understanding their influence can make them more effective in planning programs for otitis-prone children. In the future it is hoped that the developmental effects of the mild-to-moderate hearing loss associated with bouts of otitis media may be prevented by a more systematic, ecological/developmental approach to helping these children.

Acknowledgments

This research was supported by grant MCJ-420565 from the Maternal and Child Health Bureau (Title V, Social Security Act), Health Resources and Services Administration, Department of Health and Human Services.

REFERENCES

American Academy of Pediatrics, Pennsylvania Chapter. 1990. *Early childhood education linkage system (ECELS) manual.* Bryn Mawr, Penn.: ECELS/PA AAP.

Asher, S., Oden, S., and Gottman, J. 1977. Children's friendships in school settings. In L. Katz (ed.), *Current topics in early childhood education.* Vol. 1. Norwood, N.J.: Ablex.

Baumrind, D. 1977. Some thoughts about childrearing. In S. Cohen and T. Comiskey (eds.), *Child development: Contemporary perspectives.* Itasca, Ill.: F.E. Peacock.

Belsky, J. 1988. The effects of infant day care reconsidered. *Early Childhood Research Quarterly* 3:235-272.

Berman, S.A., Balkany, T.J., and Simmons, M.A. 1978. Otitis media in the neonatal intensive care unit. *Pediatrics* 62(2):198-201.

Blank, M. 1982. Language and school failure: Some speculations about the relationship between oral and written language. In L. Feagans and D. Farran (eds.), *The language of children reared in poverty.* New York: Academic Press.

Blank, M., Rose, S., and Berlin, L. 1978. *The language of learning: The preschool years.* New York: Grune and Stratton.

Bronfenbrenner, U. 1979. *The ecology of human development: Experiments by nature and design.* Cambridge, Mass.: Harvard University Press.

Cambon, K., Galbraith, J., and Kong, C. 1965. Middle ear disease in Indians of the Mount Currie reservation, British Columbia. *Canadian Medical Association Journal* 93:1301.

Capute, A.J., Shapiro, B.K., Wachtel, R.C., Gunther, V.A., and Palmer, F.B. 1986. The clinical linguistic and auditory milestone scale (CLAMS). *American Journal of Diseases in Children* 140:694-698.

Chase, C., Teele, D.W., Klein, J.O., and Rosner, B.A. 1991. Behavioral sequelae of otitis media for infants at one year of age and their mothers. Paper presented at the 5th International Symposium on Recent Advances in Otitis Media, Fort Lauderdale, Fla., May.

Children's Defense Fund. 1991. *The state of America's children.* Washington, D.C.: Children's Defense Fund.

Christie, J. 1982. Sociodramatic play training. *Young Children* 37:25-32.

Copland, F. 1987. *Early language milestone scale.* Tulsa, Okla: Modern Education Corporation.

Edelman, M. 1987. *Families in peril: An agenda for social change.* Cambridge, Mass.: Harvard University Press.

Feagans, L. 1982. The importance of the development of narratives for school-age children. In L. Feagans and D.C. Farran (eds.), *The language of children reared in poverty* (pp. 95-116). New York: Academic Press.

Feagans, L. 1986. Otitis media: A model for long term effects with implications for intervention. In J.F. Kavanaugh (ed.), *Otitis media and child development* (pp. 192-208). Parkton, Md.: York Press.

Feagans, L., Sanyal, M., Henderson, F., Collier, A., and Appelbaum, M.I. 1987. The relationship of middle ear disease in early childhood to later narrative and attention skills. *Journal of Pediatric Psychology* 12:581-594.

Feagans, L., and Blood, I. 1991. The behavioral and language sequelae of otitis media in infants and young children attending day care. Paper presented at the 5th International Symposium on Recent Advances in Otitis Media, Fort Lauderdale, Fla., May.

Feagans, L. Blood, I., Tubman, J.G. 1988. Otitis media: Models of effects and implications for intervention. In F.H. Bess (ed.), *Hearing impairment in children*. Parkton, Md.:York Press.

Feagans, L., and Manlove, E. In press. Parents, infants, & daycare teachers: Interrelationships and implications for better child care. *Journal of Applied Developmental Psychology*.

Fiellau-Nikolajsen, M. 1979. Tympanometry in 3-year-old children: Type of care as an epidemiological factor in secretory otitis media and tubal dysfunction in unselected populations of 3-year-old children. *Otolaryngology* 41:193-205.

Finkelstein, N. 1982. Aggression: Is it stimulated by daycare? *Young Children* 37:3-9.

Friel-Patti, S., and Finitzo, T. 1990. Language learning in a prospective study of otitis media with effusion in the first two years of life. *Journal of Speech and Hearing Research* 33:188-194.

Froom, J., and Culpepper, L. 1991. Otitis media in day-care children. A report from the International Primary Care Network. *Journal of Family Practice* 32: 289-294.

Giebink, G.S. 1988. Epidemiology of otitis media with effusion. In F.H. Bess (ed.), *Hearing impairment in children*. Baltimore: York Press.

Hartup, W., and Coates, B. 1967. Imitation of a peer as a function of reinforcement from the peer group and rewardingness of the model. *Child Development* 38:1003-1016.

Hill, T. 1983. The effect of self reflection on preschool children's empathetic understanding and prosocial behavior. Paper presented at the annual meeting of the Society for Research in Child Development, Detroit, April.

Hughes, R., Tingle, B., and Sawin, D. 1981. Development of empathic understanding. *Child Development* 52:122-128.

Hurwitz, E.S., Gunn, W.J., Pinsky, P.F., and Schonberger, L.B. 1991. Risk of respiratory illness associated with day-care attendance: A nationwide study. *Pediatrics* 87:62-69.

Klein, J.O. In press. Epidemiology of otitis media. Paper presented at The 102nd Ross Conference on Pediatric Research, Hearing Loss in Childhood: A Primer, Tucson, Arizona, March 1991.

Krogh, S. 1982. Encouraging positive justice reasoning and perspective taking skills. Paper presented at the annual meeting of the National Association of Early Childhood Teacher Educators, Washington, D.C., November.

Lerner, R. 1989. Developmental contextualism and the life-span view of person-context interaction. In M.H. Bornstein and J.S. Broner (eds.), *Interaction in human development*. Hillsdale, N.J.: Erlbaum.

Lerner, R., and Lerner, J. 1987. Children in their contexts: A goodness-of-fit model. In J.B. Lancaster, J. Altmann, A.S. Rossi, and L.R. Sherrod (eds.), *Parenting across the life span: Biosocial dimensions*. New York: Aldine de Gruyter.

Lim, D.J. (ed.). In press. Recent advances in otitis media: Report of the Fourth Research Conference. *Annals of Otology, Rhinology and Laryngology*.

Luloff, A., Menyuk, P., and Teele, D. 1991. The effects of persistent otitis media on the speech sound repertoire of infants. Paper presented at the 5th International Symposium on Recent Advances in Otitis Media, Fort Lauderdale, Fla., May.

Lundgren, K., Ingvarrson, L., and Olofsson, B. 1984. Epidemiologic aspects in children with recurrent acute otitis media. In D.J. Lim (ed.), *Recent advances in otitis media with effusion*. Philadelphia: B.C. Decker.

McConkey, R., and Price, P. 1986. *Let's talk: Learning language in everyday settings*. London: Souvenir Press.

Marantz, M. 1988. Fostering prosocial behavior in the early childhood classroom: Review of the research. *Journal of Moral Education* 17:27-39.

Moore, S. 1981. Unique contributions of peers to socialization in early childhood. *Theory into Practice* 20:105-108.

Morgan, G. 1987. *The national state of child care regulation 1986*. Watertown, Mass.: Work/Family Directions, Inc.

Ninio, A. 1980. Picture-book reading in mother-infant dyads belonging to two sub-groups in Israel. *Child Development* 51:587-590.

Paradise, J.L. 1980. Otitis media in infants and children. *Pediatrics* 65:917-943.

Pukander, J., Sipila, M., and Karma, P. 1984. Occurrence of risk factors in acute otitis media. In D.J. Lim (ed.), *Recent advances in otitis media with effusion*. Philadelphia: B.C. Decker.

Rogers, D.L., and Ross, D.D. 1986. Encouraging positive social interaction among young children. *Young Children* 41:12-36.

Schacter, F., Kirshner, K., Klips, B., Friedricks, M., and Sanders, K. 1974. Everyday preschool interpersonal speech usage. *Monographs of the Society for Research in Child Development* 39:1-88.

Smilansky, S. 1971. Can adults facilitate play in children?: Theoretical and practical considerations. In S. Arnaud (ed.), *Play: The child strives for reality.* Washington, D.C.: NAEYC.

Sparks, A., Thornburg, K., Ispa, J., and Gray, M. 1984. Prosocial behaviors of young children related to parental child-rearing attitudes. *Early Child Development and Care* 15:291-298.

Teale, W.H. 1984. Reading to young children: Its significance for literacy development. In H. Goelman, A.A. Oberg, and F. Smith (eds.), *Awakening to literacy.* London: Heineman Educational Books.

Teele, D.W., Klein, J.O., and Rosner, B.A. 1984. Otitis media with effusion during the first three years of life and development of speech and language. *Pediatrics* 74:291-292.

Thomas, A., and Chess, S. 1977. *Temperament and development.* New York: Brunner/Mazel.

Tough, J. 1977. *Talking and learning: A guide to fostering communication skills in nursery and infant school.* London: Word Lock Educational.

Tough, J. 1982. Language, poverty, and disadvantage in school. In L. Feagans and D.C. Farran (eds.), *The language of children reared in poverty.* New York: Academic Press.

Vaughn, B., and Waters, E. 1980. Attention structures, sociometric status, and dominance: Interrelations, behavior correlates, and relationships to social competence. *Developmental Psychology* 17:275-288.

Wallace, I.F., Gravel, J.S., and Ganon, E.C. 1991. Preschool language outcomes as a function of OME and parental linguistic styles. Paper presented at the 5th International Symposium on Recent Advances in Otitis Media, Fort Lauderdale, Fla., May.

Wells, G. 1985. Preschool literacy-related activities and success in school. In D.R. Olson, N. Torrance, and A. Hildyard (eds.), *Literacy, language, and learning.* Cambridge: Cambridge University Press.

Wendler-Shaw, P., Menyuk, P., and Teele, D. 1991. Effects of otitis media in the first year of life on language production in the second year of life. Paper Presented at the 5th International Symposium on Recent Advances in Otitis Media, Fort Lauderdale, Fla., May.

Yarrow, M., Scott, P., and Waxler, C. 1973. Learning concern for others. *Developmental Psychology* 8:240-260.

Zahn-Waxler, C., Radke-Yarrow, M., and King, R. 1979. Child-rearing and children's prosocial initiations toward victims of distress. *Child Development* 50:319-330.

Zigler, E.F., and Turner, P. 1982. Parents and day care workers: A failed partnership? In E.F. Zigler and E.W. Gordon (eds.), *Day care: Scientific and social policy issues* (pp. 174-182). Boston, Mass.: Auburn House.

Chapter 29

Parent-Infant Intervention Strategies:
A Focus on Relationships

Nancy Rushmer

INTRODUCTION

Babies learn communication and language by interacting with their parents and caregivers. For babies with hearing loss, that natural language-learning milieu is seriously diminished. Inability to hear during the early years can lead to a serious and permanent language deficit, poor reading skills, and low school performance. Although many hearing-impaired children succeed in overcoming the challenges imposed by hearing loss, the average graduate of a school for the deaf in the United States still reads below a fourth grade level (International Association of Parents of the Deaf 1985).

Why do some children with hearing loss do well and others do not so well? Many of those children who achieve academically are individuals who experienced meaningful communication and language interactions with hearing or deaf parents during the early childhood years. Many of those children with reading or academic difficulties were delayed in their introduction to language because of inadequate or absent early family services.

This chapter will address some of the elements that contribute to effective early programming for infants with hearing loss and their families. The chapter will review the timing of intervention, goals, approaches used, major program components, competencies needed by professionals, and the benefits to families of appropriate services.

EARLY INTERVENTION AND RELATIONSHIPS

Early intervention is thought to be the key to achieving success for the child with hearing loss. There are many reports of the value of early training for individual children and for graduates of specific early intervention programs. A handful of studies, however, have shown that children who had early intervention functioned no differently from their "late intervention" peers by school age (Musselman et al. 1988). When evaluating the effects of early intervention, we need to look beyond the fact that some kind of service was provided and look at the quality and appropriateness of that service. To be effective, services must be comprehensive and must be delivered by specialists competent in parent-infant habilitation and in establishing collaborative relationships with families. Effective intervention strategies are based on relationships: the professional with the family; the family with their infant. The quality of the parent-professional relationship will determine its effectiveness in supporting optimal parent-child interaction.

The ways in which parents interact with their infant have far-reaching implications for the child's later learning; therefore, the parents' needs and goals are the focus of services. The introduction of hearing loss into the parent-child relationship changes it in at least two significant ways. First, the infant is not able to respond to the parents' nurturing vocalizations and speech in ways the parents expect so they may be confused, may not feel reinforced, and may reduce their communication and interaction. Parents generally do not recognize that their baby is primarily a visual communicator and would respond if they utilized different communication strategies. Once they learn that their baby does not hear, they may feel helpless to communicate with the baby and further reduce the interaction. Second, following the diagnosis of hearing loss, parents experience a range of strong emotions. As they work through these feelings, the process of attachment can be interrupted. Loving, nurturing, and joyous interactions with their baby are difficult when parents are hurting.

During this early period neither the parents nor the infant may be contributing to the relationship in ways necessary for the infant's optimal growth. The stage is set for delay in learning language. Supporting the parent-child relationship in positive ways is a primary goal of intervention. As the family begin to understand and accept the feelings associated with the discovery of deafness in their infant, and as they acquire additional information and skills, they facilitate their child's development and learning.

The professional assists the family on an ongoing basis in defining their goals and needs for their baby. Five commonly chosen goals are (1) acquisition of a functional communication system; (2) linguistic competence, which leads to literacy; (3) social skills; (4) emotional well-being; and (5) positive self-esteem.

COMPREHENSIVE PROGRAMMING FOR FAMILIES

What does a comprehensive program for families look like? Effective programs come in all colors, shapes, and sizes. They share some common elements:

1. Focus on and adaptation to individual families, including fathers, mothers, siblings, and grandparents.
2. Activities that serve the family's expressed needs to learn information and skills at a rate and depth comfortable to them so that they may soon take over the management of their child's growth.
3. Skilled attention to emotional needs of family members as an integral part of all interactions in the intervention process.
4. A family support group.
5. Activities for siblings.
6. Sign language class, if appropriate to the approach used.
7. Introduction to and involvement with the hearing-impaired community.
8. Case manager who coordinates multidisciplinary services.
9. Other support services needed and requested by the family.

MAJOR PROGRAM COMPONENTS FOR THE CHILD

Faced with the challenge of positively affecting the parent-infant interaction, the professional must understand which elements of that interaction are affected by hearing loss and the appropriate programming content to address them. Comprehensive early intervention programs include:

1. Assessment across all areas of development: motor, cognitive, hearing, language, social-emotional, self-help.
2. Hearing aid evaluation, fitting, and beginning trial usage.

3. Auditory-verbal stimulation.
4. The use of communication strategies appropriate for infants and toddlers with hearing loss.
    a. Promoting the infant's presymbolic communication (Schuyler and Rushmer 1987).
    b. Use of motherese (Snow 1984) and fatherese.
    c. Use of nondirective language.
    d. Conversational turntaking and reciprocity.
    e. Making communication contingent on the object of the child's attention.
    f. Use of visual communication strategies.
    g. Consider the "triangle of reference" (Wood et al. 1986).
5. Incorporation of all developmental goals into intervention.

APPROACHES TO INTERVENTION

The major approaches used with infants with hearing loss are based primarily on mode of communication. They are auditory-verbal, total communication, American Sign Language, and cued speech. In the auditory-verbal approach, aided hearing is used as the primary sense for receiving linguistic information and for developing speech. In total communication, one uses speech, speech reading, aided hearing, finger spelling, and signs. Programs using total communication have varying degrees of emphasis on audition and speech. Different forms of manually coded English are used in different total communication programs. Another approach is the introduction of American Sign Language (ASL) right from the beginning. Some programs teach ASL as a first language and then later teach the child English as second language. Others offer a bilingual approach, presenting the child with both languages at different times during the day. Finally, cued speech is an oral approach using a phonemically based hand supplement to speech reading; that is, it is based on the sounds the letters make, not the letters themselves (Williams-Scott and Kipila 1987).

IS THERE A "BEST" APPROACH?

Each approach has demonstrated high degrees of success in assisting families to help their children overcome the limitations imposed by hearing loss. Each approach has also failed miserably in assisting families with that same goal. Is there a "best" approach? may be the wrong question. We might ask instead: Which approach will be best for a particular child and family? Why was a particular approach of benefit to a child? What were the characteristics of programming for those families who feel they received what they needed to meet their own goals for their child? It is helpful to look at how families measure success as well as the criteria professionals use to measure successful intervention and education.

Most studies of the effectiveness of intervention and education for children with hearing loss use literacy and academic achievement as measures of success. But families have unique goals for their children. Not everyone places a high premium on literacy and academic achievement. Clearly, determinations of the effectiveness of intervention are based on the values of the individuals making the judgment.

Of the following indicators of effectiveness, any one or all of them together have been used as criteria for determining success in helping families deal with hearing loss and promote their child's growth:

1. Parents' sense of self-confidence and competence in interacting with their child.
2. Eventual family comfort with deafness.
3. Family's acceptance of the child as a valued and cherished family member.
4. Optimal use of residual hearing.
5. Academic achievement.
6. Intelligible speech.
7. Reading at grade level.
8. A sense of positive self-esteem and personal well-being in the child.
9. Social competence and sense of personal responsibility in the child.
10. Drive to learn, acquire career/work skills, and achieve economic independence.

Geers (1985), in studying the academic achievement of groups of deaf children, stated that "no one method has been demonstrated to be the answer to the problems imposed by deafness. The answer lies not in the method but in the quality of teaching. Most deaf children require intensive, individualized instruction in order to realize their potential."

Schuyler and Rushmer (1987) reported on a group of profoundly deaf graduates of a parent-infant program whose later school achievement was studied. Those who scored at or above age level on tests of reading achievement had common histories: All had received sufficient access to spoken and/or signed language to acquire a solid foundation of symbolic language during their preschool years. In all cases their families were able to make their child's learning a family priority.

In a study of families of profoundly deaf children with high reading achievement, Bodner-Johnson (1985) learned that those families shared common characteristics. The parents viewed the hearing loss as a personal characteristic of the child; they did not focus on the handicapping nature of it. The hearing-impaired community was an important part of their lives, and the deaf child had the same rules and responsibilities as siblings. Bodner-Johnson reported that "the children's academic achievement was associated with the degree to which the parents had adapted to their child's hearing impairment...had integrated into the family schedule those activities necessitated by the hearing loss." These parents "pressed" for academic achievement. Bromwich (1978), in summarizing the UCLA Infant Studies Project, concluded that "intervention was generally effective when the infant was a high priority in the life of the family."

The best approach may be what enhances a family's ability to make their child's growth a priority and offers them the appropriate tools. The professional who contributes in ways that help the family achieve mutually pleasurable interaction goes a long way toward meeting all other goals.

COMPETENCIES NEEDED BY PARENT-INFANT SPECIALISTS

Certainly the best approach is carried out by well-prepared professionals. Specialists serving infants with hearing loss and their families come from a variety of professional training backgrounds: Education of the Deaf; Speech-Language Pathology; Educational Audiology; and Early Childhood/Special Education. Because none of these four fields of study can devote the time to sufficiently prepare the professional to specialize in infants with hearing loss and their families, further training must be obtained. Those professionals who gain Infant-Family Specialist competencies in the graduate program at Infant Hearing Resource, Portland, Oregon, require an additional year beyond their original graduate program.

Professionals are often placed in parent-infant (hearing-impaired) positions without the additional year of training in this specialty because of the limited training available and because some administrative decisions are still based on the belief that not much happens in infancy; therefore, just about anyone could do the work. This kind of decision making can cloud a child's future. The first three years are the most important in the life of the baby and his or her family. If the child is not served by professionals with the highest levels of skill in a variety of areas, the subsequent delays in learning can be irreversible. Some major areas of competency for the specialist include:

1. Knowledge of normal auditory behavior.
2. Keen ability to detect signs of hearing in a deaf child. This is critical to optimal auditory-vocal and auditory-verbal progress.
3. Complete understanding of the audiogram, characteristics of amplification systems and the acoustics of speech, in order to meet auditory-verbal goals.
4. Ability to manage the process of trial hearing aid use and evaluate the function of aids.
5. Ability to assess development across all domains: motor, cognitive, social-emotional, hearing, language, self-help.
6. Ability to advise, support, and consult with parents who are non-elective "students."
7. Skill in the "interactional approach" to intervention: use of listening, observing, modeling, and joint problem solving (Bromwich 1978).
8. Ability to counsel parents.
9. Comfort in including all family members.
10. Ability to assess family strengths and needs.
11. Ability to work with the family to draft their Individual Family Service Plan (IFSP).
12. Competence in those vocal/speech development techniques unique to the child with hearing loss.
13. Expertise in the use of adult communication strategies that promote communication and language growth in infants and toddlers, including "motherese/fatherese."
14. Knowledge of visual communication strategies used by deaf parents with their infants and the ability to communicate the use of those strategies to families with normally hearing members.
15. Skill in signed communication.
16. Skill in the sequential development of language.
17. Detailed knowledge of infant and child development.

18. Skill in promoting infant cognitive development.
19. Strategies for infants with additional special needs.
20. Ability to use play as the primary learning milieu.
21. An innate sense of playfulness and enjoyment of infants and toddlers.
22. Interdisciplinary team skills.
23. Ability to facilitate a family support group or to select an appropriate facilitator.
24. Ability to accommodate to diverse cultural practices and a variety of family styles and values.
25. Sign class instruction or hiring skills.
26. Awareness of the deaf community and culture.

The importance of each of these competencies is well known to our professions, but one in particular is recently gaining our attention: the understanding of those visual communication strategies used effectively by deaf parents with their infants. Because deaf children of deaf parents characteristically score higher than deaf children of hearing parents on tests of academic achievement and on tests of social-emotional maturity, there is justifiable interest in determining elements of the deaf parent-deaf infant interaction that might contribute to this. Research has shown clear differences in mothers' communication styles with their infants who are deaf depending on the mother's hearing status (Day et al. in press; Nienhuys et al. 1985). Visual communication strategies used by deaf parents with their infants have been noted by Launer (1982), Kantor (1982), and Harris et al. (1989). These include (1) exaggerated size of signs; (2) positive facial expression much of the time; (3) referent object brought directly into the conversational space; (4) repetition of signs as well as movement within signs; (5) prolonged gazing and eye contact; (6) up to 50% of parents' utterances include pointing; (7) Nonverbal affective acts interspersed with language, such as tickling, patting, smiling; (8) longer than normal pauses between periods of signing; (9) majority of utterances with infants consisting of one word at a time; and (10) signs made directly on the baby or on the object of the baby's attention.

PERSONAL QUALITIES OF PARENT-INFANT SPECIALISTS

Technical skill and academic knowledge will be useless to the parent-infant specialist in the absence of good interpersonal communication skills and the ability to build positive relationships. Because of the elements of counseling involved, personal characteristics desirable in counselors might be among those sought in professionals who will work well in homes with families and their infants. The specialist whose interpersonal style will promote trust may have (1) personal comfort with own and with others' expressions of strong feelings including sadness, guilt, depression, and anger; (2) the ability to feel one's own strong feelings and to allow others to feel theirs; (3) the ability to relate with warmth, empathy, respect, and positive regard; (4) openness and comfort with being known as a person; (5) ease in establishing friendships; (6) good "active" listening skills; (7) ease with relinquishing control and with giving up the role of teacher, therapist, or intervention manager for that of the consultant, adviser, and resource; and (8) a sense of playfulness.

PARENT-PROFESSIONAL RELATIONSHIP

Special care must be taken as the goal-oriented professional enters the family system. It is natural for well-intended professionals to want to fix things, to teach what we know, and to work to get the communication system going as soon as possible. It is easy to focus on the product, the goal, the child's acquisition of language and ability to hear and speak. In fact, what is needed is to focus on the present process, to attend to what each family member is feeling, thinking, and doing, what each feels would help at any given moment. This will be different for every family and for each member of the family. And it will change from visit to visit.

Just as some parents overdirect and manipulate their child in their zeal to teach communication skills, so do some adult professionals overdirect services to families. Excessive control actually impedes the language learning process for the infant. The earnest professional, anxious to meet learning objectives for the family, can get the same result. Directiveness can lead to one-way communication, from specialist to parent, and can impede family progress and learning. The effective parent-professional relationship should look like a collaboration between peers, each with valuable elements to contribute and each needing to learn from the other. The partners might share (1) goals, knowledge, and questions; (2) mutual trust and respect for the other's competence and individuality; (3) mutual enjoyment of one another; (4) playfulness; (5) joint problem solving; and (6) delight in the child.

THE SETTING FOR FAMILY SERVICES

Where does all this happen? Various combinations of home-clinic-based services are offered, depending on program philosophy, distance, cost, and money available. Home is an excellent intervention milieu; however, it is prohibitive for some programs. Paying for travel time to families' homes is expensive. Fortunately, the setting is not as important as the dynamics and content of the interactions that occur there. Intervention does need to occur in settings allowing for natural parent-infant interactions that can promote learning. This interaction centers on daily care, family routines, and play. These are the activities families engage in each day with their baby so these are the best learning environments for intervention.

Play is the primary activity through which infants and toddlers learn. It is also a positive medium for rebuilding and strengthening the parent-infant relationship. Bromwich (1978) stated: "Mutual attachment evolves through frequent playful, positive and reciprocal interaction. During play (with the parent) the infant is motivated to explore his environment and to experience objects. As the infant responds to this stimulus the parent is encouraged to provide still more interesting things to do. The parent becomes the mediator between the child and his environment." By facilitating infant learning through play, collaborative activities can facilitate parent-infant interaction, which helps promote all other learning.

THE COST

A June 1991 telephone survey of six public and private agencies serving infants and toddlers with hearing loss and their families revealed a cost range from $5,000 to $12,000 per child per year. These agencies, in different regions of the U.S., served families in a variety of ways. Families were seen from one to three times each week for a nine-, eleven-, or twelve-month year. Some of the public agencies did not have the means to account for the cost of space and overhead and so did not include these figures in their cost estimates. One of the private agencies had to include significant fund-raising costs in data. Others did not. If the hearing loss is detected soon after birth, a family might receive parent-infant programming for up to three years. The cost for a family's service over three years at these agencies can range between $15,000 and $36,000.

A review of funding sources for parent-infant services reveals that the cost is borne by public tax-supported federal or state programs, private insurance, family fees, and private philanthropy. Different programs utilized these funding sources in varying degrees.

Appropriate early intervention for infants with hearing loss is costly, but it costs society much less than other options. It costs less than (1) maintaining a late-identified, low-achieving child in an expensive special education self-contained classroom throughout his educational career; (2) graduating intelligent 18-year-olds with insufficient reading skills who cannot be employed at levels commensurate with their intellectual potential; and (3) allowing children to experience the school failure, diminished self-esteem, and sense of powerlessness that lead them to unemployment and eventual government support throughout their adult lives.

The majority of adults in the work force today who had significant hearing loss since early childhood did not have the option of early and appropriate family programming. Most of them began their language learning process at age 3 or 4 years, an age when their normal hearing peers had their language systems completely established and were sporting 1,000- to 1,500-word vocabularies. These deaf children were sent away to school before their families learned how to communicate with them or how to help them learn. The wage-earning data on these individuals suggest that insufficient education left many of them ill-prepared for economic independence. Rubin (1989) reviewed the 1984 Survey of Income and Program Participation of the U.S. Bureau of Census, which included income figures for noninstitutionalized deaf and hard-of-hearing individuals. The survey indicated that in 1984, 33% of the hard-of-hearing population and 45% of the deaf population were out of the work force and had no earnings. They received government and, in some cases, family support. The same survey showed that more than 50% of the deaf and hard-of-hearing population who *were* employed earned below poverty level ($884/month at that time). An adult with hearing loss who supports his family on Social Security Income (SSI) utilizes far more of our nation's financial resources in a lifetime than would have been spent on comprehensive early services.

This discouraging information on the minimal earning power of a large percentage of the hard-of-hearing and deaf population is not surprising in light of the data on low school achievement of the average graduates of schools for the deaf. These data would imply that earning power is related to level of education. Anecdotal reports from comprehensive early intervention programs on the progress of their graduates indicate that many of these children attend college, earn advanced degrees, and are employed at professional levels. With this advanced training their incomes approach those of their hearing peers. Welsh et al. (1988) reviewed U.S. Internal Revenue Service data accumulated through the National Technical Institute for the Deaf (NTID) of the Rochester Institute of Technology (RIT). The income of NTID graduates (with BA degrees and higher) was 93% of that of their normal hearing RIT peers. Mean income in 1982 was $15,000. The pay-off to society of an investment early in life is the likelihood that a well-trained, well-educated deaf individual will function as a productive contributor to society rather than as a recipient of tax dollars generated by his or her hearing peers.

THE FUTURE

In the coming years the question of how to best serve families of infants with hearing loss will continue to be controversial. Healthy discussion will be fueled by increased research.

1. We will see increasing evidence of the effectiveness of each of the approaches to intervention with infants and their families as well as more dissemination of the instructional techniques for the implementation of these approaches.
2. In order for the positive effects of early services to be felt by families, physicians will be called upon to evaluate the hearing of all infants from the first months of life and to refer those in question for audiologic assessment. Ideally, services for the family begin before the baby's 6-month birthday. The deleterious effects of time lost, in the United States where the average age of identification is 2½ years, are irreversible.
3. States will provide services for deaf infants within "non-categorical" nursery programs serving all children with special needs, and we will hear intense opposition from expert educators of the deaf who will question the competency of the early childhood-special educator

for the complex task of developing language and speech in a child who does not hear. Some deaf educators and deaf adults will protest that this noncategorical nursery setting followed by mainstreaming during school years, rather than being "least restrictive," may be "most restrictive" for the deaf child. For this child, "normalization" may lie not in the regular classroom with hearing peers but in classes with deaf peers taught by deaf teachers with whom the child shares a common culture.

4. In the coming years, improvements in hearing aid technology will lead to increased numbers of children utilizing hearing for auditory-verbal learning, developing intelligible speech, and communicating well with both deaf and hearing individuals.

5. We will see more data on the effective use of strategies of visual communication as a tool for parents in making their communication meaningful to the infant with hearing loss.

6. Research into the early manual babbling of deaf infants whose parents are deaf will support the position of Petito and Marentette (1991), that "the speech modality is not critical in babbling. Rather, babbling is tied to the abstract linguistic structure of language."

Most important, professionals will become better listeners. We need to listen to parents, to siblings, and to deaf adults about how to best serve them. We need to relinquish traditional control in order to relate with families as partners and consultants, a relationship more likely to maximize the family's sense of competence and control.

REFERENCES

Bodner-Johnson, B. 1985. Families that work for the hearing-impaired child. *Volta Review* 87(4):131-136.

Bromwich, R. 1978. *Working with parents and infants: An interactional approach*. Baltimore, Md.: University Park Press.

Day, P.S., Bodner-Johnson, B., and Gutfreund, M.K. 1991. In press. Interacting with infants with a hearing loss: What can we learn from mothers who are deaf? *Journal of Early Intervention*.

Geers, A. 1985. Assessment of hearing impaired children: Determining typical and optimal levels of performance. In F. Powell, T. Finitzo-Hieber, S. Friel-Patti, and D. Henderson (eds.), *Education of the hearing-impaired child*. San Diego: College Hill Press.

Harris, M., Clibbens, J., Chasin, J., and Tibbitts, R. 1989. The social context of early sign language development. *First Language* 9:81-97.

International Association of Parents of the Deaf. 1985. Today's hearing-impaired children and youth: A demographic and academic profile. The Endeavor. Silver Spring, Md.: International Association of Parents of the Deaf.

Kantor, R. 1982. Communicative interaction: Mother modification and child acquisition of American sign language. *Sign Language Studies* 36:233-282.

Launer, P.P. 1982. Early signs of motherhood: Motherese in ASL. Paper presented at ASHA Convention, Ontario, Canada.

Musselman, C.R., Wilson, A.K., and Lindsay, P.H. 1988. Effects of early intervention on hearing-impaired children. *Exceptional Children* 55:222-228.

Nienhuys, T., Horsborough, K., and Cross, T. 1985. A dialogic analysis of interaction between mothers and their deaf or hearing preschoolers. *Applied Psycholinguistics* 6:121-140.

Petito, L.A., and Marentette, P.F. 1991. Babbling in the manual mode: Evidence for the ontogeny of language. *Science*, March, 1493-1496.

Rubin, J. 1989. Income of hearing-impaired people and implications for public and private financing of non-auditory devices. Gallaudet Research Institute Working Paper, 89-5. Washington, D.C.: Gallaudet University.

Schuyler, V., and Rushmer, N. 1987. *Parent-infant habilitation: A comprehensive approach to working with hearing-impaired infants and their parents*. Portland, Oreg.: IHR Publications.

Snow, C.E. 1984. Parent-child interaction and the development of communicative ability. In R. Schiefelbusch and J. Pickar (eds.), *The acquisition of communicative competence*. Baltimore: University Park Press.

Welsh, W., Walter, G., and Riley, D. 1988. Earnings of hearing-impaired college alumni as reported by the Internal Revenue Service. *Volta Review* 90(2):69-76.

Williams-Scott, B., and Kipila, E. 1987. Cued speech: A professional point of view. In S. Schwartz (ed.), *Choices in deafness: A parents guide*. Kensington, Md.:Woodbine House.

Wood, D., Wood, H., Griffiths, A., and Howarth, I. 1986. *Teaching and talking with deaf children*. New York: John Wiley and Sons.

Chapter 30

Hearing-Impaired Children in the Schools: Integrated or Isolated?

Pamela E. Montgomery and Noel D. Matkin

INTRODUCTION

The scope of practice of the pediatric audiologist has expanded to include the early identification, assessment, and intensive habilitation of a broad spectrum of children with hearing impairment, including those with minimal hearing loss. According to Davis (1989), among others, once these children (especially those with milder degrees of hearing loss) enter school, they are often forgotten.

Ideally, each school system should have an audiologist on staff who has clinical competencies in pediatric habilitation, support from the administration, and effective communication with classroom teachers. The reality in many communities is that services are contracted with local audiologists. In other communities, the audiologist who provided the children with amplification through a private practice may be the only source of audiologic input in the development of an educational plan for the child. In this situation, a partnership with the speech-language pathologist in the school system becomes crucial.

Even in an ideal situation, many audiologists feel that their formal education in pediatric audiologic habilitation provided less experience with this population than desired. A survey of 200 working audiologists by Oyler, Oyler, and Matkin (1988) revealed that 76% of those audiologists surveyed reported their academic program requirements in pediatric habilitation were inadequate. This is a major concern in consideration of the new certificate of clinical competence (CCC) audiology requirements, which become effective in January 1993. Only 20 clock hours of supervised audiology practicum will be required in the treatment of adult and pediatric hearing disorders. However, the vast majority of these 20 hours may be with adult clients, since a minimum requirement regarding the treatment of children has not been specified.

The guidelines for defining "educationally significant" hearing loss recently generated by a task force for the state of Colorado are insightful and merit recognition (Colorado Department of Education 1991). This is especially true when one considers the growing body of research relative to mild bilateral hearing loss, such as the study completed by Blair et al. in 1985; relative to unilateral hearing loss, such as the studies by the Vanderbilt group in 1984 and by Oyler, Oyler, and Matkin in 1988; and relative to conductive hearing loss associated with recurrent otitis media as investigated by Paden et al. (1985). These guidelines, which identify children with educationally significant hearing impairment, include:

1. An average pure-tone hearing loss in the speech range (500-2000 Hz) of 20 dB HL or greater in the better ear, which is not reversible within a reasonable period of time.
2. An average high frequency, pure-tone hearing loss of 35 dB HL or greater in the better ear at two or more of the following frequencies: 2000 Hz, 3000 Hz, 4000 Hz, and 6000 Hz.
3. A permanent unilateral hearing loss of 35 dB HL or greater in the speech range (500-2000 Hz).
4. Any hearing impairment that significantly affects communication with others and where the individual requires supplemental assistance or modification of instructional methods in order to achieve optimum performance. Cases in this latter category might include the child with a fluctuating hearing loss and the hearing-impaired child with developmental delay.

Management of the school-age hearing-impaired child is a very complex topic when one considers:

A. The rules and regulations of P.L. 94-142, the federal mandate requiring a free and appropriate education for all children with special needs, including those with hearing impairment.

B. The increasingly broad spectrum of school-age children with hearing loss considered to be educationally significant. This spectrum includes not only those youngsters with bilateral sensorineural hearing loss but also those with permanent unilateral impairments and those with fluctuating hearing loss related to recurrent, and often chronic, otitis media. Traditionally, hearing impairment among children has been considered a low incidence "handicap." Yet when all of the above categories are considered, the prevalence is much greater than previously believed.

C. Most children will be mainstreamed into classroom spaces that have not been acoustically designed for hearing-impaired children. The hearing aid alone, even with preferential seating, will not provide effective support for the hearing-impaired child in noisy, reverberant teaching environments.

This chapter focuses upon three premises that merit careful consideration by both clinical and educational audiologists who work with school-age hearing-impaired children. The first premise is that many educators serving hearing-impaired children do not recognize the limitations of hearing aids or the negative impact of classroom acoustic environment as major variables affecting language acquisition, verbal communication, and academic achievement. The second premise is that many regular classroom teachers do not understand the direct relationship between the deficits imposed by the child's hearing impairment and associated academic and behavioral management problems. The third, and final, premise is that few hearing-impaired children receive comprehensive, longitudinal monitoring to assess the effects of hearing impairment on academic progress. Such ongoing assessment of progress is an essential feature of a proactive approach to educational and audiologic management.

While adhering to the above premises, the audiologic management of school-age youngsters with educationally significant hearing loss is discussed relative to preplacement considerations, classroom placement, and longitudinal monitoring.

PREPLACEMENT CONSIDERATIONS

A preplacement consideration of prime importance is audiologic input into the development of the educational management plan for each school-age child with hearing impairment. To comply with the federal mandate, an Individualized Education Plan (IEP) is to be developed on the basis of current evaluation findings of each child's current strengths and limitations.

Hearing loss may have a primary impact upon cognitive, speech-language, and social-emotional development. However, one must keep in mind a national survey by Karchner and Kirwin (1977), which indicated that approximately one out of every three youngsters with sensorineural hearing loss has at least one additional developmental disability, with a higher prevalence among males and among minority children. This finding highlights the importance of integrating audiologic findings into a matrix of performance data from other specialists rather than viewing a child's auditory status in isolation. Input from psychologists, speech-language pathologists, occupational and physical therapists, and educators is essential. Another potential variable is the estimate from the Bureau of Census that at least one-third of our pediatric clients will be from culturally diverse families by the turn of the century. The importance of teamwork becomes obvious when one considers the prevalence of young children with multiple developmental disabilities, with many coming from culturally diverse family backgrounds (Yacobacci-Tam 1987).

To effectively serve the hearing-impaired child, the audiologist must understand normal language development as well as the impact of hearing impairment upon language acquisition and verbal communication (Matkin 1986). The effect of hearing loss on a child's ability to follow the instructions of the teacher and successfully participate in verbally based classroom activities must be taken into consideration when developing audiologic recommendations. This includes the need for classroom amplification and supplemental support services.

The unaided audiogram serves as a baseline for monitoring hearing status over time, but aided audiologic results are far more important as the IEP is drafted by the evaluation team. Superimposing the aided audiogram on the dot matrix developed by Mueller and Killion (1990) is a valuable strategy. The level of expectation for auditory performance and the need for supplemental visual input in the classroom should be considered as one reviews the portions of conversational speech spectrum that are, and that are not, available to the child fitted with amplification. Use of such a visual display during a team staffing can help circumvent many of the communication problems generated by the use of the traditional audiology lexicon, which only effectively communicates with other audiologists. Figure 1 illustrates an appropriate hearing aid fitting in which the child is receiving approximately 88% of the speech spectrum. This child is a candidate for a strong auditory oral approach, with word recognition and auditory comprehension of speech being a realistic level of expectation. In contrast, figure 2 illustrates a limited aided response where the child is missing approximately 50% of the speech spectrum in conversation, most notably in the high frequency range, which is critical for reception of voiced and voiceless consonants. Such an aided audiogram may occur in children with a severe-to-profound hearing loss or with an inadequate hearing aid fitting. In such an instance, the level of expectation for auditory learning must be modified even when an optimal hearing aid fitting is made.

The second preplacement consideration is classroom acoustics. Since most hearing-impaired children will be integrated into a regular classroom for at least a portion of the school day, assessing the

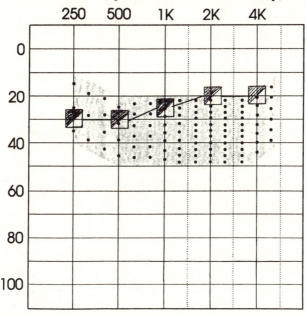

Figure 1. The Count-the-Dot Audiogram Form for Calculation of the Articulation Index from Mueller and Killion 1990, reprinted with permission The Hearing Journal. An illustration of an aided audiogram for a listener who should perceive approximately 88% of the spectrum of conversational speech.

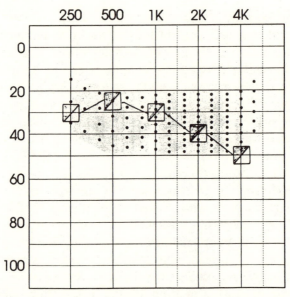

Figure 2. The Count-the-Dot Audiogram Form for Calculation of the Articulation Index from Mueller and Killion 1990, reprinted with permission The Hearing Journal. An illustration of an aided audiogram for a listener who will perceive only 38% of the speech spectrum of conversation.

youngster's auditory performance in competition, as well as in quiet, is essential. The classic study by Finitzo-Hieber and Tillman (1978) clearly demonstrated the negative impact of noise and reverberation on aided word recognition among school-age children. While the adverse effects of the acoustic environment upon the hearing-impaired child are well recognized among audiologists, this crucial concern often is not considered as a primary issue during the development of the IEP to be implemented in a classroom that may have little acoustic treatment and is noisy and reverberant.

An effective and easy-to-use method for improving the signal-to-noise ratio in noisy, reverberant classrooms is the addition of a personal FM system to assist the hearing-impaired child in these settings. Too often, when asking school administrators for funding to purchase such systems, requests are made by citing the research literature. It is far more effective to advocate with the school system for the provision of personal FM units when aided scores in quiet and in noise for the *specific* child under study can be highlighted and discussed. A practical method for obtaining such scores, even in a child as young as 3 years of age, is the use of speech spectrum noise as a competing signal.

In the University of Arizona hearing clinics, a signal-to-noise ratio of +5 is maintained and word recognition scores are obtained with developmentally appropriate materials such as Phonemically Balanced Kindergarten (PBK-50) word lists, Word Intelligibility by Picture Identification (WIPI), Northwestern University Children's Perception of Speech Test (NUCHIPS) or, as a last resort, with informal tests using a variety of familiar toy objects. Figure 3 illustrates the findings for a child with a unilateral hearing loss when tested in quiet and then in a monaural indirect condition in competition. Sound field testing in quiet, while using familiar objects, resulted in correct identification of nine out of ten objects. When competing noise was added, and the child was asked to identify the same objects, the child's performance dropped dramatically. Only four out of the ten objects were identified correctly, and the youngster's response time lengthened significantly. Another benefit of environmental testing in noise is education of parents regarding the impact of noise on their child's ability to listen. Often, they are astounded by the results of such tests and are much better prepared to advocate for their child with school administrators for appropriate classroom placement and supplemental assistive listening devices.

The third preplacement consideration is observation in the classroom prior to placement of the hearing-impaired child. The goal of such an observation is twofold. First, knowledge of the acoustics in the classroom is essential because decisions are made relative to the need for use of a personal FM system. Numerous studies have documented the high noise levels in many educational settings, with signal-to-noise levels approaching 0 dB, particularly in the lower grades. Yet, as noted by Olsen (1977), hearing-impaired children require a signal-to-noise ratio of +15 to +20 dB for optimal auditory performance. Ideally, ambient noise levels inside the classroom should not exceed a sound level reading of 35 dB-A, whereas maximum noise levels outside the classroom should not exceed 65 dB-A. Finally, the ambient noise level at a building site should not exceed 70 dB-A (Fourcin 1980).

In reality, options regarding a choice of classrooms may be limited, and in many instances the hearing-impaired child may have classes in several different locations during the course of the school day. Existing classrooms can be modified acoustically, but this strategy may be fiscally

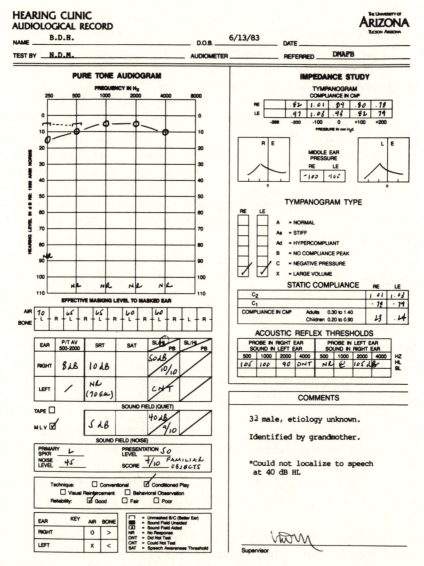

Figure 3. The audiologic findings for a 3-year-old child with a profound unilateral hearing loss whose sound field performance in noise shows a marked decrement.

prohibitive if there are only a few children with hearing impairment mainstreamed in a school building. In such an instance, the provision of assistive listening devices to supplement personal amplification becomes a crucial issue.

The second goal during the classroom observation is the assessment of the appropriateness of the teacher's communication style and classroom management strategies relative to the needs of the hearing-impaired child. A survey form consisting of 12 key questions published by Ling and Ling (1978) is useful in focusing attention on important considerations. The teacher's ability to meet the requirements of the child with hearing impairment, while at the same time considering all members of the class, should be assessed. Also, the teacher's creativity in contriving situations that promote speech and language development is a crucial element. The ideal teacher proceeds from known to unknown, familiar to unfamiliar, simple to complex, and easy to difficult. Finally, the creative teacher supplements auditory instruction with visual support since the hearing-impaired child needs a multimodality focus to provide optimal learning experiences (Ling and Ling 1978).

The fourth preplacement consideration is the inclusion of parents in the decision-making process. Too often, when the IEP team discusses school-age children and classroom placement, parental input is not considered. As part of the IEP process, a survey of family needs should be completed yearly. Such a survey should address family concerns regarding child development, hearing impairment, communication, and the community services available for children with hearing impairment. As an example, the Tucson Catalina Foothills School District has developed a questionnaire to provide parents with an opportunity to contribute information regarding student placement. The questionnaire begins on a positive note by asking the parents to discuss two or three things they treasure about their child. The parents are then asked the following questions:

1. Describe how you believe your child learns best.
2. Describe pertinent information about your child's social/emotional needs.
3. What are two or three goals you have for your child this year, academically or socially?
4. What are your expectations of the school, in terms of helping your child meet these goals?

A cover letter is enclosed explaining the process of classroom placement as the collaborative effort between parents, administration, grade level teachers, special area teachers, and specialists with the goal of optimal placement of all students (Prosnitz 1991). In addition, the resource specialist meets with all parents of children with special needs to gather parental input prior to writing the IEP goals for the following year. Booklets, videotapes, handouts, and daily log books, as well as referral to family support groups, may be used to supplement such face-to-face conferences.

Differences in family systems influence decision making. Traditional role models and family structures do not characterize many parents needing support services. The two-parent family pictured in much of the early intervention literature represents only a minority of households in the United States. These differences must be recognized and respected as services are delivered.

CLASSROOM PLACEMENT CONSIDERATIONS

As noted earlier, classroom placement considerations are our second major area of concern. Most regular classroom teachers have had minimal, if any, experience in integrating a hearing-impaired child into the daily classroom routine and in managing amplification systems. Since children fitted with glasses are considered to have corrected vision, it is not surprising to find that a teacher may perceive the youngster fitted with binaural amplification or an FM system as having "corrected hearing." This fact was highlighted by Paul and Young (1975), who found that half of the classroom teachers they surveyed did not appreciate the relationship between a child's hearing loss and academic difficulties. As a consequence, unrealistically high levels of expectation may be set. Problems in auditory attention, auditory comprehension, and classroom participation may be perceived as behavioral problems rather than limitations imposed by the hearing loss, even when the student is aided.

In sharp contrast, studies of the "hearing aid effect" suggest that in some instances the visible presence of hearing aids or FM units may stigmatize the child, not only among peers but with the teacher. As a result, unrealistically low levels of expectation may become a prophecy of self-fulfillment, and thus an obstacle to optimal classroom achievement. When either of these possibilities is considered, the need for an ongoing teacher in-service program becomes readily apparent.

Since responsibility for using and monitoring amplification in the classroom may be viewed as burdensome and even threatening by some teachers, orientation and ongoing support in the optimal use of amplification is a vital first step in a teacher in-service program.

During the early school years, before the child uses reading to acquire new information, he must follow the teacher's verbal instruction during the majority of classroom activities. For this reason, consultation with the teacher about the child's current level of language function is essential. This can be done by the educational audiologist or, more commonly, by the speech-language pathologist. Use of a developmental profile to visually highlight a hearing-impaired child's strengths and limitations relative to his chronological age across language domains enhances communication with teachers during in-service conferences. Without such visual supplements, the specialized terminology used in reporting speech-language test results creates a barrier to effective communication with teachers and parents.

The teacher needs to understand the impact of hearing loss on self-esteem since a hearing-impaired child's behavior may be the most visible sign of the impairment. General and specific strategies for managing hearing-impaired children are needed in the four major areas of audition, cognition, language skills, and socialization. The interested reader is referred to the work of Davis (1989) and to the curriculum supplement of the Test of Auditory Comprehension (TAC) for examples of effective classroom teaching strategies. The guidelines for teachers developed by Matkin and Sturgeon (1980) may appear simplistic to audiologists. However, in our experience, most classroom teachers welcome such information since use of such guidelines facilitates the integration of the child with a hearing loss into the activities of the regular classroom (see Appendix A).

Just as the teacher should function as part of the child's support system, the audiologist needs to become an effective part of the support system for the classroom teacher (Davis 1989). In-service education is not enough. The audiologist and the classroom teacher need to form a collaborative partnership. The audiologist can help the teacher learn about hearing loss, while the teacher can assist the audiologist in evaluating the effect of the hearing loss on academic performance as well as the effectiveness of aural rehabilitation efforts. With such an exchange of knowledge, the need for consistent use of amplification, the need for support services to supplement classroom instruction, and the need for use of compensatory management strategies in the classroom are more readily appreciated and accepted by the classroom teacher.

LONGITUDINAL MONITORING CONSIDERATIONS

Finally, the third major consideration is longitudinal monitoring since it is essential to determine whether or not our recommendations are making a difference in the child's performance. Once a hearing-impaired child is evaluated, personal and educational amplification is acquired, classroom placement is made, and support services are in place, it is imperative for the managing audiologist to implement a systematic and consistent longitudinal monitoring plan. Assuring that adequate achievement occurs over time is an essential feature of a comprehensive, proactive audiologic plan. At a minimum, school-age children should be scheduled for annual evaluations, while more frequent monitoring is needed during the preschool years.

The rationale for ongoing audiologic evaluations is readily apparent. Although recurrent middle ear dysfunction with conductive hearing loss and progressive sensorineural impairments are less frequently encountered in school-age children than among preschoolers, such changes can and do occur. Electroacoustic modifications of the child's amplification systems and more intensive support services will be needed if decrements in hearing cannot be reversed by medical and surgical treatment.

Ongoing evaluation of the child's hearing aids, including their physical condition, electroacoustic function, and ear mold fit, is the second monitoring goal. Public Law 94-142 clearly states:

Each public agency shall insure that the hearing aids worn by deaf and hard of hearing children in school are functioning properly (Federal Register 1977).

Yet, a national survey reported by Reichman and Healey (1989) revealed that only 54% of programs provide daily monitoring and listening checks of the children's hearing aids.

With the increased use of personal FM units interfaced with hearing aids in the educational setting, it is mandated that the function of these systems also be assessed. A field study by Bess et al. (1984) revealed that the malfunction rate among classroom amplification units is alarmingly high, approaching 50%. The national survey by Reichman and Healey revealed that 42% of programs do not have a daily monitoring program to assure that educational amplification units are functioning adequately (1989). It seems ironic that monitoring plans are not in place when it is assumed that the majority of mainstreamed hearing-impaired children will use *aided* auditory input as a primary channel for comprehending classroom instruction.

The third component of monitoring is obtaining input from the primary classroom teacher before an audiologic evaluation and amplification assessment are undertaken. Far too often, audiologists draw conclusions and generate recommendations without knowledge of the child's performance in the classroom. When one considers the paperwork demands on teachers, it is not reasonable to request a detailed narrative report relative to the child's classroom performance. However, the use of a teacher rating scale, such as the Screening Instrument for Targeting Educational Risk (SIFTER) (Anderson 1989), can provide the managing audiologist with key information while requiring minimal time and effort from the teacher.

A further advantage of using such a screening instrument is that the child's performance profile across the five key areas of academics, attention, communication, class participation, and school behavior can be monitored on a yearly basis (figure 4). When a child's SIFTER profile is characterized by one or more areas of deficit, the audiologist not only has the responsibility to review the adequacy of audiologic management but has a relatively objective basis to take a proactive stance and call for a review of the current IEP.

The fourth component of annual monitoring is review of the findings from an annual speech-language evaluation. Results of such evaluations are helpful in determining the effectiveness of amplification in the development of auditory language comprehension. Another clinical strategy that provides essential information is the annual administration of the Test of Auditory Comprehension (TAC) (1977). While the tradition of administering tests of word recognition during the audiologic evaluation has merit, it is difficult to track growth in auditory skills longitudinally with only scores on a single word recognition task. Plotting a youngster's profile of performance across a variety of auditory subtests graded in difficulty, and then comparing the child's performance

Content Area	Total Score	Pass	Marginal	Fail
Academics	13	15 14 (13) 12 11 10	9 8	7 6 5 4 3
Attention	9	15 14 13 12 11 10 (9)	8 7	6 5 4 3
Communication	12	15 14 13 (12) 11	10 9 8	7 6 5 4 3
Class Participation	13	15 14 (13) 12 11 10 9	8 7	6 5 4 3
School Behavior	14	15 (14) 13 12 11 10	9 8	7 6 5 4 3

Figure 4. The SIFTER (Anderson 1989) profile for a 6-year-old child with a moderate bilateral hearing loss whose performance in a mainstream classroom is perceived as adequate across all domains. Reprinted with the permission of PRO-ED.

to that of other children of the same age and with a similar degree of hearing loss, is well worth the time and effort required. As mentioned earlier, an especially appealing feature of the TAC is the accompanying curriculum guide, which suggests intervention strategies based on the test findings.

Ideally, the fifth component of the monitoring program is direct observation of the hearing-impaired child in the classroom. Time constraints and scheduling difficulties are recognized as hindrances, but in our experience there is no substitute for direct observation. This observation should focus on the child's interactive skills with his teachers and peers in classroom activities, his specific learning strategies, and his use of amplification (Ross and Calvert 1977).

The information gathered during the monitoring activities described above forms the basis for the review of current classroom placement and the development of IEP goals for the next school year. Determination of the appropriateness of classroom placement or the need for modification of the existing placement should be one focus of the IEP review. As the child reaches the high-school level, IEP goals should be expanded to include prevocational counseling while keeping the limitations imposed by the hearing loss in mind. Finally, active inclusion of parents during yearly evaluations is essential. Ongoing education, guidance, and counseling are needed by most parents throughout their child's school years (Matkin 1988). Different questions and concerns develop as children mature and move through the educational system. Unfortunately, parent support services often are viewed by clinicians as a primary responsibility *only* during the preschool years.

In conclusion, audiologists should ensure that mainstreamed hearing-impaired children are, in fact, effectively integrated into the classroom. Without the audiologist's participation in teacher education, IEP development, and longitudinal monitoring, the school-age child with a hearing loss may be isolated, not integrated.

REFERENCES

—. 1977. Education of handicapped children: Implementation of Part B of the education of the handicapped act. *Federal Register* 42:42474-42518.

Anderson, K. 1989. *Screening instrument for targeting educational risk* (SIFTER). Austin, Tex.: PRO-ED.

Bess, F., Sinclair, J., and Riggs, D. 1984. Group amplification in schools for the hearing impaired. *Ear and Hearing* 5(3):138-144.

Blair, J.C., Peterson, M.E., and Veihweg, S.H. 1985. The effects of mild sensorineural hearing loss on academic performance of young school-age children. *Volta Review* 87:87-93.

Colorado Department of Education. 1991 in press. Effectiveness Indicators for Audiological Services, 1-18.

Davis, D.S. 1989. *Otitis media: Coping with the effects in the classroom.* Curriculum adaptations and classroom strategies for the child with hearing loss. Stanhope, N.J.: Hear You Are, Inc.

Finitzo-Hieber, T., and Tillman, T.W. 1978. Room acoustics effects on monosyllabic word discrimination ability for normal and hearing impaired children. *Journal of Speech and Hearing Research* 21:440-458.

Fourcin, A.J. 1980. Design of educational facilities for the deaf children. *British Journal of Audiology* Suppl. 3:1-24.

Karchner, M.A., and Kirwin, L.A. 1977. *The use of hearing aids by hearing impaired students in the United States.* Washington, D.C.: Office of Demographics Studies, Gallaudet College.

Ling, D., and Ling, A. 1978. *Aural habilitation: The foundations of verbal learning in hearing impaired children,* chapter 13 (pp. 278-279). 1st ed. Washington, D.C.: Alexander Graham Bell Association for the Deaf.

Matkin, N.D. 1986. The role of hearing in language development. In J. Kavanaugh (ed.), *Otitis media and child development.* Parkton, Md.: York Press.

Matkin, N.D. 1988. Key considerations in counseling parents of hearing-impaired children. *Seminars in Speech and Language* 9(3):209-222.

Matkin, N.D., and Sturgeon, J.A. 1980. Guidelines for the classroom teacher serving the hearing-impaired child. University of Arizona, Children's Hearing Clinic, Tucson, Ariz. Unpublished.

Minnesota child development inventory. 1974. Behavior Science Systems, Inc., Box 1108, Minneapolis, Minn. 55458.

Mueller, G., and Killion, M. 1990. The count-the-dot audiogram form for calculation of the articulation index. *Hearing Journal* 43(9):14-17.

Olsen, W.O. 1977. Acoustics and amplification in classrooms for the hearing impaired. In F.H. Bess (ed.), *Audiology, education, and the hearing impaired child*, chapters 8 and 9. St. Louis: C.V. Mosby Co.

Oyler, R.F., Oyler, A.L., and Matkin, N.D. 1988. Unilateral hearing loss: Demographics and educational impact. *Language, Speech and Hearing Services in Schools* 19(2):201-210.

Paden, E., Novak, M., and Kuklinski, A. 1985. Otitis media and phonological delay: An avoidable relationship. Paper presented at ASHA Convention, Washington, D.C.

Paul, R., and Young, B. 1975. The child with mild sensorineural hearing loss: The failure syndrome. Paper read at International Congress of the Deaf, Tokyo.

Prosnitz, E. 1991. Personal correspondence to Pam Montgomery.

Reichman, J., and Healey, W.C. 1989. Amplification monitoring and maintenance in schools. *Asha* 31(11):43-45.

Ross, M., and Calvert, D. 1977. Guidelines for auditory programs in educational settings for hearing impaired children. *The condition of hearing aids worn by children in a public school program*. HEW Publication no. OE77-05002. Washington, D.C.: United States Government Printing Office.

Test of auditory comprehension. 1977. Fireworks Publications, Box 9747, North Hollywood, Calif. 91609.

Yacobacci-Tam, P. 1987. Interacting with the culturally different family. *Volta Review* 89(5):46-58.

Appendix A

Guidelines for the Classroom Teacher Serving the Hearing-Impaired Child

Noel D. Matkin, Ph.D. and Joann Sturgeon, M.A.
University of Arizona, Children's Hearing Clinic.

Classroom Seating. Hearing-impaired children should be assigned seats away from hall or street noise and not more than 10 feet from the teacher. Such seating allows the child to better utilize residual hearing, the hearing aid, and visual cues (speechreading, gestures, etc.). Flexibility in seating—movable desks and group arrangements—all enable the hearing-impaired child to observe and actively participate in class activities.

Look and Listen. Children, even those with minimal hearing loss, function much better in the classroom if they can better look and listen.

Check Comprehension. Consistently ask children with a hearing loss questions related to the subject under discussion to make certain that they are following and understanding the discussion. Many hearing-impaired children smile and nod "yes" when they do not understand.

Rephrase and Restate. Encourage hearing-impaired children to indicate when they do not understand what has been said. Rephrase the question or statement since certain words contain sounds that are not easily recognized by either speechreading or aided hearing. Also, most hearing-impaired children have some delay in language development and may not be familiar with key words. By substituting words, the intended meaning may be more readily conveyed.

Pre-tutor Child. Have hearing-impaired children read aloud on a subject to be discussed in class so they are familiar with new vocabulary and concepts, and thus more easily follow and participate in classroom discussion. Such pre-tutoring is an important activity that the parents can undertake.

Involve Resource Personnel. Inform resource personnel of planned vocabulary and language topics to be covered in the classroom so that tutoring can supplement classroom activities during individual therapy.

List Key Vocabulary. Before discussing new material, list key vocabulary on the blackboard. Then build the classroom discussion around this key vocabulary.

Visual Aids. Visual aids help hearing-impaired children by providing the association necessary for learning new concepts.

Individual Help. The child with impaired hearing needs individual attention. When possible provide individual help in order to fill gaps in language and understanding stemming from the child's hearing loss.

Write Instructions. Hearing-impaired children may not follow verbal instructions accurately. Help them by writing assignments on the board so they can be copied in a notebook. Also, use a buddy system by giving a classmate with normal hearing the responsibility for making certain the hearing-impaired child is aware of the assignments made during the day.

Encourage Participation. Encourage participation in activities such as reading, conversation, story telling and creative dramatics. Reading is especially important, since information and knowledge gained through reading help compensate for what is missed because of the hearing loss. Again, parents can assist the child through participation in local library reading programs and modeling in the home.

Monitor Efforts. Remember that children with impaired hearing become fatigued more readily than other children because of the continuous strain resulting from efforts to keep up with and compete in classroom activities.

Inform Parents. Provide the parents of hearing-impaired children in your class with consistent input so that they understand the child's successes and difficulties.

S-P-E-E-C-H. The following mnemonic device, developed by Robert Peddicord, entitled "SPEECH" has been found helpful by teachers and parents when communicating with hearing-impaired children.

S = State the topic to be discussed.
P = Pace your conversation at a moderate speed with occasional pauses to permit comprehension.
E = Enunciate clearly, without exaggerated lip movements.
E = Enthusiastically communicate, using body language and natural gestures.
CH = Check comprehension before changing topics.

Monitor Hearing Aids. Many children with impaired hearing are wearing hearing aids which are in poor repair. The school audiologist or speech-pathologist can give you information about how the hearing aid works and guidance for checking its daily function. Ideally, a battery tester and a hearing aid stethoscope will be available for the daily hearing aid check. Also, a small supply of fresh batteries should be kept at school.

Appendix 1

Joint Committee on Infant Hearing
1990 Position Statement

The following expanded position statement was developed by the Joint Committee on Infant Hearing and approved by the American Speech-Language-Hearing Association (ASHA) Legislative Council (LC 40-90) in November 1990.[1] Joint Committee member organizations that approved this position statement and their respective representatives who prepared this statement include the following: American Speech-Language-Hearing Association—Fred H. Bess, chair, Noel D. Matkin, and Evelyn Cherow, ex officio; American Academy of Otolaryngology-Head and Neck Surgery—Kenneth M. Grundfast, co-chair; American Academy of Pediatrics—Allen Erenberg and William P. Potsic; Council on Education of the Deaf (A.G. Bell Association for the Deaf, American College of Educators of the Hearing Impaired, Convention of American Instructors of the Deaf, and the Conference of Educational Administrators Serving the Deaf)—Lita Aldridge and Barbara Bodner-Johnson; Directors of Speech and Hearing Programs in State Health and Welfare Agencies—Thomas Mahoney. Consultants: Alan Salamy and Gregory J. Matz. Ann L. Carey, 1988-1990 vice president for professional and governmental affairs, was the ASHA monitoring vice president.

I. BACKGROUND

The early detection of hearing impairment in children is essential in order to initiate the medical and educational intervention critical for

---

[1] Reproduced with permission, Joint Committee on Infant Hearing. 1991. 1990 position statement. *Asha* 33(suppl. 5):3-6.

developing optimal communication and social skills. In 1982, the Joint Committee on Infant Hearing recommended identifying infants at risk for hearing impairment by means of seven criteria and suggested follow-up audiological evaluation of these infants until accurate assessments of hearing could be made (ASHA 1982). In recent years, advances in science and technology have increased the chances for survival of markedly premature and low birth weight neonates and other severely compromised newborns. Because moderate to severe sensorineural hearing loss can be confirmed in 2.5% to 5.0% of neonates manifesting any of the previously published risk criteria, auditory screening of at-risk newborns is warranted (Hosford-Dunn, Johnson, Simmons, Malachowski, and Low 1987; Jacobson and Morehouse 1984; Mahoney and Eichwald 1987; Stein, Ozdamar, Kraus, and Paton 1983). Those infants who have one or more of the risk factors are considered to be at increased risk for sensorineural hearing loss.

Recent research and new legislation (P.L. 99-457) suggest the need for expansion and clarification of the 1982 criteria. This 1991 statement expands the risk criteria and makes recommendations for the identification and management of hearing-impaired neonates and infants. The Joint Committee recognizes that the performance characteristics of these new risk factors are not presently known; further study and critical evaluation of the risk criteria are therefore encouraged. The protocols recommended by the Committee are considered optimal and are based on both clinical experience and current research findings. The Committee recognizes, however, that the recommended protocols may not be appropriate for all institutions and that modifications in screening approaches will be necessary to accommodate the specific needs of a given facility. Such factors as cost and availability of equipment, personnel and follow-up services are important considerations in the development of a screening program (Turner 1990).

II. IDENTIFICATION

A. Risk Criteria: Neonates (birth-28 days)

The risk factors that identify those neonates who are at-risk for sensorineural hearing impairment include the following:

1. Family history of congenital or delayed onset childhood sensorineural impairment.
2. Congenital infection known or suspected to be associated with sensorineural hearing impairment such as toxoplasmosis, syphilis, rubella, cytomegalovirus and herpes.
3. Craniofacial anomalies including morphologic abnormalities of the pinna and ear canal, absent philtrum, low hairline, etcetera.
4. Birth weight less than 1500 grams (~ 3.3 lbs.).
5. Hyperbilirubinemia at a level exceeding indication for exchange transfusion.
6. Ototoxic medications including but not limited to the aminoglycosides used for more than 5 days (e.g., gentamicin, tobramycin, kanamycin, streptomycin) and loop diuretics used in combination with aminoglycosides.
7. Bacterial meningitis.
8. Severe depression at birth, which may include infants with Apgar scores of 0-3 at 5 minutes or those who fail to initiate spontaneous respiration by 10 minutes or those with hypotonia persisting to 2 hours of age.
9. Prolonged mechanical ventilation for a duration equal to or greater than 10 days (e.g., persistent pulmonary hypertension).
10. Stigmata or other findings associated with a syndrome known to include sensorineural hearing loss (e.g., Waardenburg or Usher's Syndrome).

B. Risk Criteria: Infants (29 days-2 years)

The factors that identify those infants who are at-risk for sensorineural hearing impairment include the following:

1. Parent/caregiver concern regarding hearing, speech, language and/or developmental delay.
2. Bacterial meningitis.
3. Neonatal risk factors that may be associated with progressive sensorineural hearing loss (e.g., cytomegalovirus, prolonged mechanical ventilation and inherited disorders).
4. Head trauma especially with either longitudinal or transverse fracture of the temporal bone.

5. Stigmata or other findings associated with syndromes known to include sensorineural hearing loss (e.g., Waardenburg or Usher's Syndrome).
6. Ototoxic medications including but not limited to the aminoglycosides used for more than 5 days (e.g., gentamicin, tobramycin, kanamycin, streptomycin) and loop diuretics used in combination with aminoglycosides.
7. Children with neurodegenerative disorders such as neurofibromatosis, myoclonic epilepsy, Werdnig-Hoffmann disease, Tay-Sachs disease, infantile Gaucher's disease, Niemann-Pick disease, any metachromatic leukodystrophy, or any infantile demyelinating neuropathy.
8. Childhood infectious diseases known to be associated with sensorineural hearing loss (e.g., mumps, measles).

III. Audiologic Screening

Recommendations for Neonates and Infants

A. Neonates

Neonates who manifest one or more items on the risk criteria should be screened, preferably under the supervision of an audiologist. Optimally, screening should be completed prior to discharge from the newborn nursery but no later than 3 months of age. The initial screening should include measurement of the auditory brainstem response (ABR) (ASHA 1989). Behavioral testing of newborn infants' hearing has high false-positive and false-negative rates and is not universally recommended. Because some false-positive results can occur with ABR screening, ongoing assessment and observation of the infant's auditory behavior is recommended during the early stages of intervention. If the infant is discharged prior to screening, or if ABR screening under audiologic supervision is not available, the child ideally should be referred for ABR testing by 3 months of age but never later than 6 months of age.

The acoustic stimulus for ABR screening should contain energy in the frequency region important for speech recognition. Clicks are the most commonly used signal for eliciting the ABR and contain energy in the speech frequency region (ASHA 1989). Pass criterion for ABR screening is a response from each ear at intensity levels 40 dB nHL or less. Transducers designed to reduce the probability of ear-canal collapse are recommended.

If consistent electrophysiological responses are detected at appropriate sound levels, then the screening process will be considered complete except in those cases where there is a probability of progressive hearing loss (e.g., family history of delayed onset, degenerative disease, meningitis, intrauterine infections or infants who had chronic lung disease, pulmonary hypertension or who received medications in doses likely to be ototoxic). If the results of an initial screening of an infant manifesting any risk criteria are equivocal, then the infant should be referred for general medical, otological, and audiological follow-up.

B. Infants

Infants who exhibit one or more items on the risk criteria should be screened as soon as possible but no later than 3 months after the child has been identified as at-risk. For infants less than 6 months of age, ABR screening (see II A.) is recommended. For infants older than 6 months, behavioral testing using a conditioned response or ABR testing are appropriate approaches. Infants who fail the screen should be referred for a comprehensive audiologic evaluation. This evaluation may include ABR, behavioral testing (> 6 months) and acoustic immittance measures (see ASHA 1989 Guidelines, for recommended protocols by developmental age).

IV. EARLY INTERVENTION FOR HEARING-IMPAIRED INFANTS AND THEIR FAMILIES

When hearing loss is identified, early intervention services should be provided, in accordance with Public Law 99-457. Early intervention services under P.L. 99-457 may commence before the completion of the evaluation and assessment if the following conditions are met: (a) parental consent is obtained, (b) an interim individualized family service plan (IFSP) is developed, and (c) the full initial evaluation process is completed within 45 days of referral.

The interim IFSP should include the following:

A. The name of the case manager who will be responsible for both implementation of the interim IFSP and coordination with other agencies and persons;

B. The early intervention services that have been determined to be needed immediately by the child and the child's family.

These immediate early intervention services should include the following:

1. Evaluation by a physician with expertise in the management of early childhood otologic disorders.

2. Evaluation by an audiologist with expertise in the assessment of young children, to determine the type, degree, and configuration of the hearing loss, and to recommend assistive communication devices appropriate to the child's needs (e.g., hearing aids, personal FM systems, vibrotacile aids).

3. Evaluation by a speech-language pathologist, teacher of the hearing-impaired, audiologist, or other professional with expertise in the assessment of communication skills in hearing-impaired children, to develop a program of early intervention consistent with the needs of the child and preferences of the family. Such intervention would be cognizant of and sensitive to cultural values inherent in familial deafness.

4. Family education, counseling and guidance, including home visits and parent support groups to provide families with information, child management skills and emotional support consistent with the needs of the child and family and their culture.

5. Special instruction that included:
   a. the design and implementation of learning environments and activities that promote the child's development and communication skills.

b. curriculum planning that integrates and coordinates multidisciplinary personnel and resources so that intended outcomes of the IFSP are achieved; and,

c. ongoing monitoring of the child's hearing status and amplification needs and development of auditory skills.

V. FUTURE CONSIDERATIONS FOR RISK CRITERIA

Because of the dynamic changes occurring in neonatal-prenatal medicine, the committee recognizes that forthcoming research may result in the need for reversion of the 1990 risk register. For example, the committee has concerns about the possible ototoxic effects on the fetus from maternal drug abuse; however, present data are insufficient to determine whether the fetus or neonate are at risk for hearing loss. In addition, yet-to-be-developed medications may have ototoxic effects on neonates and infants. Therefore, the committee advises clinicians to keep apprised of published reports demonstrating correlations between maternal drug abuse and ototoxicity and between future antimicrobial agents and ototoxicity. Clinicians should also take into account the possible interactive effects of multiple medications administered simultaneously. Finally, the committee recommends that the position statement be examined every 3 years for possible revision.

REFERENCES

American Speech-Language-Hearing Association. 1989. Guidelines for audiologic screening of newborn infants who are at-risk for hearing impairment. *Asha* 31(3):89-92.

Early intervention program for infants and toddlers with handicaps: Final regulations. 1989. *Federal Register*, 54, no. 119, June 22, pp. 26306-26348.

Hosford-Dunn, H., Johnson, S., Simmons, B., Malachowski, N., and Low, L. 1987. Infant hearing screening: Program implementation and validation. *Ear and Hearing* 8:12-20.

Jacobson, J., and Morehouse, R. 1984. A comparison of auditory brainstem response and behavioral screening in high risk and normal newborn infants. *Ear and Hearing* 5(4):245-253.

Joint Committee on Infant Hearing. 1982. Position statement. *Asha* 24(12):1017-1018.

Mahoney, T.M., and Eichwald, J.G. 1987. The ups and "downs" of high risk hearing screening: The Utah statewide program. In K.P. Gerkin and A. Amochaev (eds.), *Seminars in Hearing* 8(2):155-163.

Stein, L., Ozdamar, O., Kraus, N., and Paton, J. 1983. Follow-up of infants screened by auditory brainstem response in the neonatal intensive care unit. *Journal of Pediatrics* 63:447-453.

Turner, R.G. 1990. Analysis of recommended guidelines for infant hearing screening. *Asha* 32(9):57-61.

SUGGESTED READING

EARLY INTERVENTION

Early intervention program for infants and toddlers with handicaps: Final regulations. 1989. *Federal Register* 54, no. 119, June 22, pp. 26306-26348.

Levitt, H., McGarr, N., and Geffner, D. 1987. *Development of language and communication skills in hearing impaired children.* ASHA (Monograph no. 26). Rockville, Md.: American Speech-Language-Hearing Association.

Ling, D. 1981. Early speech development. In G. Mencher and S.E. Gerber (eds.), *Early management of hearing loss* (pp. 310-335). New York: Grune and Stratton.

McFarland, W.H., and Simmons, F.B. 1981. The importance of early intervention with severe childhood deafness. *Pediatric Annals* 9:13-19.

A Report to the Congress of the United States. 1988. The Commission on Education of the Deaf: *Toward equality: Education of the deaf.*

EARLY IDENTIFICATION OF HEARING IMPAIRMENT IN NEONATES AND INFANTS

Alberti, P., Hyde, M., Riko, K., Corbin, H., and Fitzhardinge, P. 1985. Issues in early identification of hearing loss. *Laryngoscope* 95(4):373-381.

American Academy of Pediatrics. 1986. Committee on Fetus and Newborn. Use and abuse of the Apgar score. *Pediatrics* 78:1148.

American Speech-Language-Hearing Association. 1989. Guidelines for audiologic screening of newborn infants who are at-risk for hearing impairment. *Asha* 31(3):89-92.

American Speech-Language-Hearing Association. 1990. Guidelines for infant hearing screening—Response to Robert G. Turner's analysis. *Asha* 32(9):63-66.

Bergman, I., Hirsch, R.P., Fria, T.J., Shapiro, S.M., Holzman, I., and Painter, M.J. 1985. Cause of hearing loss in the high-risk premature infant. *Journal of Pediatrics* 106:95-101.

Bess, F.H. (ed.). 1988. *Hearing impairment in children*. Parkton, Md.: York Press.

Brummett, R.E. 1981. Ototoxicity resulting from the combined administration of potent diuretics and other agents. *Scandinavian Audiology* Suppl. 14:215-224.

Brummett, R.E., Traynor, J., Brown, R., and Himes, D. 1975. Cochlear damage resulting from kanamycin and furosemide. *Acta Otolaryngologica* 80:86-92.

Brummett, R.E., Fox, K.E., Russell, N.J., and Davis, R.R. 1981. Interaction between aminoglycoside antibiotics and loop-inhibiting diuretics in the guinea pig. In S. Lerner, G. Matz, and J. Hawkins (eds.), *Aminoglycoside ototoxicity* (pp.67-77). Boston: Little, Brown.

Church, M.W., and Gerkin, K.P. 1988. Hearing disorders in children with fetal alcohol syndrome: Findings from case reports. *Pediatrics* 82:147-154.

Coplan, J. 1987. Deafness: Ever heard of it? Delayed recognition of permanent hearing loss. *Pediatrics* 79:206-213.

Elssman, S., Matkin, N., and Sabo, M. 1987. Early identification of congenital sensorineural hearing impairment. *The Hearing Journal* 40:13-17.

Gerkin, K.P. 1984. The high risk register for deafness. *Asha* 26(3):17-23.

Gerkin, K.P., and Amochaev, A. (eds.). 1987. Hearing in infants: Proceedings from a national symposium. *Seminars in Hearing* 8:77-187.

Gorga, M., Reiland, J., Beauchaine, K., Worthington, D., and Jesteadt, W. 1987. Auditory brainstem responses from graduates of an intensive care nursery: Normal patterns of response. *Journal of Speech and Hearing Research* 30:311-318.

Gorga, M., Kaminski, J.R., and Beauchaine, K.A. 1988. Auditory brainstem responses from graduates of an intensive care nursery using an insert earphone. *Ear and Hearing* 9:144-147.

Halpern, J., Hosford-Dunn, H., and Malachowski, N. 1987. Four factors that accurately predict hearing loss in 'high risk' neonates. *Ear and Hearing* 8:21-25.

Hendricks-Muñoz, K.D., and Walton, J.P. 1988. Hearing loss in infants with persistent fetal circulation. *Pediatrics* 81(5):650-656.

Hosford-Dunn, H., Johnson, S., Simmons, B., Malachowski, N., and Low, L. 1987. Infant hearing screening: Program implementation and validation. *Ear and Hearing* 8:12-20.

Hyde, M., Riko, K., Corbin, H., Moroso, M., and Alberti, P. 1984. A neonatal hearing screening research program using brainstem electric response audiometry. *Journal of Otolaryngology* 13:49-54.

Jacobson, J., and Morehouse, R. 1984. A comparison of auditory brainstem response and behavioral screening in high risk and normal newborn infants. *Ear and Hearing* 5(4):245-253.

Joint Committee on Infant Hearing. 1982. Position statement. *Asha* 24(12):1017-1018.

Kahlmeter, O., and Dahlager, J.I. 1984. Aminoglycoside toxicity—A review of clinical studies published between 1975 and 1982. *Journal of Antimicrobial Chemotherapy* 13(suppl. A):9-22.

Kaka, J., Lyman, C., and Kllarskl, D. 1984. Tobramycin-furosemide interaction. *Drug Intelligence and Clinical Pharmacy* 18:235-238.

Lary, S., Briassoulis, G., DeVries, L., Dubowitz, L., and Dubowitz, V. 1985. Hearing threshold in preterm and term infants by auditory brainstem response. *Journal of Pediatrics* 107:593-599.

Mahoney, T.M., and Eichwald, J.G. 1987. The ups and "downs" of high risk hearing screening: The Utah statewide program. In K.P. Gerkin and A. Amochaev (eds.), *Seminars in Hearing* 8(2):155-163.

Matkin, N.D. 1984. Early recognition and referral of hearing impaired children. *Pediatrics in Review* 6:151-158.

Matz, G. 1990. Clinical perspectives on ototoxic drugs. *Annals of Otology, Rhinology, and Laryngology* 99:39-41.

Naulty, C.M., Weiss, I.P., and Herer, G.R. 1986. Progressive sensorineural hearing loss in survivors of persistent fetal circulation. *Ear and Hearing* 7:74-77.

Nield, T.A., Schrier, S., Ramos, A.D., Platzker, A.C.G., and Warburton, D. 1986. Unexpected hearing loss in high-risk infants. *Pediatrics* 78:417-422.

Northern, J.L., and Downs, M.D. 1984. *Hearing in children.* 3d ed. Baltimore: Williams and Wilkins.

Salamy, A., Eldridge, L., and Tooley, W.H. 1989. Neonatal status and hearing loss in high-risk infants. *Journal of Pediatrics* 114:847-852.

Schwartz, D.M., Pratt, R.E., and Schwartz, J.A. 1989. Auditory brainstem responses in preterm infants: Evidence of peripheral maturity. *Ear and Hearing* 10:14-22.

Stein, L., Ozdamar, O., Kraus, N., and Paton, J. 1983. Follow-up of infants screened by auditory brainstem response in the neonatal intensive care unit. *Journal of Pediatrics* 63:447-453.

Surgonski, N., Shallop, J., Bull, M.J., and Lemons, J.A. 1987. Hearing screening of high risk newborns. *Ear and Hearing* 8:26-30.

Turner, R.G. 1990. Analysis of recommended guidelines for infant hearing screening. *Asha* 32(9):57-61.

DIAGNOSIS AND MANAGEMENT

Bess, F.H. (ed.). 1988. *Hearing impairment in children*. Parkton, Md.: York Press.

Clark, T.C., and Watkins, S. 1985. *The SKI*Hi model: Programming for hearing impaired infants through home intervention*. Logan, Utah: SKI*Hi Institute.

Dodge, P.R., Davis, H.D., Feigin, R.D., Holmes, S.J., Kaplan, S.L., Jubelirer, D.P., Stechenberg, B.W., and Hirsh, S.K. 1984. Prospective evaluation of hearing impairment as a sequela of acute bacterial meningitis. *New England Journal of Medicine* 311:869-874.

Fitzgerald, M.T., and Bess, F.H. 1982. Parent/infant training for hearing impaired children. *Monographs in Contemporary Audiology* 3:1-24.

Gravel, J.S. (ed.). 1989. Assessing auditory system integrity in high-risk infants and young children. *Seminars in Hearing* 10:213-290.

Hosford-Dunn, H., Simmons, B.F., Winzelberg, J., and Petroff, M. 1986. Delayed onset hearing loss in a two-year old. *Ear and Hearing* 7:78-82.

Matkin, N.D. 1988. Key considerations in counseling parents of hearing-impaired children. In R.F. Curlee (ed.), *Seminars in Speech and Language* 9(3):209-222.

Mencher, G.T., and Gerber, S.E. 1981. *Early management of hearing loss*. New York: Grune and Stratton.

Ross, M., and Giolas, T.G. (eds.). 1978. *Auditory management of hearing impaired children*. Baltimore: University Park Press.

Thompson, G., and Wilson, W.R. 1984. Clinical application of visual reinforcement audiometry. In T. Mahoney (ed.), *Seminars in Hearing* 5:85-89.

Thompson, M., Atcheson, J., and Pious, C. 1985. *Birth to three: A curriculum for parents, parent trainers, and teachers*. Seattle, Wash.: University of Washington Press.

United States House of Representatives 99th Congress, 2d session. Report 99-860. *Report accompanying the education of the handicapped act amendment of 1986*.

Appendix 2

Consensus Statement
Screening Children for Auditory Function

In June 1991, the Division of Hearing and Speech Sciences, Vanderbilt University School of Medicine, and the Bill Wilkerson Center cosponsored the International Symposium on Screening Children for Auditory Function in Nashville, Tennessee. This symposium was designed to discuss and debate current issues concerned with the early identification and intervention of children with hearing impairment. Following the symposium Maternal and Child Health Bureau (MCHB) funded the development of a consensus statement on screening children for auditory function. The multidisciplinary team who prepared the statement consisted of representatives from several professional organizations. The organizations and their respective representatives include the following: James W. Hall III, Ph.D., American Academy of Audiology; Stephen Epstein, M.D., American Academy of Otolaryngology—Head and Neck Surgery; Elizabeth S. Ruppert, M.D., American Academy of Pediatrics; Donna McCord Dickman, Ph.D., Alexander Graham Bell Association for the Deaf, Inc.

THE PROBLEM

Each year in the United States, about 4,000 children are born deaf or with a profound hearing loss. Approximately 37,000 additional children are born with milder degrees of hearing loss (greater than 35 dB), which can still interfere with development of communication. For almost all of these children, the hearing loss is due to sensorineural (inner ear or auditory cranial nerve) disorders and is permanent. Modern intensive care has produced better chances for survival of very-low-birth-weight infants but has also led to much greater likelihood of neurodevelopmental handicaps including hearing disorders. Approximately one million school-age children have hearing loss. In many cases, the hearing loss is congenital and permanent, but for other children of any age the hearing loss is related to recurrent otitis media and can be corrected with appropriate medical or surgical therapy. Otitis media is second only to preventive health care visits as the most frequent reason for office visits to physicians serving children. Over 80% of children experience acute otitis media by the age of 3 years, with a peak rate of occurrence between the 7th and 12th month after birth.

Hearing loss, regardless of etiology, affects speech and language development of infants and young children. Communication deficits may initially occur within the first six months of life. Hearing loss in preschool- and school-age children interferes with educational development. Early identification of hearing loss, with prompt and appropriate intervention and management, is essential if the child is to reach his or her communicative and educational potential. Although hearing screening is now mandated by 16 states and federal legislation (Public Law 99-457) mandates interventional assistance for handicapped children from birth to 3 years, early identification and intervention remain an ideal and not a reality. At this time, the average age of identification of hearing loss in the United States is 2½ years, and initial detection of serious hearing loss in children is sometimes delayed until the preschool- and even school-age years. Multiple factors continue to conspire against early intervention of hearing impairment, ranging from limited financial resources to inadequate parental and professional appreciation of current screening techniques and the impact of hearing loss on development.

Maintenance of high-risk registers is useful in identification of some children with hearing impairment. Experience has shown, however, that most of these at-risk children do not have a hearing impairment. Conversely, more than 50% of children who do have hearing impairment are not detected by a high-risk register approach. Appreciation of these two limitations of high-risk registers has led to increased interest in hearing screening of all newborn infants, including those at risk and those who are not at risk. Commercially available automated auditory brainstem response hearing screening techniques have contributed to this interest. Proposed federal legislation (HR 2089) for hearing screening of all babies at birth is perhaps the best example of the seriousness of this concern.

RESEARCH PRIORITIES

Hearing screening procedures separate children into groups with a high versus low probability of having a hearing disorder. Rigorous evidence on the performance of hearing screening procedures is lacking for all age groups, from newborn infants to the school-age population. As an example, performance characteristics of the high-risk register, which has a 20-year history, are still undefined. Recent advances in technology have yielded procedures, among them automated auditory brainstem response and otoacoustic emissions, that may play a role in hearing screening of all infants, although documentation is lacking. Even the statistics on prevalence of hearing impairment in the general population are not known. The product of such research—precise guidelines for screening—must then be coupled with a well-designed strategy for formation of public policy, including public awareness of the problem, legislative action, and implementation of funded programs for early identification and intervention of hearing impairment.

CLINICAL PROTOCOLS

Effective screening for auditory function in children requires a coordinated effort by parents, teachers, trained volunteers, and a variety of health care professions, including audiology, neonatology, otolaryngology—head and neck surgery, pediatrics, and speech pathology. A multidisciplinary team is also needed for prompt and successful implementation of medical and nonmedical management of hearing impairment in children. The first step is education of these groups on the importance of early identification of hearing impairment, available screening techniques, and treatment options. National legislation, state legislation, and independent medical and nonmedical resources must be utilized in this effort.

In consultation with pediatricians, *audiologists* will be responsible for supervision of newborn hearing screening programs and initiation of appropriate management. However, even perfect newborn hearing screening programs are inadequate for early detection of delayed onset and acquired hearing impairment in children. Monitoring a child's hearing at periodic and regular intervals during the first five years of life is the responsibility of *pediatricians* and *primary care physicians*. Key ages to formally screen hearing and language development include 6 months, 15 to 18 months, and 2, 3, 4, and 5 years. All children with a developmental delay or developmental disability should have a formal audiologic evaluation at the time the developmental delay or disability is disclosed. Finally, because noise induced hearing loss is preventable and its occurrence increases with age, auditory screening in adolescents should be inseparably joined with a preventive health education message.

Pediatricians and *other primary care physicians serving children* should be familiar with high-risk criteria for infant hearing impairment, administer formalized developmental screening tests with referral for audiologic assessment as indicated, administer screening pure-tone audiometry and tympanometry with referral to audiology and otolaryngology—head and neck surgery as indicated, advocate for the early diagnosis and treatment of congenitally hearing-impaired infants, and collaborate and coordinate with audiologists, educators of the deaf, early intervention specialists, and otolaryngologists—head and neck surgeons in developing comprehensive family focused early intervention plans for all congenital hearing-impaired children.

A VISION

All infants born with a hearing impairment will be identified in the newborn period by the year 2000. Infants and young children with acquired hearing losses will be detected within two months of the onset. Infants and young children not at high risk will be screened for hearing loss as a routine component of preventive health care (American Academy of Audiology in press).

REFERENCE

American Academy of Audiology. In press. Vision/mission statement. *Audiology Today*.

Appendix 3

Newborn Hearing Screening with Auditory Brainstem Response: Programs and Protocols

James W. Hall III and Charlotte H. Prentice

INTRODUCTION

Establishing and maintaining a newborn hearing screening program can be difficult and even frustrating but also rewarding. For audiologists, newborn hearing screening is both a unique and a challenging clinical activity. It is unique because no other profession is adequately prepared by education or training to identify, evaluate, and manage hearing-impaired infants. Newborn hearing screening is challenging because it requires such diverse clinical skills, ranging from expertise in ABR measurement and interpretation (frequently under adverse test conditions) to the ability to obtain valid behavioral and immittance audiometry findings (often from difficult-to-test patients) to knowledge of habilitation and rehabilitation approaches (from amplification to parent-infant stimulation strategies) to the ability to coordinate a multidisciplinary team management effort. In addition to these clinical challenges, the audiologist is faced with financial difficulties associated with running most hospital-based newborn hearing screening programs. In view of the increasing number of states with legislation requiring early identification of hearing impairment and potential federal legislation, such as the House of Representatives bill mandating hearing screening of all newborn infants, audiologists in medical settings, private practice, and community clinics across the United States must be prepared to accept the responsibility for proposing, establishing, and implementing effective hearing screening and audiologic follow-up programs. The information in this appendix is presented as a starting point for this effort. More detailed information on the topic is available in a recent textbook (Hall 1992).

IMPLEMENTATION OF A NEONATAL AUDITORY SCREENING PROGRAM

INTRODUCTION

Successful implementation of any new clinical program requires considerable planning and preparation. Minimally, there must be a proposal (usually written), public relations efforts, financial arrangements (mechanisms for billing and reimbursement for services), assurance of an adequate number of technically skilled personnel, proper equipment, and a thorough understanding of the appropriate clinical knowledge. Adequate clinical skill may be the single requirement that comes to mind in anticipating a new program. However, other factors, outlined above, are equally important for a successful screening program. In addition, no screening program is complete, or will be effective, unless there is a well-organized system for follow-up auditory evaluation and management of hearing-impaired infants.

PERSONNEL

Staff are usually needed to (1) identify infants at risk for hearing impairment, (2) perform the screening procedure and interpret and report the results, (3) conduct follow-up audiologic assessment and management of hearing-impaired infants, (4) examine infants for otologic pathology, and (5) carry out clerical duties. Who should be on staff? If all infants admitted to the intensive care nursery (ICN) are to be screened, then little or no staff time will be spent in identifying at-risk infants. Before proposing this policy, that is a "standing order" for hearing screening of all infants admitted into the neonatal ICN, estimation of the proportion who will meet risk criteria is advisable. This proportion is likely to vary considerably from one institution to the next. If less than 85% to 90% of infants in the neonatal ICN actually meet one or more risk criteria, then the apparent advantage of bypassing the initial chart review will be more than offset by the disadvantage, in terms of both time and unnecessary charges to patients, of automatically screening 15% or more of infants who would not need to be screened on the basis of chart review. This issue is addressed in chapter 10 of this book.

With most screening programs, an ongoing register of infants at risk for hearing impairment must be maintained by screening personnel. The most common approach is to identify infants at risk by routinely reviewing medical charts in search of risk factors. Among the types of persons who may be chosen to carry out this task are audiologists, nurses, or volunteers. Each choice presents advantages and disadvantages. Audiologists typically understand why they are conducting the chart review and are often involved in subsequent screening and follow-up testing. Having a single person coordinate a screening program offers definite advantages. On the other hand, this task takes audiology staff away from other responsibilities. Nurses are experienced with medical terminology and certainly are familiar with medical records but most often have no time to devote to chart review. For both audiologists and nurses, someone is paying relatively good wages for an activity that may not be associated with a fee (financial and billing concerns are noted below). Volunteers are the least expensive alternative for the chart-reviewing task but also the least appropriate alternative in terms of consistency of effort, medical background, and knowledge of the reasons for newborn auditory screening. The authors have documented a substantial increase in the proportion of infants meeting risk criteria as chart reviewers gain experience. In the interest of consistency and public relations in the newborn units, a single chart reviewer or only a few trained individuals are preferable to many.

In most settings and with most equipment, audiologists or trained technicians actually conduct the auditory screening. Newborn auditory screening with conventional ABR can be extremely challenging and should not be undertaken by inexperienced or unskilled persons. Of course, highly trained personnel are not essential if the equipment is an automated screener (e.g., the ALGO-1), although specific skills, such as electrode application, are still necessary. Screening with this device is done in many hospitals by nursing staff, technicians, or volunteers. The reader is referred to the chapter by Yellin and Wurm (chapter 11) for more information on the possible role of volunteers in newborn hearing screening.

The time required to fulfill clerical duties is often underestimated in planning a newborn auditory screening program. As the number of infants requiring screening and/or follow-up testing mounts, there is a correspondingly progressive increase in all types of paperwork, including billing, record keeping, data base maintenance, and correspondence. Telephone communication also must be considered. These activities are time consuming and generate expenses without generating revenue. Computer support for infant data management and word processing is almost essential. In the authors' experience, this clerical requirement is the most difficult issue to address in implementing a newborn screening program with limited staff and a shoestring budget.

How many staff members are needed? In order to determine staffing requirements, the amount of time needed to meet each of these responsibilities must first be estimated. This staffing assumption, in turn, depends to a large extent on the estimated caseload of infants. A rough estimate of the proportion of infants who are likely to meet risk criteria for a particular nursery can be determined from a "trial" chart review period (e.g., several days). Reasonable estimates on average test times can be determined similarly (a few "dry run" tests in the ICN) or by speaking with staff conducting screenings in other programs. The number of follow-up contacts to parents of infants who do not pass the screening or who are discharged or back transported from the hospital before screening must also be taken into account. With hospital neonatology statistics on the total number of infants admitted to the hospital areas of interest (usually intensive care and intermediate or special care nurseries) and information from the literature on screening failure rates and incidence of serious hearing impairment, it is possible to calculate the number of infants per unit of time (e.g., a week or month) who will probably need to be chart reviewed, screened, and followed up and managed audiologically.

Finally, there are ancillary personnel who must be available to meet the medical, educational, parental, and communicative needs of hearing-impaired infants. These professionals, who are vital members of the hearing screening team and must be committed to the objectives of the program, include pediatricians, otolaryngologists, speech-language pathologists, parent-infant specialists, and social workers.

EQUIPMENT

There are two basic approaches to meeting equipment needs. One is to utilize an evoked response system that will also be used for other clinical measurements. This approach is attractive because it takes advantage of existing equipment, which, presumably, is familiar to staff clinicians and generates revenue in other ways. The major limitation is that the equipment may become overutilized by the newborn screening. Scheduling conflicts quickly develop when, for example, the evoked response system is being used in the clinic, surgical intensive care unit, or operating room for an entire morning on a day when several infants are about to be discharged. One solution to this problem is to schedule most newborn screening for after hours, such as in the evening. In this way, the same equipment is exploited without conflicts in usage. An added positive feature of this arrangement is the possibility that the nursery will be less hectic and the babies more available than during daytime hours. Another limitation of employing clinical equipment is that conducting single channel ABR recordings at a screening intensity level may be a vast underutilization of an expensive instrument. Also, such equipment is often large and difficult to regularly transport to the ICN.

The alternative approach is to dedicate an ABR instrument to newborn screening. If the equipment is purchased specifically for newborn screening, it is more likely to be portable, simple to operate, and inexpensive. The system may even be designed for screening and offer automated data collection and analysis, such as the ALGO-1 (available from Natus, Inc.). With this approach, newborn screening does not interfere with other evoked response services. Valuable transportation and travel time can be saved by storing the equipment in or near the nurseries. The dedicated system approach is probably most appropriate, budget permitting, in major hospitals with busy clinical schedules having large numbers of at-risk infants.

ENLISTING THE SUPPORT OF NEONATOLOGY

Once the availability of personnel and equipment necessary to consistently screen at-risk infants has been verified, the next important step in implementing a newborn auditory screening program is to secure the support of neonatologists, neonatal nurses, ward clerks and, in short, anyone essential to the success of a screening program. The best approach is to submit a written proposal to the person in charge of the neonatal nurseries, usually the Chief of Neonatology and/or the Director of Newborn Nurseries. The most important objective in developing the proposal is to provide information that the neonatology staff wants to

MC 0003 (7/91)

HEARING RISK CRITERIA CHART REVIEW RECORD

⊗ Vanderbilt University Hospital

NEWBORN AUDITORY SCREENING PROGRAM

Nursery: NICU _____   IN _____   NN _____

Name: _____ , _____ Sex: _____ VUH #: _____
                          LAST   FIRST

Date of Birth: _____ Gestational Age (wks): _____

Home Address: _____

City: _____ Cty: _____ State: _____ Zip: _____

Telephone #: (_____) _____ Mother's Name: _____

Father's Name: _____ Chart Reviewer: _____ Date: _____

Transported From: _____ To: _____ Date: _____

Insurance: Private _____   Medicaid _____   Physician: _____

(Circle the risk factor(s) and comment as indicated)

1. Family history of hearing impairment: _____

2. Congenital perinatal infection (e.g. cytomegalovirus, rubella, herpes, toxoplasmosis, syphilis): _____

3. Anatomic malformation of head, face or neck (e.g. dysmorphic appearance, cleft palate, abnormalities of pinna, preauricular tags/pits): _____

4. Low birth weight (<1500 grams). Specify: _____

5. Hyperbilirubinemia (requiring exchange transfusion): _____

6. Bacterial meningitis, especially H. flu: _____

7. Severe asphyxia   Apgar of 0-3 at 5 minutes: _____

                        No spontaneous respiration by 10 minutes: _____

                        Hypotonia persisting to 2 hours of age: _____

8. Mechanical ventilation > 10 days: (PPH) _____

9. Ototoxic medications (e.g. aminoglycosides + lasix) specify: _____

10. Syndrome with SNHL (e.g. Waardenburg, Usher's, etc): _____

Other information: _____ IVH   _____ hydrocephalus   Other: _____

ALGO-1:   Right ear LR _____   SWPS _____   Comment: _____

            Left ear LR _____   SWPS _____   Comment: _____

Audiologist: _____   Date: _____

Figure 1. An example of a form used for chart review of infants who may be at risk for hearing loss.

have. Keep in mind, for example, that neonatology staff is usually less interested in exactly how the ABR data will be collected, analyzed and interpreted, and more concerned about which infants are to be screened, the safety of these infants, the possible interruption of ongoing nursing care, cost of the screening, and what will be done with the results.

NEWBORN HEARING SCREENING TEST PROTOCOL

Chart review. The first component of test protocol is the method for determining which infants will be screened. An example of a form used for chart review of infants who may be at risk is shown in figure 1. A primary objective of chart review is, of course, to identify which infants are at risk by careful inspection of available medical records. The frequency with which chart reviews should be done depends upon the volume of births and admissions to the ICN and intermediate nursery for the hospital as well as discharge policies. When there is adequate and regular communication with the neonatal discharge nurse or equivalent person, daily or weekend chart review may not be necessary. For infants meeting one or more of these criteria, however, it is also important to accurately document information in the upper portion of this sheet, which ranges from birth information (e.g., date of birth, gestational age) to biographical information (hospital unit number, parent's or caregiver's name[s], address, telephone number). This information is essential for efficient follow-up communication with family of infants who do not pass the screening or those infants who are discharged to home or back transported to another hospital before the screening could be carried out.

ABR measurement parameters. Guidelines for stimulus and acquisition parameters in newborn auditory screening with ABR are summarized in table 1. Rationale for selection of each of these specific parameters is summarized within the table and explained in detail elsewhere (Hall 1992). One must certainly adopt an adaptive and flexible strategy in newborn auditory screening, as in other auditory evoked response applications. No one test protocol or strategy will invariably be successful with all infants and in all test settings.

Problems with screening. Some problems commonly encountered in newborn screening, and possible solutions, are listed in table 2. These are largely generic problems, that is, they are virtually unavoidable and independent of the newborn population to be screened, the equipment used, or clinical skills of the tester.

Table 1
Auditory Brainstem Response Measurement Parameters for
Newborn Auditory Screening, with Primary Rationale
(see Hall 1992 for detailed discussion of each ABR measurement parameter)

Parameter	Selection	Rationale
Stimulus		
transducer	Infant Tubephone	prevents ear canal collapse; comfortable
type	click	produces robust response
duration	0.1 msec	conventional for generating onset response
rate	37.1/sec	faster rate reduces test time; odd number reduces interaction with 60 Hz electrical artifact
polarity	rarefaction	usually produces optimal response; condensation or alternating may be used
intensity	35 dB HL	adequate for ruling out serious hearing impairment while minimizing over-referral rate; intensity level of 0 dB nHL RE: adult click threshold may actually be greater in smaller infant ear canal
ear	monaural	test each ear separately to identify unilateral hearing impairment
Acquisition		
gain	X100,000	enhance typically small amplitude response
artifact reject	yes	to reject from signal averaging excessive myogenic and electrical artifact
analysis time	15 msec	long enough to encompass even abnormally delayed response at low stimulus intensity levels in premature infants

Table 1 (continued)

Parameter	Selection	Rationale
filter settings high pass	30 Hz	low enough cutoff to pass low frequency energy, which contributes to infant ABR
low pass	1500 Hz	little ABR energy falls above this cutoff; high frequency electrical interference may be reduced
60 Hz notch	no	notch filter tends to distort response latency without minimizing harmonics of 60 Hz electrical interference
number of sweeps	variable	number of sweeps needed is defined by signal (response)-to-noise ratio, and may range from several hundred to 4000 or more depending on test conditions (e.g., intensity level, amount of electrical and myogenic interference)
electrode array* inverting	Fz	high forehead positive electrode yields a response from infants that is comparable to the vertex (Cz) electrode site
noninverting	nape	back of neck negative electrode site contributes to larger wave V amplitude and eliminates need to move inverting electrode to test ear side; stimulus ipsilateral earlobe is, however, an acceptable alternative for the inverting electrode site

* More than one electrode array may be used. Care should be taken not to record the ABR with only a contralateral (Fz-to-contralateral ear) array from infants since a response may not be detected.

Overall newborn screening protocol. The sequence of steps in a newborn auditory screening program is illustrated in figure 2. This particular flowchart was developed for the screening program at

Vanderbilt University Hospital. Details will, of course, vary among programs. Infants screened are those in the ICN and intermediate nursery with one or more of the 1990 Joint Committee risk criteria as identified by chart review (discussed in Appendix 1). Infants admitted directly to the normal nursery are referred for auditory screening only upon physician request if clinical findings suggest possible hearing impairment. Examples of such clinical indications in otherwise healthy newborn infants are family history of hearing loss and obvious ear deformities. Pamphlets or brochures providing information on development of hearing, speech and language, risk factors, available resources for hearing evaluation and management of hearing impairment in children, and other pertinent facts are distributed to parents or caregivers of all infants admitted to the hospital, including those in the normal nursery.

The hearing screening of infants who are identified as at risk for hearing impairment is then delayed until the final few days before hospital discharge to home or back transport to another hospital. Whenever possible, screening is carried out while the infant is in the hospital. A policy of routinely recalling infants to the hospital for screening in the weeks or months after they are discharged, rather than

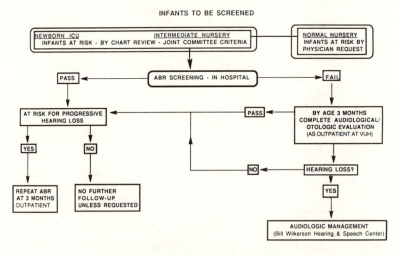

Figure 2. Vanderbilt University Medical Center Audiology/Otolaryngology Neonatal Hearing Screening Protocol. Flowchart illustrating the sequence of steps in a newborn auditory screening program.

Table 2

Summary of Potential Factors Contributing to Incorrect (False) Failures for Newborn Screening with Auditory Brainstem Response and Guidelines for General Solutions*

Factor	Solution
prematurity	defer screening until postconceptional age of 40 weeks whenever possible
transient middle ear dysfunction	otologic management, immittance measurement; bone conduction stimulus for follow-up ABR assessment
neurologic disease involving auditory CNS	identify at-risk infants during chart review; analyze latency of wave I rather than wave V
imprecise earphone placement	insert Tubephone for infants*
collapsing ear canal	insert Tubephone for infants*
inappropriate stimulus rate	use a rate consistent with normative data whenever possible; appreciate effect of rate on ABR latency and amplitude*
excessive ambient noise	use infant Tubephone; remove infant to treatment room; test in sound-treated room if feasible; discontinue test if necessary*
excessive movement artifact	perform screening with infant sleeping (e.g., after feeding); pause or abort recording; increase number of sweeps averaged to improve signal-to-noise ratio; return to test at another time*
small wave V	extend high pass filter setting to 30 Hz; use noncephalic inverting electrode site (e.g., nape)*
poor waveform morphology	slow the stimulus rate; alter the stimulus polarity; rule out myogenic interference; increase number of sweeps averaged

* The ALGO-1 automated infant ABR screening device incorporates a comparable solution to these measurement problems.

on-site hospital screening after birth, typically produces an unacceptably high proportion of infants that do not get screened and/or are lost to follow-up altogether. There are at least three reasons for delaying screening until just before discharge. First, premature infants are given time to develop neurologically and auditorally before the screening. Second, infants who might die before discharge are not screened. Mortality among infants at risk for hearing impairment in the ICN may be as high as 10%. It is clearly advisable to avoid, whenever possible, screening an infant who is not likely to survive. Along this line, for at-risk infants who do survive their hospital stay, one must also defer contacting parents/caregivers regarding follow-up audiologic testing until an attempt has been made to assure that they did not die during the time interval after leaving the hospital. Third, potentially ototoxic medical therapies are more likely to have had their effect by hospital discharge. If hearing is screened within days of birth, there is a possibility that infants subsequently receiving ototoxic drugs and developing a permanent hearing impairment after the screening will leave the hospital having passed the screening. Identification of the hearing loss could then be significantly delayed.

The exact timing of the screening is best determined not by clinical schedule but by the infant's daily routine and activities in the nursery. As for the former, an infant is most likely to be a peaceful and cooperative patient soon after feeding. On the day the screening is scheduled, therefore, the tester should contact the infant's nurse and set up a screening "appointment" after one of the feeding times. As a rule, an earlier feeding time during the day is advisable, so that another feeding time later in the day can be used as a back-up test time in the event that the first screening attempt is unsuccessful. Although screenings late in the hospital discharge day are sometimes unavoidable, for the sake of the tester they should be prevented if possible. Another factor to consider in determining when the screening will be done is the nursery schedule in general and, in particular, the infant's schedule. One should avoid screening during physician rounds or at times when other procedures (e.g., ultrasonography) are scheduled. Infants are often discharged from the hospital on short notice. At that time, the attending physician should have information on whether screening was carried out and, if so, the outcome of screening. A report of screening outcome should immediately be inserted in the infant's medical record, complete with appropriate recommendations and signed by the audiologist responsible for the testing. Figure 3 shows an example of a screening report.

Charging for hearing screening services. Immediately before or after screening is attempted, a signed physician order is obtained, and a copy is inserted into the infant's medical record. Billing for the hearing screening is initiated on the day that the service is rendered, assuming that valid results are obtained and a report is generated. The charge is submitted with a modified ABR current procedural terminology (CPT) code (for simplified auditory brainstem response). According to an informal nationwide survey of 16 audiologists by the authors, ABR hearing screening charges range from $55 to over $200. As a rule, the lower charges involve automated ABR screening techniques or an operator controlled pass-fail procedure at a single stimulus intensity level whereas the higher charges involve a full diagnostic ABR for each infant. One should avoid the use of "hearing screening" CPT codes, which imply a simple pure-tone screening procedure and are associated with a low charge. A diagnostic code for sensorineural hearing loss is typically appropriate for newborn hearing screening, even if the ultimate outcome of screening and follow-up audiometry confirms apparently normal hearing status. Some audiologists performing hearing screening use diagnosis codes associated with the infant's risk factor.

Follow-up protocol. As indicated in the left portion of the flowchart (figure 2), routine follow-up audiologic testing is waived for infants passing the hospital hearing screening bilaterally (both ears pass), unless they are at risk for progressive hearing loss. *Follow-up testing at 3 months (postterm) always consists of a battery of procedures, including ABR, acoustic immittance measurement, and behavioral audiometry.* The "cross-check principle" (Jerger and Hayes 1976) is regularly applied in infant hearing evaluation. Factors putting an infant at risk for progressive hearing loss (e.g., CMV, family history, rubella), were discussed in detail above. As discussed in chapter 10 of this book, over a third of infants at risk for hearing loss by the 1990 Joint Committee criteria may be at risk for progressive hearing loss. If there is a risk factor for progressive hearing loss, the infant is recalled for complete follow-up audiologic assessment at three months and periodically thereafter until serious hearing impairment is confidently ruled out. The parents/caregivers of all infants, including those passing the screening and not at risk for progressive hearing loss, are given pamphlets or

MC 0006 (7/91)

NEWBORN AUDITORY SCREENING REPORT

AUDIOLOGY SERVICE/OTOLARYNGOLOGY

⊘ The Vanderbilt Clinic
Room 1501
Nashville, TN 37232-5555
(615) 322-6180

Date of screening: _____

Name: _____, _____ Sex: _____

Birthdate: _____ Gestational age: _____ VUH #: _____

Referring Physician: _____

POTENTIAL RISK FACTOR (S):

_____ Family history of hearing loss   _____ Bacterial meningitis

_____ Congenital perinatal infection   _____ Asphyxia

_____ Head/neck deformity   _____ Mechanical Ventilation

_____ Birth weight less than 1500 grams   _____ Ototoxic medications

_____ Hyperbilirubinemia   _____ Syndrome

                                                _____ Physician order

SCREENING PROTOCOL:

Test: auditory brainstem response (ABR)

Equipment: _____ ALGO-1   _____ Bio-Logic Traveler

Stimulus parameters: type: click   rate: 37/.sec;

                       intensity: 35 dB nHL   mode: monaural

Test site: _____ ICU   _____ Intermediate Nursery

             _____ Normal Nursery   _____ Audiology facility

SCREENING RESULTS:

_____ Pass: peripheral hearing sensitivity is within or near normal limits bilaterally in the 1000 to
4000 Hz region

_____ Refer: _____ right ear fail   _____ left ear fail

_____ Incomplete: _____ right   _____ left

RECOMMENDATIONS:

_____ No further testing is required at this time. Retest only if a change in hearing is suspected.

_____ Follow up audiologic testing in 3 months. Did not pass auditory screening.

_____ Follow up audiologic testing in 3 months. At risk for progressive hearing loss _____.

_____ Follow up audiologic testing in 6 months. At risk for progressive hearing loss (ototoxic meds).

Audiologist: _____   Date: _____

Figure 3. An example of a screening outcome report. This report should be inserted into the infant's medical record, complete with appropriate recommendations and signed by the audiologist responsible for the testing.

brochures urging audiologic testing if the infant later shows any of the signs of hearing impairment (e.g., delayed communicative milestones, middle ear infection, perinatal infection). Information on newborn hearing brochures that are appropriate for parents and caregivers can be obtained from the American Academy of Audiology (call toll free at 800-AAA-2336).

Infants failing the hospital screening, or infants who are discharged prior to successful completion screening, are recalled for complete audiologic evaluation at 3 months of age, whenever possible, but no later than 6 months of age. Again, chronological age here is defined beginning with 40 weeks gestational age. For a term infant, thus, the follow-up testing would be scheduled for 3 months after birth. However, for an infant born at 32 (vs. 40) weeks, that is, 8 weeks (2 months) prematurely, follow-up testing would not be scheduled until 5 months after birth. It is clear from these calculations that one must, at the time of chart review, document accurate information on gestational age and date of birth. In some cases, premature infants who failed the hospital screening or were discharged without being screened return for follow-up testing by 3 months posthospital discharge when, according to calculated gestational age plus chronological age, they are barely past term. The policy in these instances is to first repeat an ABR screening, usually in a sound-treated room. Infants passing this screening are followed in the same manner as are hospital screening "passes" (see figure 2). The charge for a full audiologic assessment is thus avoided. If the infant fails this second screening, done under ideal conditions, then we proceed with complete follow-up audiologic assessment.

The initial follow-up audiologic evaluation, according to our screening program protocol, can be done by any qualified audiologist. An attempt is made to recall infants to our hospital, if possible, to assure that the testing is complete and proper recommendations are made. Sedation is also available at the hospital clinic if necessary for ABR assessment. Infants aged 3 months or less (RE: term birth) are generally not sedated, but older infants may require sedation for complete ABR evaluation. Recalling the infant to an outpatient clinic without medical support for administration of sedation can lead to further delays in management of hearing impairment if the results of behavioral testing are equivocal and unsedated ABR evaluation fails. Whenever there are appropriate test facilities near the infant's hometown, arrangements are usually made to schedule the initial assessment there. In fact, when implementing a newborn screening program, it is valuable to develop a network of referral centers for pediatric hearing evaluation and management that are within the catchment area for at-risk infants.

The most important single component in the entire newborn auditory screening program—initiation of audiologic management—is shown in the lower right portion of the flowchart in figure 2. Audiologic, otologic, and educational management of infants whose initial follow-up testing (at or about 3 months of age whenever possible) confirms hearing impairment should begin as soon as possible. This management is best coordinated by a facility that offers all relevant services, especially hearing aid dispensing, parent-infant stimulation, aural rehabilitation, and speech-language therapy. A precise definition of the hearing impairment (i.e., complete pure-tone and speech audiometry findings) is almost never obtained at this time and, in fact, may not be available for months or even years. Nonetheless, audiologic management is begun immediately on the basis of audiometric data at hand. Just as the "cross-check principle" guides pediatric audiologic assessment, there is a "follow-up principle" that guides pediatric audiologic management. Namely, pending medical or surgical treatment, audiologic management is initiated as soon as a serious hearing impairment is confirmed.

Infants who yield normal findings upon follow-up audiologic assessment are then released from further testing, unless again they are at risk for progressive hearing loss. The initial follow-up test session, however, provides a good opportunity to verify that parents/caregivers both have and understand information on communicative developmental milestones and illnesses that, in the future, might pose additional risk to hearing.

Problems with follow-up testing. The biggest problem with follow-up testing is actually getting infants back to a test facility so that the testing can be carried out. The reasons for poor compliance with recommendations for follow-up testing are multiple and varied. Some are easily explained. For example, letters recommending follow-up testing are returned as undeliverable and attempts to contact parents by telephone are foiled by disconnected or unlisted numbers. Most other reasons are also understandable. Hearing impairment in general is less visible and apparent than, for instance, visual impairment. Many infants at risk for hearing impairment are, during their hospital stay, at risk as well for life-threatening medical problems. Parents may be simply happy to have their child home and thriving, and may not be as concerned as parents of normal nursery graduates about possible hearing impairment. Difficulty in transporting infants from outlying areas or financial concerns certainly contribute to reduced follow-up of screening failures. Finally, there are a wide range of socioeconomic and education factors among parents of some at-risk infants that contribute to poor return rates for follow-up testing. A systematic, varied, and aggressive approach for communicating with parents/caregivers of infants is required. A letter is a good starting point. A telephone call is a logical second step for those parents who do not respond within a reasonable time to the letter. One should during the telephone conversation attempt to identify any potential concerns about the follow-up testing, such as transportation or financial problems. At each step in the follow-up process, the infant's pediatrician should be kept informed. After parents, pediatricians are the next line of support in early detection of hearing impairment. Our follow-up rate has increased from less than 40% to almost 70% by coordinating audiologic assessment with other follow-up clinic visits, such as the six-month visit to the clinic for low-birth-weight babies.

REFERENCES

Hall, J.W. III. 1992. *Handbook of auditory evoked responses*. Needham Heights, Mass.: Allyn and Bacon.

Jerger, J.F., and Hayes, D. 1976. The cross-check principle in pediatric audiometry. *Archives of Otolaryngology* 102:614-620.

Author Index

Only authors cited at length are included in this index.

Bailey, D. B., 388-90, 391, 392
Baumeister, A. A., 351
Bess, F. H., 41, 42
Blood, I., 436
Bodner-Johnson, B., 468
Bromwich, R., 468, 472
Bronfenbrenner, U., 439-40, 441, 442
Bruner, J., 411

Clinton, Bill, 262
Clinton, Hillary Rodham, 262
Connor, L. E., 305
Crandell, C., 52-53
Crosby, P. B., 343-47

Darley, F., 300-301
Davidson, D., 305-6, 307
Downs, M. P., 62-67, 281, 283, 351-52

Eilers, R. E., 250, 252, 256

Feagans, L., 436
Fiellau-Nikolajsen, M., 46, 299
Finitzo, T., 436
Folsom, R. C., 250
Friel-Patti, S., 436

Geers, A., 467

Haggard, M. P., 47, 273-74
Halpern, J., 90-92, 99
Heller, J. W., 49-52, 56-57, 315, 321, 322-23
Holland, W. W., 3-4
Hosford-Dunn, H., 90-92, 99

Hughes, E., 47

Keith, R. W., 373, 374, 375
Killion, M., 480, 481, 482
Koebsell, K. A., 315, 321, 322-23
Kuklinski, A., 477-78

Lamme, L. L., 411
Lerner, R., 441-43
Ling, A., 485
Ling, D., 485
Longhurst, Tom, 335-36
Lopez, C., 250, 252
Lous, J., 299, 303, 304

Malachowski, N., 90-92, 99
Margolis, R. H., 49-52, 56-57, 315, 317, 321, 322-23
Matkin, N. D., 280-81, 477-78
McConkey, R., 447, 451-52
McWilliam, P. J., 391
Miskiel, E., 250, 252, 256
Morrow, L. M., 410, 411
Moses, K. L., 401
Mueller, G., 480, 481, 482
Murphy, N. J., 305

Ninio, A., 411
Northern, J. L., 41, 44-45, 46, 62-67, 281, 283, 306
Novak, M., 477-78

Olmstead, R. W., 34-35
Oyler, A. L., 477-78
Oyler, R. F., 477-78

Packer, A. B., 411
Paden, E., 477-78
Piaget, J., 413, 414, 415, 418, 421
Price, P., 447, 451-52
Primus, M. A., 249-50, 252-53

Quinn, J., 413-14

Ramig, Peter, 335-36
Roeser, R. J., 44-45, 46, 47, 52-53, 306
Roush, J., 40, 46, 53, 305-6, 307
Rubin, J., 473-74
Rubin, K., 413-14
Rushmer, N., 467-68

Sackett, D. L., 3-4, 8
Schow, Ronald, 348
Schuyler, V., 467-68
Simeonsson, R. J., 391

Tait, C., 46
Teele, D., 53-56
Teele, J. H., 53-56
Tharp, R., 405
Thompson, G., 249-50, 252-53
Turner, R. G., 96-98

Wald, E. R., 33-34
Weber H., 254, 282
Wetzel, R., 405
Widen, J. E., 250, 252, 254-55, 256
Winton, P. J., 391, 395
Wolery, M., 388-90, 392

Subject Index

Page numbers in bold indicate material in figures and tables.

ABR. *See* Auditory brainstem
response (ABR)
Acoustic admittance testing
as diagnostic tool, 324
measures for, 318-20
Acoustic immittance. *See* Immittance
measurements; Immittance
screening
Acoustic otoscope, **54**
Acoustic reflectometry, 53-56
Acoustic reflex (AR)
as indicator of middle ear
status, 48, 50, 318-20
test, sensitivity of, 319-20
test, specificity of, 319-20
tympanometry and, 40, 41, 46, 53
Acute otitis media (AOM). *See also*
Otitis media with effusion (OME)
age as factor in, 32, 33, 36
asymptomatic, 31
breast-feeding and, 33
complications of, 34-36
consequences of, 41
day care and, 33-34
definitions of, 31
hearing loss associated with, 31,
34-36
nonsuppurative, 35-36
prevalence of, 31, 32
risk factors for, 32-34
suppurative, 35
ventilating tubes in, 34
Advisory Council for Hearing-Impaired
Infants (Maryland), 108-9
Advocacy Committee for the Early
Identification of Hearing loss in

Children, 107, 109
AIDS, 118.
Alexander Graham Bell Association for
the Deaf, 107, 331
American Academy of Family Practice,
107
American Academy of Neonatology,
107
American Academy of Otolaryngology-
Head and Neck Surgery, 107
American Academy of Pediatrics, 107,
275
American Academy of Public Health
Physicians, 107
American Medical Association, 2
American Public Health Association,
276-77
American Sign Language, 466
American Speech-Language-Hearing
Association (ASHA)
guidelines of, (1975), 275; (1979),
40-41, **43**, 46; (1985), 49, 277,
282-83; (1990), 49-50, **51**, 52-53,
56, 57, 127, 277
Apgar score, as risk factor, 92, 157,
160
Arkansas, Infant Hearing Program in,
261-71
Children's Hearing and Speech
Clinic and, 262
follow-up in, 263-66
program development, 262-65
socio-economic factors in, 261-62,
269-70
screening procedures in, 263, 265-69
volunteers in, 263-65

531

Audiometry. *See also* Behavioral
  audiometry; Behavioral
  observational audiometry (BOA);
  Immittance measurements; Visual
  reinforcement audiometry (VRA)
  in assessing auditory processing,
    71-75
  for preschool-age screening, 283-84
  pure-tone and, 46, **74**
Auditory brainstem response (ABR)
    testing
  bone conducted click stimuli for,
    129-30
  click-evoked, 129-30, 132-33, 134
  criteria used for, 80
  as diagnostic procedure, 128,
    137-40, 176, **177**
  evaluation of, 132-37
  high-risk questionnaire and, 105-6,
    172-74
  for infants, 127-40, 210-11, 229-32
  in locating dysfunction, 134-37, 139
  maturation and, 130-32, 137-38,
    200-3
  methodology, 128-34
  for neonates, 127-40, 244, 517, **518,
    519, 521**
  normative latency-intensity functions
    and, **131**
  pure-tone audiogram and, 132-34
  for sensorineural hearing loss,
    229-32
  Wave I latency, 133-34
  Wave V latency, 133-34
Auditory Figure Ground Subtest, 375

Behavioral assessment of hearing
  catch-trials in, 182-87
  design for neonatal, 181-83
  goal of, 183
  NEST as test environment for,
    183-85
  in older children, 244
  orienting as factor for, 182-89
  techniques for, 245-47

test-trials in, 182-87
Behavioral audiometry, reliability of,
    245. *See also* Behavioral
    observation audiometry (BOA)
Behavioral observation audiometry
    (BOA)
  with ABR screening, 175
  as screening tool for young children,
    245
  stimuli used in, 192-94, 245
  visual inspection in, 194-98, 209
Benzyl alcohol, as risk factor, 235-36
Bilateral middle ear disorder, 48
Bill Wilkerson Hearing and Speech
    Center, 39, 507
Birthweight, as risk factor, 17, **19**,
    20-22, 92, 147, 155-56, 236,
    261-62
BOA. *See* Behavioral observation
    audiometry
Bronchopulmonary dysplasia, 22-23

Canadian Task Force on the Periodic
    Health Examination, 3, 4
Centers for Disease Control report, 437
Central auditory processing disorder
    (CAPD). *See also* Hearing loss;
    Selective Auditory Attention Test
    (SAAT)
  diagnosis of, 67-76
  as learning disability, 63-64
  as public health problem, 62-70, **69**
  remediation, 361
  screening for, 61-64, 66-76, 362-63
Cerumen management, 52-53, 57
Cheers for Ears (Northwest Ohio
    screening program), 287-93
Children's Hearing and Speech Clinic
    (Arkansas), 262
Children's Hospital Medical Center
    (Ohio), 176-78
"Children's Preschool Vision and
    Hearing Screening and
    Follow-Up," 276-77

Classification of audiograms by
sequential testing (CAST), 255-57.
See also Visual Reinforcement
Audiometry (VRA)
Click stimuli in acoustic testing, 192-94
Clinical Linguistic and Auditory
Milestone Scale, 450-51
CMV. *See* Cytomegalovirus
Coagulase-negative staphylococcus,
23-24
Colorado task force guidelines, 478
Communication. *See also* Hearing loss,
impact of
definition, 407-8, 410
disorders, impact of, 374
language and speech in, 408-10
significance of, 374
between parents and hearing-
impaired children, 464-66
Competing Sentence Test, 67-68
Conductive hearing loss, due to MEE,
34, 35
Competing Word Subtest, 375-76
Count-the-Dot Audiogram, **481, 482**
Crib-O-Gram, 164, 210
Curriculum for 3-5 years, 421-26
Cytomegalovirus, 23, 146, 158, 172

Deaf students. *See* Hearing-impaired
children
Dichotic Sentence Identification (DSI)
Test, 71

Early identification of hearing loss
importance of, 106-9, 138-39, 208-9,
257, 361, 508
protocol for, **87**
Early Language Milestone Scale (ELM),
281-82, 450
Effusion, 31. *See also* Otitis media with
effusion (OME)
EOAE, evoked otoacoustic emissions.
See Otoacoustic hearing screening
in newborns
Equivalent ear canal volume, as measure

of acoustic admittance, 318
Escherichia coli, 23

Family service plans, 419-20, 465-66,
472-74
Fifth International Symposium on Otitis
Media, 436
Filtered Speech Test, 67-68
Filtered Word Test, 375
FM systems, signal-to-noise ratio and,
65-66, 482, 483, 486, 488-89
Food and Drug Administration,
investigation of otitis media, 32
Fourth International Symposium on
Recent Advances in Otitis Media
(1989), report of, 47-49
Furosemide, 22-23, 236-37

Genetic causes of deafness, autosomal
recessive, 178
Gestational age as risk factor, 158
Gram-negative enteric bacteria, 23
Greater Boston Otitis Media Study
Group, 32-34, 35
Group B beta-hemolytic streptococcus,
23

Haemophilus species, 23
Handicapped Children's Education
Program, 385-86
Head Start, as early intervention, 385-86
Healthy People 2000, 113, 114
Hearing aids
coupled to FM, 488-89
fitting, 481
Hearing-impaired children. *See also*
Hearing loss
classroom acoustics for, 481-85
communication with parents, 106-9,
138-39, 208-9, 257, 361, 508
continuing monitoring of, 488-91
early identification of, 106-9,
138-39, 208-9, 257, 361, 508
educational placement of, 479-87

Hearing-impaired children — *continued*
  FM systems for, 482, 483, 486,
    488-89
  hearing assessment of, 480-81
  Individualized Education Plan (IEP)
    for, 479-82, 486, 489
  multiple handicaps among, 480
  parents/school relationship, 485
  teachers of, 485, 486-88, 489
Hearing loss. *See also* Hearing-impaired
    children; Sensorineural hearing
    loss
  autosomal recessive, 178
  cost, 473-74
  educationally significant, 478
  genetic, 178
  guidelines to identify infants at risk
    for. *See* High-risk infants
  impact on development and
    communication skills, 6-7, 41,
    63-65, 171, 191, 207-9, 257, 298,
    299-300, 463, 480, 508
  intervention strategies, 65-66,
    387-90, 393-95, 466-72
  risk factors, 79-81, **80**. *See* High-risk
    infants
  TORCH syndrome and, 146
Hearing screening in Montana
  ADEPT Model for, 342-47
  Commission on Aging and
    Vocational Rehabilitation, 333
  Department of Health and, 332, 333
  Easter Seal Society and, 333
  funding of, 333, 335-36, 339-40,
    346-47
  Office of Public Instruction and,
    333, 342-43, 346-47, 348
  organization of, 336-42
  promotion for, 348-51
  public/private partnership in, 339-44,
    351-53
  regional nature of, 332-36
  service delivery models, **339, 340,
    341**
  University of Montana and, 332, 341

U.S. WEST Foundation and, 331,
    335, 336, 339, 342-43, 345-47,
    349-51, 352
Herpes simplex virus, 23, 146, 172
High-risk children (above 8 years),
    306-7
High-risk infants, criteria for *See also
    under* Joint Committee on Infant
    Hearing
  asphyxia, 148, 157, 158, 160
  bacterial meningitis, 147-48
  congenital infections, 146
  cost of screening, 87-92, **91** (mv)
  craniofacial anomalies, 146-47, 158
  family history, 146, 172
  hyperbilirubinemia, 92 147
  low birth weight, 92, 147, 155-56,
    236, 262
  ototoxic medications, 148-49, 160,
    161, 173, 236-37
  prolonged ventilation, 149, 160
  questionnaire for, 172-74
  stigmata of syndrome, 149
High-risk register (HRR), 79-81,
    92-102, 508-9. *See also under*
    Joint Committee on Infant Hearing
Hirtshals Procedure for immittance
    screening, 303
Histograms, 186-87

Illinois Department of Health, screening
    program of, 284
Immittance measurements, instruments
    for, 53-55, 56
Immittance screening
  ASHA guidelines for, (1979) 302;
    (1990) **43**, 49-53, 279, 303-5, 323,
    324, 325
  International Symposium on Otitis
    Media guidelines for, 47-49
  for middle ear disease, 39-57, 48-49,
    302-5, 309, 315-29
  Nashville guidelines for, 39-40, **42**,
    302-3, 304
  in preschool testing, 283-84

Immittance screening — *continued*
    and pure tone, 308
    Roeser-Northern guidelines for,
        44-45, 46, **47**
    in school hearing screening
        programs, 46, 47, 302-5
Individualized educational plan (IEP),
    419-20, 479-82, 486, 489, 490
Infants. *See* Hearing-impaired children;
    High-risk infants; Neonatal
    screening
Intensive care unit. *See* Neonatal
    intensive care unit (NICU)
International Symposium on Screening
    Children for Auditory Function
    (Nashville, 1991), consensus
    statement, 507-510
Intervention, early
    approaches to, 466-72
    definition, 385
    family-centered services for, 390-93,
        395, 404-5, 419-20, 472, 474-75
    family system as learning
        environment, 400-407, 464-68,
        472
    goals of, 387-90
    normalizing experiences, 389,
        393-95
Intubation as risk factor, 92

Joint Committee on Infant Hearing
    position statement (1990), 495-501
    recommended high-risk register,
        79-81, **80**, 108-9, 209-10
    risk criteria of 1974, 263
    risk criteria of 1982 and 1990, 26,
        129, 145-61, 163, 164, 165, 175,
        229-30, 236, 279-80
Junior League of Toledo (Ohio), 288,
    289, 290

Labyrinthitis, 34
Language and speech tests, 67-68,
    71-73, 281-82, 364, 365, 366,
    375-76, 450-51, 483, 487, 489,

490. *See individual test names*
Literacy, early, 410-12
Listeria monocytogenes, 23
Little Rock Hearing & Speech Clinic,
    265

Magee-Womens Hospital, 229, 234
Mainstreaming hearing-impaired
    children, 392-93, 478, 481-82
Mastoiditis, 35
Medicaid eligibility for children, 273
"Middle Ear Disease and Language
    Development," 275
Middle ear disease. *See* Central auditory
    processing disorder (CAPD); Otitis
    media; Screening
Middle ear effusion. *See* Effusion; Otitis
    media with effusion (OME),
Montana Educational Hearing
    Conservation Program, 331-53
Multiple handicaps among
    hearing-impaired children, 480
Myringotomy, 316-17

National Association for the Education
    for Young Children, 394-95
National Council of Jewish Women —
    Dallas Section, 166-68
National Technical Institute for the
    Deaf, 474
Neonatal Environment for Sensitivity
    Testing (NEST). *See under*
    Behavioral assessment of hearing
Neonatal hyperbilirubinemia, 25-26
Neonatal infections, 23-24, 173
Neonatal intensive care unit (NICU).
    See also Auditory Brainstem
    Response (ABR) testing;
    Vanderbilt NICU
    ABR testing in, 127-40
    hearing loss in graduates of, 158
Neonatal screening
    ABR measurement, 517, **518**, **519**,
        521
    equipment for, 514-15

Neonatal screening — *continued*
  false negative results, **521**
  follow-up, 523-27
  Ohio program for, 171-79
  at Parkland Memorial Hospital
    (Dallas), 163-68
  personnel for, 512-14
  prioritization of infants for, **164**, 165
  protocol for, 517, 519-27
  use of volunteers in, 165-68, 513
Neonatal sepsis, 23-24, 173
Neonates. *See also* Neonatal screening
  ABR testing of, 127-40
  acoustic reflexes in, testing of, 105-9
NEST, **184**. *See under* Behavioral
  assessment of hearing.
Neurosensory Center of Houston, 66,
  70-75
NICU. *See* Neonatal Intensive Care Unit
  (NICU)
Noisemakers, use of in testing, 281-82
Northwest Ohio Easter Seal Society,
  287-89, 290, 292
Northwestern University Children's
  Perception of Speech Test, 483

Observer-based psychoacoustic
    procedure (OPP)
  compared to VRA, 246
  as hearing-screening tool, 245, 246
Ohio
  infant screening in, 171-79
  preschool screening in, 287-93
OM. *See* Otitis media
OME. *See* Otitis media with effusion
  (OME)
Ossicular discontinuity, 34
Otitis media (OM). *See also* Acute otitis
    media; Otitis media with effusion
    (OME)
  consequences for development,
    435-37
  day-care/school setting and, 449-54
  developmental/contextual perspective
    on, 441-43

ecological perspective on, 439-41
effect on parental relations, 436
health care setting for, 443-46
home setting and, 446-49
language development and, 450-52
macrosystem interaction, 455
prevalence, 435, 437
risk factors for, 437-39
school system policies and, 455
social development and, 452-54
workplace policies and, 454-55

Otitis media with effusion (OME). *See
    also* Effusion; Otitis media
  diagnosis of, 315
  prevalence of, 298-99
  screening for, 47
  social factors and, 299
  surgical procedures for, 316-17
Otoacoustic hearing screening in
    newborns
  age as factor, **198**
  cost efficiency of, 212, 222, 224
  definition of, 212-13
  in Denmark, 191-204
  feasibility, 211, 220-21, 223-24
  in neonates, **214**
  procedure for, 212-20
  purpose of, 211
  recording of, **213**
  stimuli used in, 192-94, 201
  structural development and, 202
  oxygen tension and, 202-3, 204
  tympanometry and, 193-97, 199-202,
    328
  validity of, 211-212, 221-22
Otoscopic inspection of ear, 52, 57,
    318-19, 320; correlation with
    tympanometry, 320-22, 328
Ototoxic medication, 22, 24, 92,
    148-49, 156-58, 236-37
Oxygen tension in neonatal blood, 203-4

Parents
  interaction with hearing-impaired
    child, 464-66

Parents — *continued*
  professionals and, 471-72
Parent-infant specialists, 468-72
Parkland Memorial Hospital, infant
    screening in, 163-69
Peabody Picture Vocabulary Test, 68,
    436
Pediatric Speech Intelligibility (PSI)
    Test, 71-73
Pennsylvania State University Health
    and Daycare Project, 437, 444
Periventricular-intraventricular
    hemorrhage (P-IVH), 24-25
Petrositis, and AOM, 35
Phonemically Balanced Kindergarten
    word lists, 483
Physicians, knowledge of pediatric
    hearing loss and, 105-9, 280-81
Play as learning, 412-17, 472
Prematurity, prevention of, 26
Preschool-age child screening
    American Academy of Pediatrics
      Policy Statement on, 275
    challenges in, 273-74
    identification audiometry as method
      for, 282-84
    middle ear screening of, 278. *See
      also* Central Auditory Processing
      Disorder (CAPD), screening for
    Ohio program for, 287-93
    protocols (U.S. Dept. Health &
      Human Services), 274-75
    purpose, 278
    role of primary care giver, 280-81
    strategies for, 277-78
    use of volunteers in, 165-69, 263-66,
      288-93
    VRA as method for, 282
President's Committee on Mental
    Retardation, report of, 113-14
Program Information for Primary Care
    Physicians, 108
Protocols for Screening and Assessment
    of Preschool Children, 274-75
Psychiatric patients

auditory disorders in, 373-74, 379-81
    relation of learning disabilities,
      373-74
Public Law 94-142, (Right to Education
    Act), 393, 418, 420, 488
Public Law 99-457, 257, 273, 288, 386,
    388, 393, 508
Public policy and hearing-impaired
    children
    formulation of, 111-13, 115-18,
      121-23
    politics of, 113-15
    problems in, 118-20
Pure-tone screening
    ASHA (1975, 1985) guidelines,
      301-2, 306
    for middle ear disorders, 46, 305-7,
      308, 309
    evaluating, 300-302
    sensitivity of, 306, 309
    specificity of, 306, 309

Rapidly Alternating Speech Test, 67-68
Randomized controlled trial (RCT), 7-8,
    11
Receiver Operation Characteristic
    (ROC), 186-87, **319**
Referral
    ASHA criteria for, 49, **50**
    problems in, 40, 41, 46
Reflectometry. *See* Acoustic
    reflectometry
Regionalization of prenatal care, 17-18
Rhode Island Hearing Assessment
    Project (RIHAP), 207-24
Right to Education Act, 393, 418, 420,
    488. *See also* Public Act 99-457
Risk factors
    definition and interpretation of, 82,
      85
    evaluation of, 85-92, 98-101
    as predictors of hearing loss, 81-85,
      84-85, 209-10, 229, **230**
Rubella, 23, 146

Rural Speech and Hearing Outreach
  Program (Montana), 331-32, 336,
  337-39, 343, 349, 351-52

SCAN. *See* Screening Test for Auditory
  Processing Disorders
Screening. *See also under* Auditory
  brainstem response (ABR) testing;
  Immittance screening
  age as factor in, 243-44, 298-99
  alternative procedures for neonatal,
    209-211
  with BOA, 209
  community projects for, 165-69
    261-71, 287-93
  concept of, 2-4
  by Crib-O-Gram, 164, 210
  definition, 3-4, 61-62, 243, 283
  economic concerns in, 11-13, 93-95
  evaluation, **9**
  follow-up on, 10, 139-40, 160, 167,
    169
  by high-risk questionnaire, 105-6,
    172-73
  by high-risk register, 79-81. 92-102,
    209-10, 508-9
  interpretation of tests, 67-70, 175-78
  of infants, 18-19, 244
  neonatal, 105-9, 244. *See also*
    Neonatal screening
  preschool, 5, 273-85, 287-93
  principles of, 1, 4-14
  protocols for, **96, 97, 98**, 302-6,
    509-10
  psychiatric patients, 373-81
  sensitivity of, 8-10, 301, 304
  school-age, 297-309, 315-29
  specificity of, 8-10, 301, 304
  tests, evaluation of, 2-3, 4, 8-10,
    200-203, 322-26
  of well babies, 167-68
"Screening for Hearing Impairment,"
  276-77
Screening Instrument for Targeting
  Educational Risk, 489, **490**

Screening Test for Auditory Processing
  Disorders, 68-69, 375-79
Selective Auditory Attention Test
  (SAAT)
  criteria for screening, **362**
  description of, 363-65
  scores in, 364-65, 367-68
  usefulness of, 366-69
Sensorineural hearing loss
  ABR screening for, 229-32
  asymmetrical hearing loss in, 232-33
  benzyl alcohol and, 235-36
  bilirubin and, 236
  clinical variables in, **231-32**
  in otitis media, 31, 34-36, 41
  ototoxic medications and, 236-27
  prevalence in neonates, **233**, 234-36
  risk factors for, 229-30, 235-37
  symmetrical hearing loss in, 232-33
Signal Detection Test, 182-83, 185-89
Signal-to-noise (S/N) ratio, 65-66, 196,
  482, 483, **484**
Speech and language tests, 67-68,
  71-73, 281-82, 364, 365, 366,
  375-76, 450-51, 483, 487, 489,
  490. *See individual test names*
Staggered Spondaic Word Test, 67-68
State of Maryland Program to Identify
  Hearing Impaired Infants, 107-9
Syndromes associated with hearing loss,
  174
Synthetic Sentence Identification (SSI)
  Test, 71

Test of Auditory Comprehension (TAC),
  487, 489-90
TORCH syndrome, infections
  comprising, 146
Toxoplasmosis gondii, 23, 146
Transitioning from birth to 3 to 5 years,
  417-21
Treatment. *See* Intervention
Treponema pallidum, 23
Tucson Catalina Foothills School
  District questionnaire, 485-86

Tympanometry
  acoustic reflex measurement and, 41, 48, 50, 53
  criterion for positive acoustic admittance, **324**
  with hand-held tympanometer, 56-57
  otoscopy and, 320-22, 329
  and presence of EOAE, 199-200
  protocol for, **316**
  as screening tool, 40, 41, 46, 48, 49-50, **51**
  variables in ears with no MEE, **321**
  width as indicator of acoustic admittance, **325**, **326**, 327, 328

Unilateral middle ear screening, 48-49
University of Arizona hearing clinics, 483
U.S. Preventive Services Task Force, 3, 4, 276
Usher's syndrome, 149

Vancomycin, 24
Vanderbilt NICU
  experience with Joint Committee risk criteria, 150-61
  flowchart for infant screening, 519, **520**
  hearing screening at, 18-26, 149-50
  screening statistics, **151, 152, 153, 154, 155, 156, 157, 159**
Vanderbilt University School of Medicine, 1977 symposium, 39-42, 46
Vater syndrome, 156
Very-low-birth-weight neonates (VLBW)
  handicaps of, **21**
  hearing loss in, 20-22
  survival rates of, 17, **19**, 20
Visual inspection of ear, 52, 57
Visual reinforcement audiometry (VRA)
  as screening tool, 247, 252-54
  compared to BOA, 247-48
  conditioning criteria in, 248-51
  procedures for, 254-57

threshold-search in, 251-52
VRA. *See* Visual reinforcement audiometry (VRA)

Waardenburg's syndrome, 149
Wechsler Intelligence Scale for Children, 366
Word Intelligibility by Picture Identification (WIPI) Test, 364, 365, 366, 483
World Health Organization (WHO), 4